ANTIBIOTICS AND ANTIBIOSIS IN AGRICULTURE

Published Proceedings of Previous Easter Schools in Agricultural Science

SOIL ZOOLOGY*
Edited by D.K.McE. Kevan (Butterworths, London, 1955)

THE GROWTH OF LEAVES*
Edited by F.L. Milthorpe (Butterworths, London, 1956)

CONTROL OF THE PLANT ENVIRONMENT*
Edited by J.P. Hudson (Butterworths, London, 1957)

NUTRITION OF THE LEGUMES*
Edited by E.G. Hallsworth (Butterworths, London, 1958)

THE MEASUREMENT OF GRASSLAND PRODUCTIVITY*
Edited by J.D. Ivins (Butterworths, London, 1959)

DIGESTIVE PHYSIOLOGY AND NUTRITION OF THE RUMINANT*
Edited by D. Lewis (Butterworths, London, 1960)

NUTRITION OF PIGS AND POULTRY*
Edited by J.T. Morgan and D. Lewis (Butterworths, London, 1961)

ANTIBIOTICS IN AGRICULTURE*
Edited by M. Woodbine (Butterworths, London, 1962)

THE GROWTH OF THE POTATO*
Edited by J.D. Ivins and F.L. Milthorpe (Butterworths, London, 1963)

EXPERIMENTAL PEDOLOGY*
Edited by E.G. Hallsworth and D.V. Crawford (Butterworths, London, 1964)

THE GROWTH OF CEREALS AND GRASSES*
Edited by F.L. Milthorpe and J.D. Ivins (Butterworths, London, 1965)

REPRODUCTION IN THE FEMALE MAMMAL*
Edited by G.E. Lamming and E.C. Amoroso (Butterworths, London, 1967)

GROWTH AND DEVELOPMENT OF MAMMALS*
Edited by G.A. Lodge and G.E. Lamming (Butterworths, London, 1968)

ROOT GROWTH*
Edited by W.J. Whittington (Butterworths, London, 1968)

PROTEINS AS HUMAN FOOD
Edited by R.A. Lawrie (Butterworths, London, 1970)

LACTATION*
Edited by J.R. Falconer (Butterworths, London, 1971)

PIG PRODUCTION
Edited by D.J.A. Cole (Butterworths, London, 1972)

SEED ECOLOGY
Edited by W. Heydecker (Butterworths, London, 1973)

HEAT LOSS FROM ANIMALS AND MAN: ASSESSMENT AND CONTROL
Edited by J.L. Monteith and L.E. Mount (Butterworths, London, 1974)

MEAT
Edited by D.J.A. Cole and R.A. Lawrie (Butterworths, London, 1975)

PRINCIPLES OF CATTLE PRODUCTION*
Edited by Henry Swan and W.H. Broster (Butterworths, London, 1976)

LIGHT AND PLANT DEVELOPMENT
Edited by H. Smith (Butterworths, London, 1976)

PLANT PROTEINS
Edited by G. Norton (Butterworths, London, 1977)

**These titles are now out of print*

Antibiotics and Antibiosis in Agriculture

with special reference to synergism

M. WOODBINE, Ph.D., M.Sc., F.R.I.C., F.I.Biol.
Department of Applied Biochemistry and Nutrition
University of Nottingham

BUTTERWORTHS
LONDON - BOSTON
Sydney - Wellington - Durban - Toronto

The Butterworth Group

United Kingdom	**Butterworth & Co (Publishers) Ltd** London: 88 Kingsway, WC2B 6AB
Australia	**Butterworths Pty Ltd** Sydney: 586 Pacific Highway, Chatswood, NSW 2067 Also at Melbourne, Brisbane, Adelaide and Perth
Canada	**Butterworth & Co (Canada) Ltd** Toronto: 2265 Midland Avenue, Scarborough, Ontario, M1P 4S1
New Zealand	**Butterworths of New Zealand Ltd** Wellington: 26–28 Waring Taylor Street, 1
South Africa	**Butterworth & Co (South Africa) (Pty) Ltd** Durban: 152–154 Gale Street
USA	**Butterworth (Publishers) Inc** Boston: 19 Cummings Park, Woburn, Mass. 01801

First published 1977

ISBN 0 408 70917 0

BRITISH LIBRARY CATALOGING IN PUBLICATION DATA

Easter School in Agricultural Science, 25th,
University of Nottingham, 1976
Antibiotics and antibiosis in agriculture.
1. Antibiotics in veterinary medicine – Congresses
2. Antibiotics in agriculture – Congresses
I. Title II. Woodbine, Malcolm
636. 089′5′329 SF918.A5 77–30021

ISBN 0–408–70917–0

Typeset and produced by Scribe Design, Chatham, Kent
Printed in Great Britain by Butler & Tanner, Frome, Somerset

PREFACE

The Easter Schools in Agricultural Science began in 1953 with one organized by E.G. Hallsworth on 'micropedology'. The success of this venture encouraged the development of successive Easter Schools in the Faculty of Agricultural Science and this is the 25th – all those published have been under the Butterworths imprimatur.

The ideas for the 25th Easter School follow up firstly that of the First International Conference on 'The Use of Antibiotics in Agriculture', held in Washington in 1955 and published as *Publication 397* of the National Academy of Science – National Research Council, in 1956. Secondly, that of the Second International Conference, also held at Sutton Bonington and as the Ninth Easter School, in 1962 and published under the title *Antibiotics in Agriculture,* in 1962.

The prospect of a Third International Conference and 25th Easter School in Agricultural Science on 'Antibiotics in Agriculture' was based on the view that the updating of earlier topics could be regarded as either a good thing in itself (not having been done before in the Easter School series) or as losing some appeal by virtue of repetition. The programme was designed to meet these views then by giving an opportunity for updating the 1956 and 1962 volumes and, at the same time, to introduce a new aspect by inviting contributors and topics for discussion to give 'special reference to synergic aspects'. Synergic aspects could be regarded as operating either within the inhibition of micro-organisms or during their possible subsequent resuscitation (which may be attempted as a check on the efficacy of the initial inhibitory measures).

As with the previous volume, no attempt was made to cover every aspect of the use of antibiotics in agriculture and the volume contains broad surveys, critical evaluations, and the interpolation of special topics. The contributions are as the authors prepared them, in the due hope that any editorial blanket is conspicuous by its absence and that the final volume is a pleasure to refer to, or to read.

Finally, those attending the Easter School considered that another be held – possibly in 1982 – under the title 'Antibiotics in Agriculture: Benefits and Malefits'.

MALCOLM WOODBINE

ACKNOWLEDGEMENTS

Any symposium or conference needs both general and financial support in order for it to be organized at all. A very deep 'thank you', therefore, to the following.

For financial help:

Abbott, S.A., Agriculture and Veterinary Products Division, Brussels
Beecham Research International, Brentford, Middlesex
The Boots Co. Ltd, Agricultural Division, Nottingham
Difco Laboratories Ltd, West Molesey, Surrey
Foundation for Microbiology (Dr. Byron Waksman, President), U.S.A.
Glaxo Research Ltd, Greenford, Middlesex
Lilly Research Centre Ltd, Windlesham, Surrey
Merck, Sharp and Dome, Merck and Co. Inc., Rockway, N.J., U.S.A.
RHM Research Ltd, High Wycombe, Buckinghamshire
Roche Ltd, Welwyn Garden City, Hertfordshire
Sigma (London) Chemical Co. Ltd
The Wellcome Trust, London

To colleagues Dr. Alan Seaman, Mr. Lindsey Wood, Mr. David Fowler, Mr. Alan Sims and Mrs. Julie Wortley for manning all the servicing involved in the meeting and the volume; to Mr. Ian Higginson (and the domestic staff); Miss Nancy Rhodes (and library colleagues); Mr. Tony Whitting (and administrative colleagues); Mrs. Doreen Borrows, Mrs. José Newcombe and Mrs. Lynda Siddall for the secretarial work and to my daughter Barbara Woodbine for her help on the references and indexing.

CONTENTS

I Introduction

1 **BETA-LACTAM ANTIBIOTICS: PERSPECTIVE AND PROSPECTIVE** 3
F.P. Doyle, *Beecham Pharmaceuticals, Betchworth*

2 **ANTIBIOTICS BY THE THOUSAND: AN OVERVIEW FROM THE U.S.A.** 15
D. Perlman, *School of Pharmacy, University of Wisconsin, U.S.A.*
C.K.A. Martin, *Gesellschaft Für Molekularbiologische Forschung mbH, Stockheim über Braunschweig, West Germany*

II The Context of Synergism

3 **A SYNERGIC PERSPECTIVE** 27
M. Woodbine, *Department of Applied Biochemistry and Nutrition, University of Nottingham, Sutton Bonington*

4 **SYNERGY IN CHEMOTHERAPY** 57
F. O'Grady, *Department of Microbiology, University of Nottingham, City Hospital, Nottingham*

5 **SYNERGY OF TRIMETHOPRIM AND SULPHONAMIDES: HISTORY AND CURRENT STATUS** 64
S.R.M. Bushby, *Wellcome Research Laboratories, Research Triangle Park, U.S.A.*

6 **TRIMETHOPRIM PLUS SULPHAMETHOXAZOLE: SYNERGIC OR ANTAGONISTIC COMBINATION?** 82
D. Greenwood, *Department of Microbiology, University of Nottingham, City Hospital, Nottingham*

7 **SYNERGIC ACTIVITIES OF PENICILLIN COMBINATIONS** 89
R. Sutherland, *Beecham Pharmaceuticals, Betchworth*

III Antibiotics, Antibiosis and Food

8 NISIN AND ITS APPLICATIONS 103
Ewa Lipińska, *Institute of Dairy Industry, Warsaw, Poland*

9 STRESS EFFECTS AND FOOD MICROBIOLOGY 131
Z.J. Ordal and L.D. Witter, *Department of Food Science and Microbiology, University of Illinois, U.S.A.*

10 STAPHYLOCOCCI IN CHEESE 139
A. Seaman and M. Woodbine, *Department of Applied Biochemistry and Nutrition, University of Nottingham, Sutton Bonington*

11 THE EFFECTS OF SO_2 AND CO_2 ON THE GROWTH OF *MICROBACTERIUM THERMOSPHACTUM*, A SPOILAGE ORGANISM FROM SAUSAGES 157
D. Welsby, *Kerry Cooperative Creameries, Listowel, Eire*
A. Seaman and M. Woodbine, *Department of Applied Biochemistry and Nutrition, University of Nottingham, Sutton Bonington*

12 RECOVERY AND REVIVAL OF MICROBIAL CELLS, ESPECIALLY THOSE FROM ENVIRONMENTS CONTAINING ANTIBIOTICS 174
J.E.L. Corry, *Metropolitan Police Forensic Science Laboratory, London*
H. van Doorne, *Department of Pharmacy, University of Leiden, The Netherlands*
D.A.A. Mossel, *Department of Food Microbiology, University of Utrecht, The Netherlands*

IV Antibiotics, Antibiosis and Animals

13 THE USE OF ANTIBIOTICS IN THE VETERINARY FIELD IN THE 1970S 199
G.C. Brander, *Beecham Pharmaceuticals, Tadworth*

14 FARM ANIMAL DISEASE: VETERINARIAN AND ANTIBIOTICS 210
B. Martin, *Kilmarnock, Scotland*

15 INTRAMAMMARY THERAPY: ITS ACHIEVEMENTS AND LIMITATIONS 217
J.K.L. Pearson, *Department of Agriculture, Stormont, Belfast, Northern Ireland*

16 **TRIMETHOPRIM–SULPHONAMIDE SYNERGY IN SALMONELLA THERAPY** 229
G. White, *Wellcome Research Laboratories, Berkhamsted*

17 **THE DEVELOPMENT OF BETA-LACTAM ANTIBIOTICS FOR THE TREATMENT OF BOVINE MASTITIS** 232
Anne M. Harris and P.W. Muggleton, *Glaxo Research Ltd, Greenford*

18 **DETECTION OF ANTIBIOTIC RESIDUES IN SLAUGHTERED ANIMALS** 239
Ann McCracken, *Department of Agriculture, Stormont, Belfast, Northern Ireland*

19 **NON-SPECIFIC RESISTANCE TO INFECTION IN RELATION TO MASTITIS** 245
K.G. Hibbitt and A.W. Hill, *Institute for Research on Animal Diseases, Compton, Newbury*

V Antibiotics, Antibiosis and Feed

20 **A MECHANISM OF GROWTH PROMOTION: NON-LETHAL FEED ANTIBIOTIC INDUCED, CELL WALL LESIONS IN ENTERIC BACTERIA** 259
J.R. Walton, *Veterinary Field Station, University of Liverpool, Wirral*

21 **CHEMICAL CONTROL OF CROP CONSERVATION**
A.R. Drysdale, *B.P. Nutrition (U.K. Ltd), Witham, Essex*

VI Practical Considerations

22 **CHEMICALS AND HEAT AS ASCOPORE ACTIVATORS** 275
V.M. Palmer and J.J. McEvoy, *Department of Industrial Microbiology, University College, Dublin, Eire*

23 **SOME FUNDAMENTAL REFLECTIONS ON 'ANTI-MICROBIAL POTENCY'** 284
A.J. Zwart Voorspuij, *Municipal Hospital, Dordrecht, The Netherlands*

24 **SYNERGISM EXHIBITED: TOO SIMPLE A TECHNIQUE?** 296
Jane, C. Fisher, Angela C. Leaman, R.J.L. Paulton, A. Seaman and M. Woodbine, *Department of Applied Biochemistry and Nutrition, University of Nottingham, Sutton Bonington*

25 **STUDIES IN THE BIOAVAILABILITY, PHARMACOKINETICS AND RESIDUES OF SEMISYNTHETIC PENICILLINS IN RELATION TO THEIR VETERINARY APPLICATION** 307
J.F. Buswell and G.H. Palmer, *Beecham Pharmaceuticals, Tadworth*

VII Public Health Aspects

26 **ANTIBIOTICS, ANIMALS AND MAN – AN APPRAISAL OF A CONTENTIOUS SUBJECT** 315
A.H. Linton, *Department of Bacteriology, University of Bristol, Bristol*

27 **ANTIBIOTIC RESISTANCE IN BACTERIA AND ASSOCIATED PROBLEMS IN FARM ANIMALS BEFORE AND AFTER THE 1969 SWANN REPORT** 344
H. Williams Smith, *Houghton Poultry Research Station, Huntingdon*

LIST OF PARTICIPANTS 359

INDEXES 363
Organism 363
Author 365
Subject 379

I

INTRODUCTION

1

BETA-LACTAM ANTIBIOTICS: PERSPECTIVE AND PROSPECTIVE

F.P. DOYLE
Beecham Pharmaceuticals, Betchworth

This being the first paper of the Easter School, the title was chosen with a view to giving a broad overview of the topics to be covered. Many experts will cover later, and in detail, various properties of penicillins, cephalosporins, sulphonamides, etc. and, in particular, several aspects of synergistic combinations of these and other antibacterial substances.

As an erstwhile chemist, this contribution will naturally be biased towards the structural aspects of the beta-lactam antibiotics rather than their biological properties. There will be ample opportunity later to explore the biology in more detail. In view of the word 'perspective' in the title, we should perhaps remind ourselves that 50 years ago very few medicines of any type were available and doctors had to depend upon aspirin, kaolin, sulphur, and a few alkaloids. Farm livestock were also denied any of the benefits that several contributors will be discussing and which veterinarians now take for granted.

When the Beecham Group Ltd first became interested in pharmaceutical research, in 1947, Penicillin G had already become the wonder-drug of the 20th century owing to the work of Chain, Florey, and the industrial expertise of Chas, Pfizer and others in the U.S.A. It led the way to the avalanche of antibacterial secondary mould metabolites, which for a number of years diverted most Companies' attention away from beta-lactam antibiotics to the seemingly more attractive amino glycoside, macrolide, and peptide mould metabolites. Interest in beta-lactams was, however, continued and later revitalized by the work of three groups of workers:

(1) In the early 1950s, Eli Lilly in the U.S.A. and Biochemie in Austria, developed the acid-stable and orally absorbed Penicillin V;

(2) in the late 1940s, Sir Howard Florey and colleagues at Oxford, and subsequently Glaxo and Eli Lilly, with the N.R.D.C., started the long haul to the cephalosporins;

(3) and in 1957, Beecham isolated 6-aminopenicillanic acid (6-APA) in sufficient quantities to establish its usefulness as a source of new semi-synthetic penicillins.

Semi-Synthetic Penicillins

Figures 1.1 to *1.5* show the range of the penicillins that became available during the period 1959–70 – having been derived mainly by Beecham workers from 6-APA. Some of their more interesting antibacterial properties are also indicated.

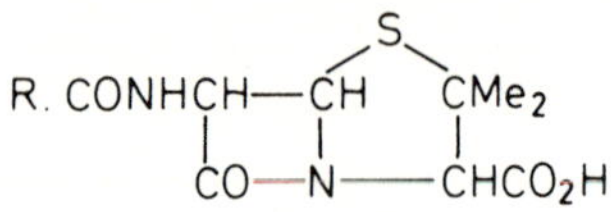

Approved name	U.K. trade name	R
Methicillin	Celbenin	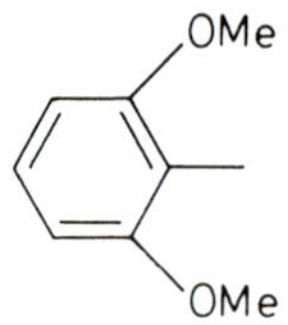
Naficillin	–	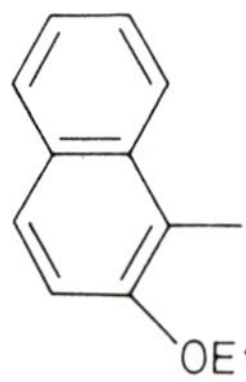
Oxacillin	–	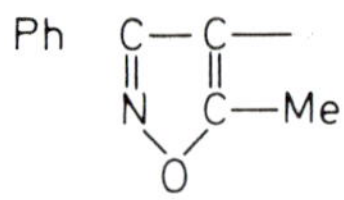
Cloxacillin	Orbenin	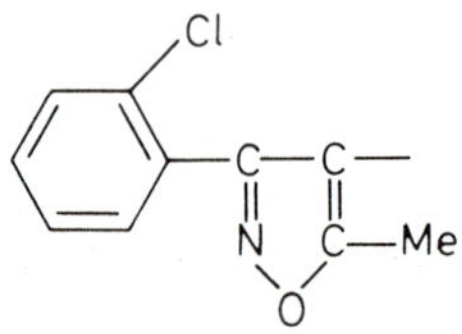
Dicloxacillin	–	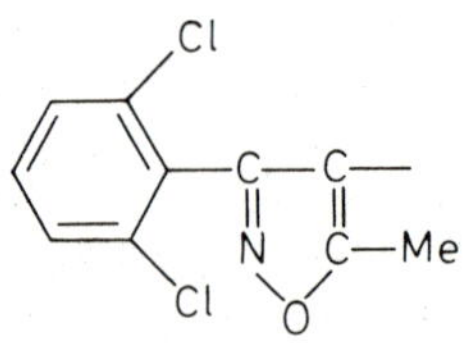
Flucloxacillin	Floxapen	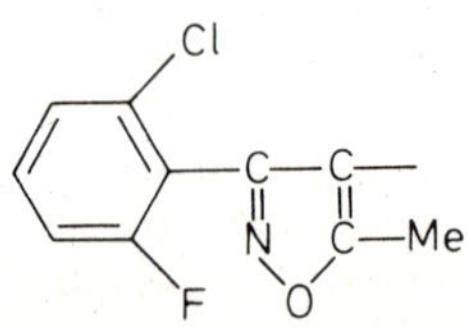

Figure 1.1 Penicillinase-resistant penicillins

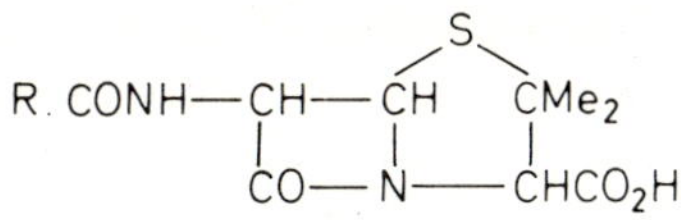

Approved name	U.K. trade name	R
Phenethicillin	Broxil	PhOCH(Me)—
Propicillin	Brocillin	PhOCH(Et)—
Phenbenicillin	Penspek	PhOCH(Ph)—
Clometicillin	Rixapen	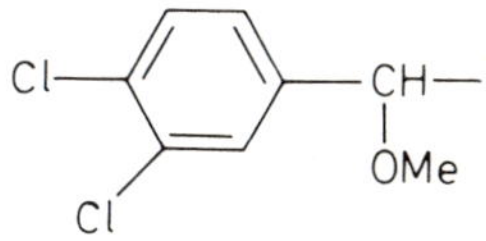

Figure 1.2 Penicillins active against Gram-positive organisms

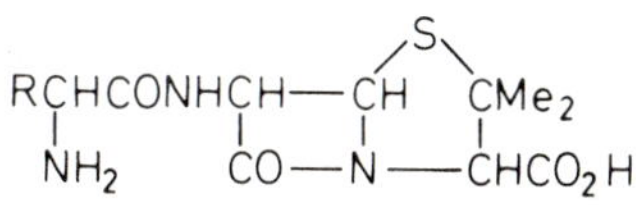

Penicillin	R	Peak Blood Levels μgml^{-1} 500mg oral dose	Peak Blood Levels μgml^{-1} 250mg oral dose
PENBRITIN Ampicillin	Ph	5·0	2·3
BRL 2333	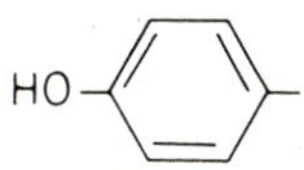	10·7	5·5

Figure 1.3

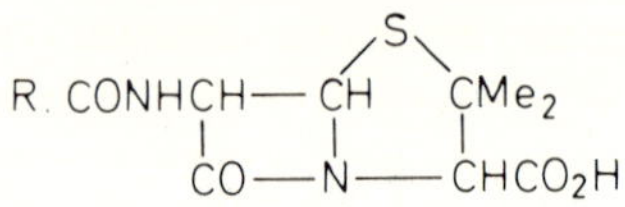

Approved name	U.K. trade name	R
Carbenicillin	Pyopen	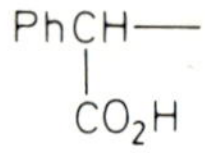
Ticarcillin	–	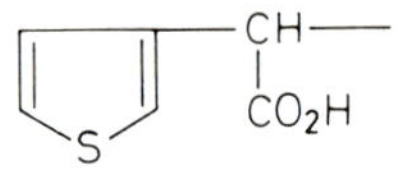
Sulbenicillin	–	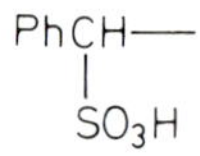

Figure 1.4 Anti-pseudomonas penicillins

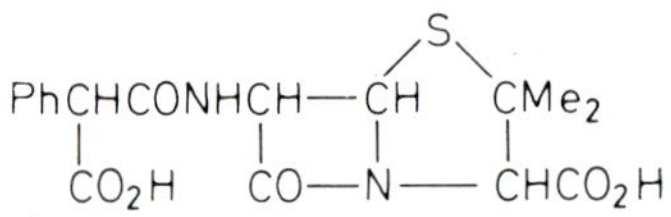

Organism	M.I.C. $\mu g ml^{-1}$	
	Carbenicillin	Ampicillin
Pseudomonas	50–100	>500
Ampicillin Resistant Proteus	5–10	>50
Other gram –ve bacteria	5–10	2·5–5·0

Figure 1.5

During the period since 1970 further progress has been achieved which, although not as dramatic as the original developments, is nevertheless significant in its own right. One such area has been the development of pro-drug forms of some of the more active penicillins.

The pro-drug idea has been around for a number of years but only relatively recently has it been used deliberately in the development of improved versions of active pharmaceutical substances. [For a full review, *see* 'Pro-Drugs as Novel Drug Delivery Systems' by T. Higuchi and V. Stella, American Chemical Society Symposium Series 14, published 1975.]

Pro-drugs may be of four different types:

(1) A labile derivative of an active molecule which gives improved properties for pharmaceutical formulation (e.g. improved long-term stability). Insoluble salts and derivatives of penicillins that hydrolyse readily in the stomach (e.g. hetacillin, *Figure 1.6*) are examples of this type.

(2) A derivative of an active molecule that shows improved oral absorption over the parent molecule but is rapidly hydrolysed either during or after absorption to give the active molecule. The penicillin esters, pivampicillin, talampicillin, and carfecillin, are examples of this type (*Figures 1.7* and *1.8*).

(3) A compound that undergoes metabolism to give a new structure with improved properties.

(4) A biologically inactive compound that preferentially penetrates to an active site and is then converted at the site by hydrolytic enzymatic change to an active molecule. This would be a highly desirable objective but has so far proved difficult to achieve in clinical practice.

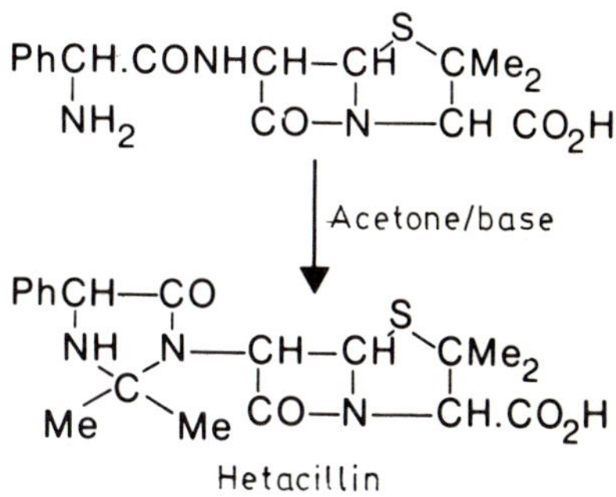

Figure 1.6

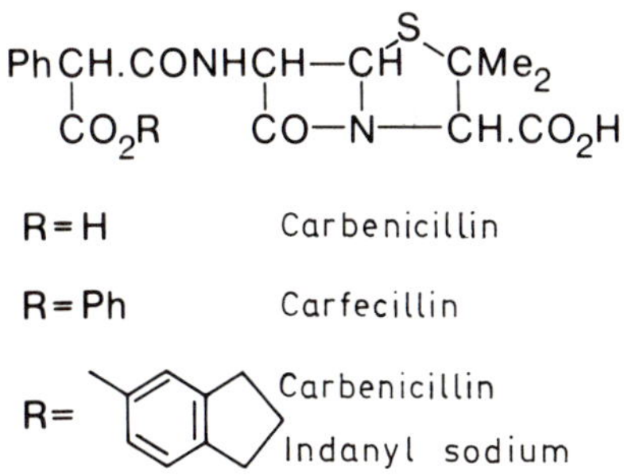

Figure 1.7

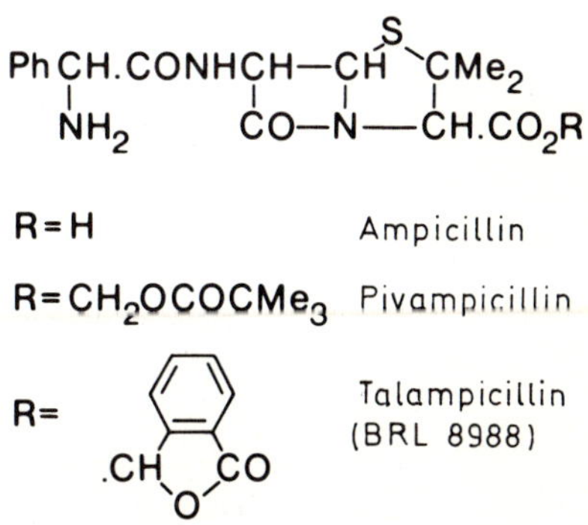

Figure 1.8

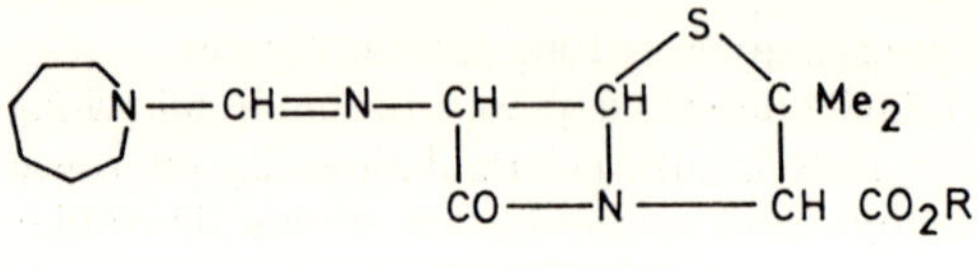

I Orally administered form: R = $CH_2OCOCMe_3$
II Active hydrolysis product: R = H

	Concentrations (μgml^{-1}) producing 50% inhibition in vitro	
Bacterium	II	Ampicillin
Sensitive Staph.	5	0.025
Strep. faecalis	>100	0.8
E. coli	0.1	2
Kleb. pneumoniae	0.65	26

Leo, Netherlands Pat. Appl. 7016435

Figure 1.9

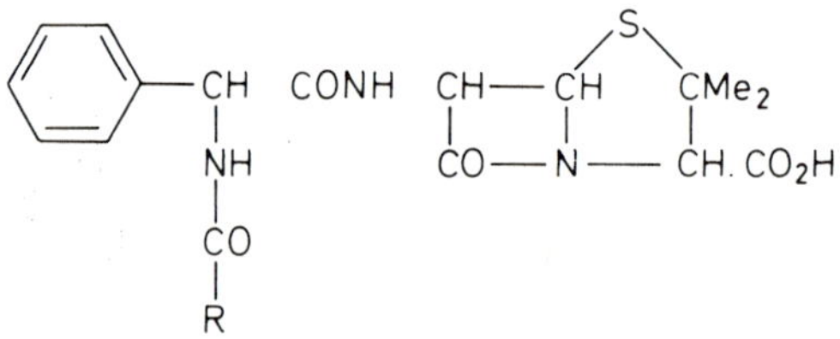

AMPICILLIN DERIVATIVES Compound	R	Anti-Pseudomonas activity μgml^{-1}
Bayer 6907	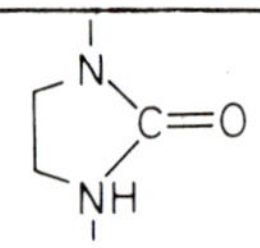	12·5
Bristol BL-P 1654	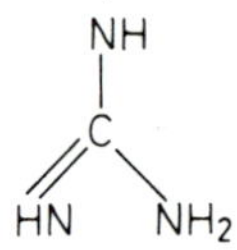	12·5
Sumitomo PC-904	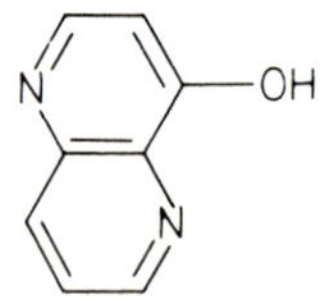	2·5
Ticarcillin	–	25
Ampicillin	–	>250

Figure 1.10

The penicillin, pivmecillinam (*Figure 1.9*) is an interesting recent development in view of both its structure (not an acyl derivative of 6-APA) and its spectrum of activity, which is shifted very much towards activity against Gram-negative organisms. Possible synergistic combinations of the pivaloyloxymethyl ester of mecillinam and amoxycillin were discussed at the ICAAC meeting in Washington last autumn by Roche Laboratories. Such a combination combines the pro-drug approach with the idea of synergistic combinations, about which, no doubt, a good deal more will come later.

Before leaving the penicillins, some products described very recently might be referred to which can be looked upon as derivatives of ampicillin with modified spectra, particularly the acquisition of antipseudomonas activity (*Figure 1.10*).

Cephalosporins

Later contributors to the Easter School, particularly those from Glaxo Laboratories, will also be covering the subject of novel cephalosporins, but a brief review here of the cephalosporins currently available, or in development, is in order (*Figures 1.11* to *1.15*). A particular advantage of the cephalosporins is of course their inbuilt resistance to staphylococcal penicillinase. A disadvantage is the infrequency with which oral absorption occurs in the series, most of those currently available being formulated for parenteral administration.

Recent publications from Merck, and Lilly, have also described some beta-lactam-containing metabolites (*Figure 1.16*) closely related to the cephalosporins but isolated from *Streptomyces* fermentations.

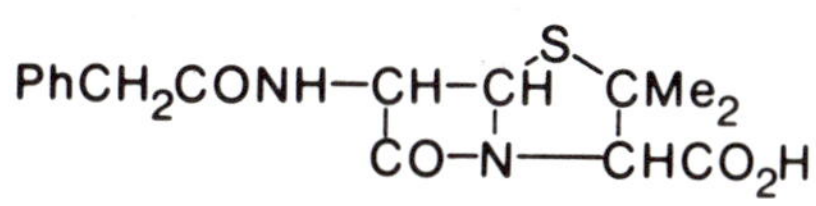

Penicillin G

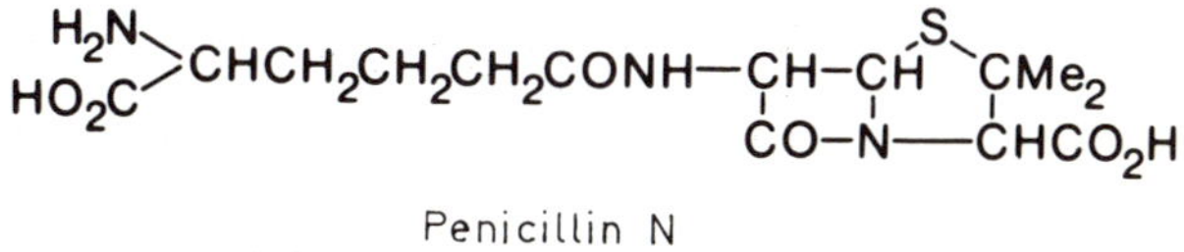

Penicillin N
(Cephalosporin N)

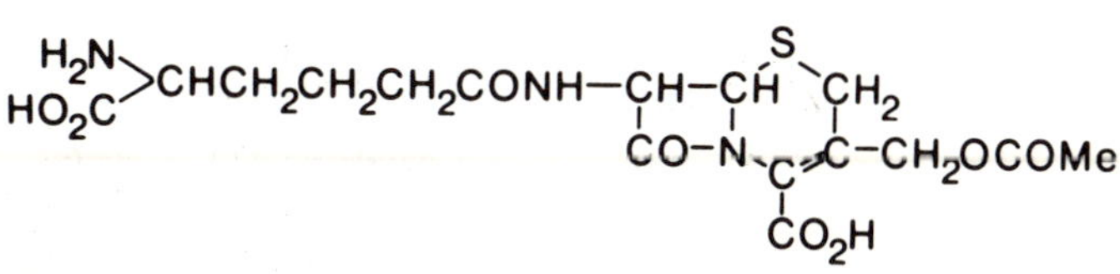

Cephalosporin C

Figure 1.11

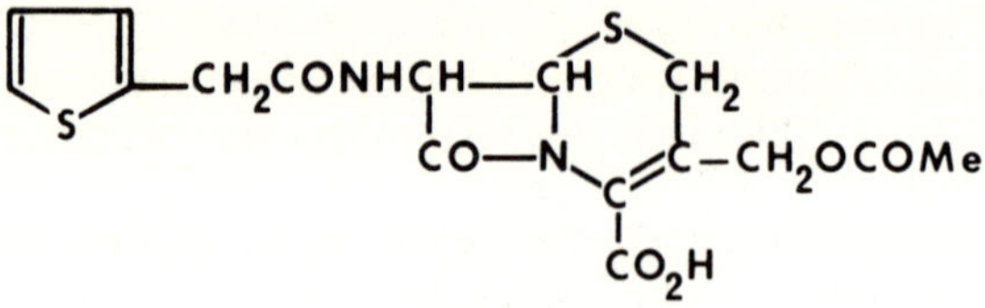

Cephalothin

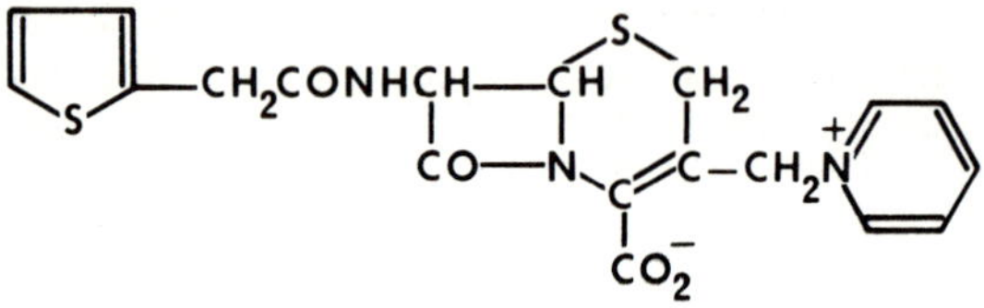

Cephaloridine

Figure 1.12

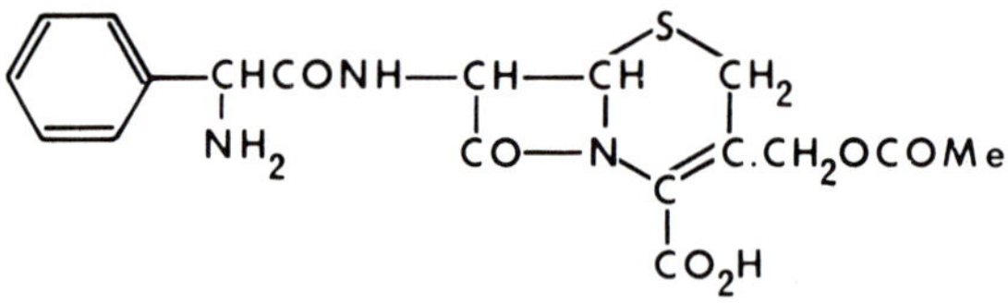

Cephaloglycine

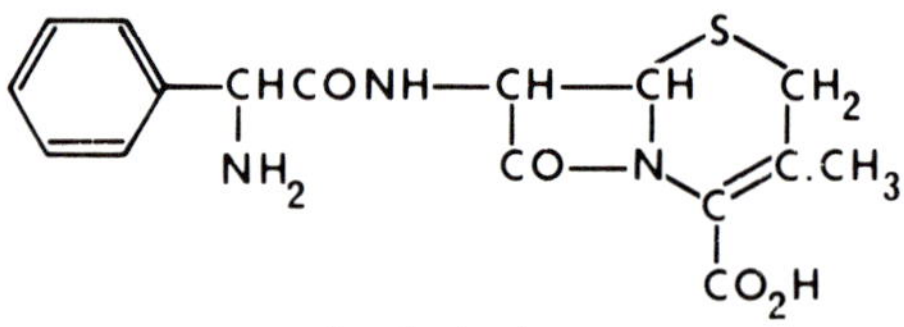

Cephalexin

Figure 1.13

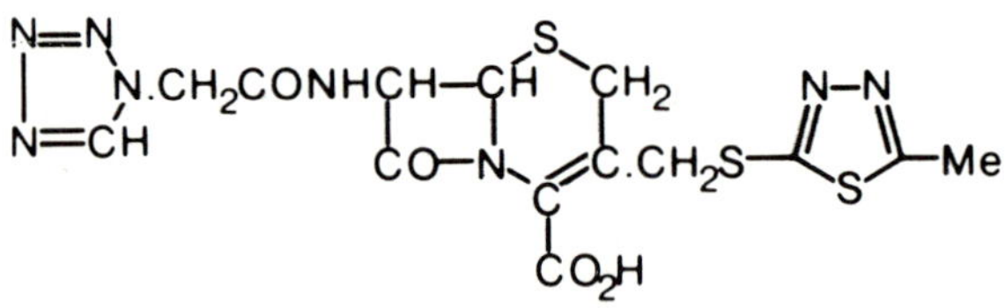

Cefazolin (Fujisawa)

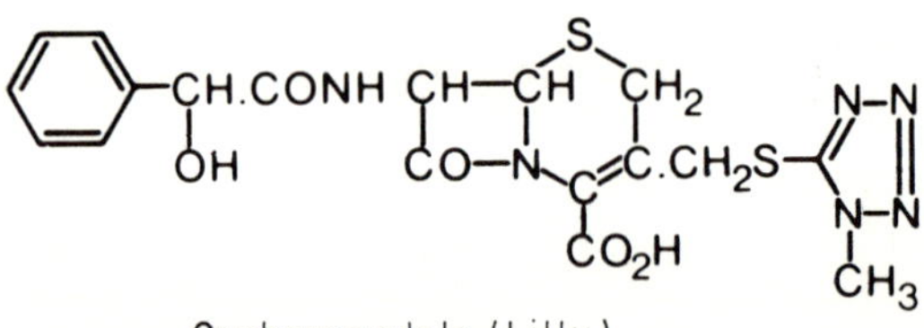

Cephamandole (Lilly)

Figure 1.14

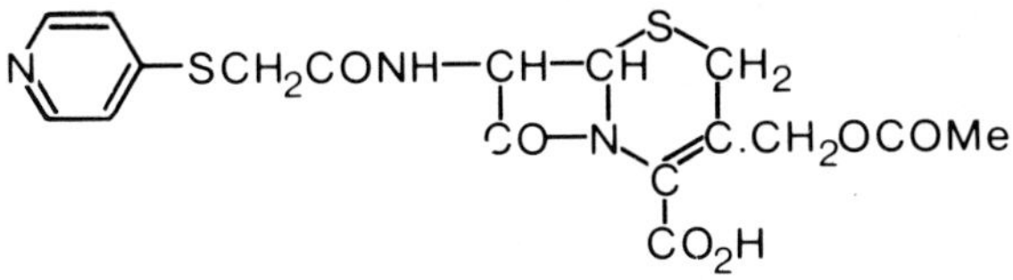

Cephapyrin (Bristol)

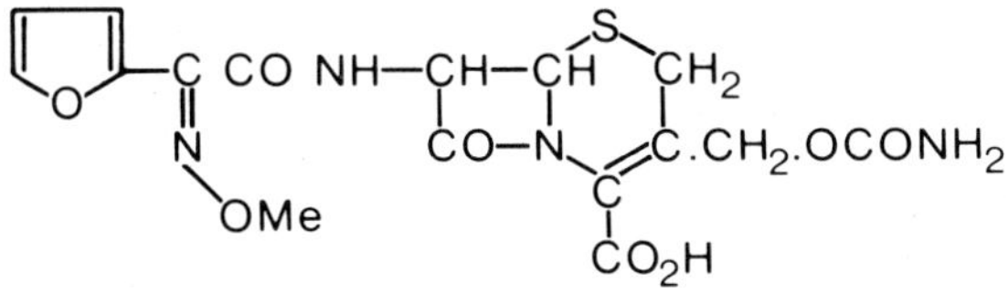

Cefuroxime (Glaxo)

Figure 1.15

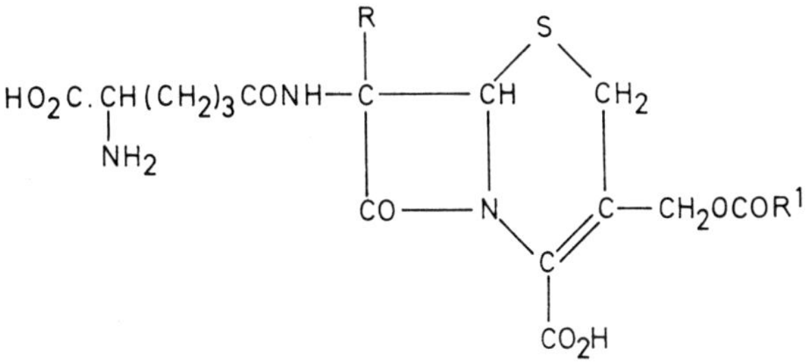

Proposed name	R	R^1	Reported by
–	H	NH_2	Lilly, 1971
–	OMe	Me	Lilly, 1971
Cephamycin C	OMe	NH_2	Lilly, Merck, 1971
Cephamycin B	OMe	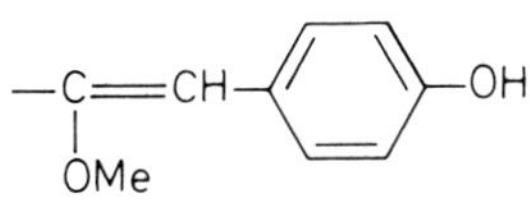	Merck, 1971
Cephamycin A	OMe	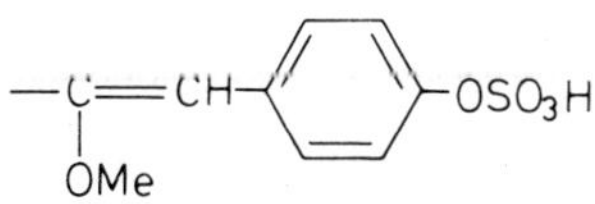	Merck, 1971

Figure 1.16 Beta-lactam antibiotics from streptomyces fermentations

Where Do We Go From Here?

From what has been described so far, it may be realized that the position today is one of having a wide range of beta-lactam antibiotics for both oral and injectable use for the treatment of most of the common bacterial diseases. All these compounds act by specifically inhibiting bacterial cell wall synthesis and are, therefore, virtually non-toxic to human cells because of their apparent inability to penetrate such cells. [It is, perhaps, not surprising therefore that the beta-lactam antibiotics are ineffective against organisms with more complicated cell walls such as the mycobacteria of tuberculosis or leprosy.]

It is fair to ask, at this point, where do we go from here – and a number of scientists in industry, the universities, and government agencies, have posed this question in various forms. It is obvious, however, that neither medical nor veterinary practice will give much thanks for yet more variants on the penicillin and cephalosporin theme, unless a significant advantage can be shown from a cost, activity, or toxicity point of view.

Penicillins and cephalosporins are already very active against most organisms and are relatively non-toxic. It is true that both can give rise to allergic phenomena but even this has now been minimized by more careful use of the compounds coupled with higher levels of purity.

One drawback to the more extended use of beta-lactam antibiotics is the presence, in some strains of some bacteria, of lactamases which will destroy the beta-lactam ring of the compounds before they have had an opportunity to exert their effect on the building enzyme systems of the cell wall. Cephalosporins of course have an inbuilt resistance to one particular enzyme (staph. penase) but are still susceptible to the beta-lactamases from some Gram-negative organisms.

Synergistic Combinations

When discussing synergism I believe we should define very carefully what we mean, since synergism can appear to mean different things to different people in different situations.

One type of antibacterial synergism is concerned with the use of two antibacterial substances acting on entirely different targets in the bacterial cell. This applies particularly to the sulphonamide-trimethoprim combination successfully developed by Roche Products, and Burroughs Wellcome, and which is the subject of later papers.

A second type is concerned with a double attack on an enzyme cascade system associated with a particular cell function, e.g. cell wall synthesis. The recently described combination of a deuterated fluorinated phenylalanine with a pentadione derivative of cycloserine, by the Merck workers, is an example of a combination that works on this basis.

Another type on which my own laboratories have been working for some years is concerned with the idea, referred to earlier, of inhibiting the beta-lactamase enzyme system present in some bacteria, which can destroy the antibiotic before it has a chance to exert its antibacterial effect. My colleague, Mr. Sutherland, will be referring later to the synergistic activities of penicillin combinations which act in this way: one penicillin inhibiting the enzyme which inactivates the other (e.g. cloxacillin and ampicillin or amoxycillin).

For a number of reasons it would obviously be more desirable to have a synergist with weak or non-existent antibacterial activity, and a number of such compounds have recently been described either specifically or by implication and are shown in *Figures 1.17* and *1.18*. *Figure 1.19* shows the effect of small amounts of one of these (the Beecham compound, clavulanic acid) on the antibacterial activity of ampicillin.

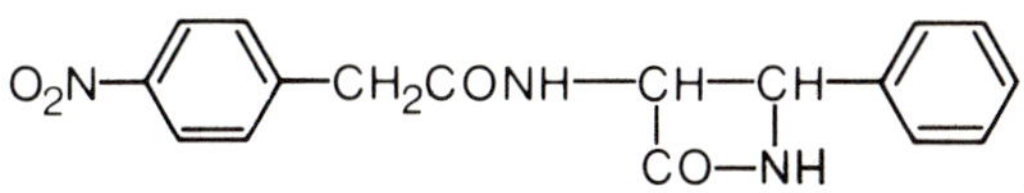

Enzyme inhibitor
(Allen and Hanbury Patent 1970)

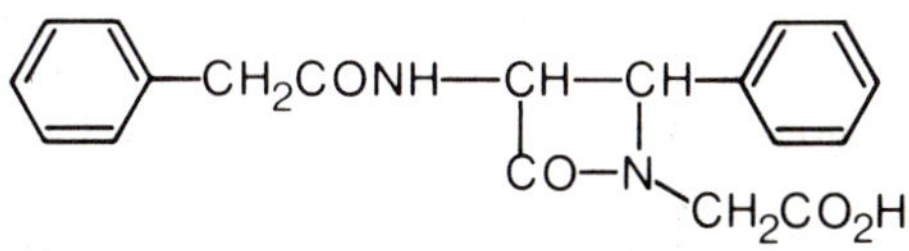

Azetidinone
(Baer and Mertes 1973)

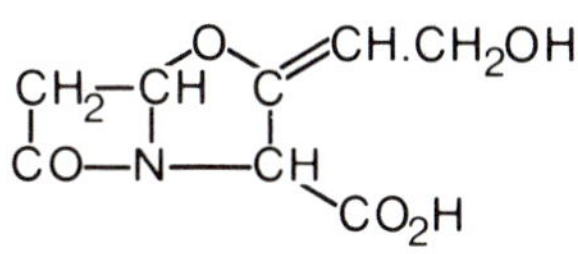

Clavulanic acid
(Beecham Patent 1974)

Figure 1.17

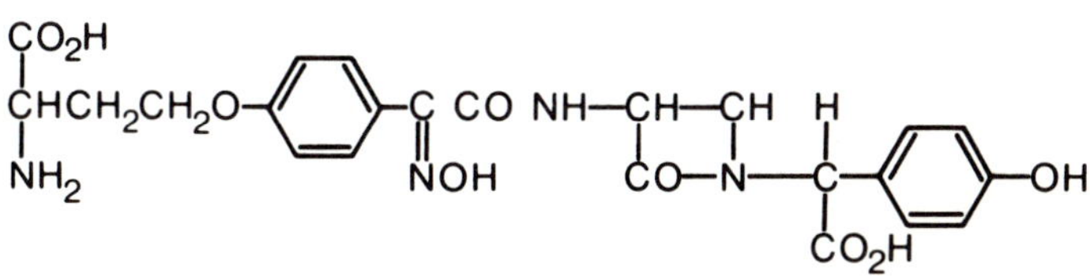

Nocardicin A
(FR 1923 Fujisawa 1975)

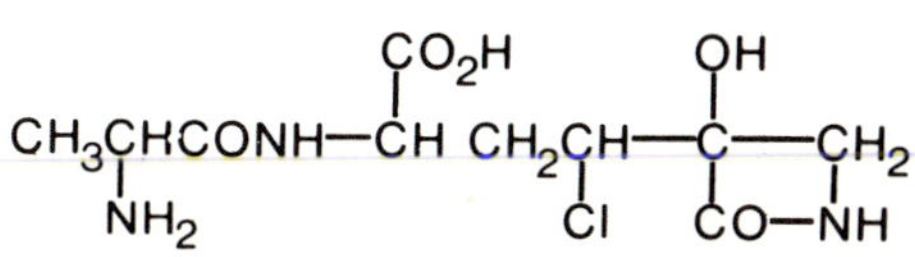

Azetidinone ex. Streptomyces
(J. Antibiotics 1975)

Figure 1.18

Organism	M.I.C. Ampicillin alone ($\mu g\ ml^{-1}$)	M.I.C. Ampicillin + 1 $\mu g\ ml^{-1}$ of clavulanic acid ($\mu g\ ml^{-1}$)
E. coli B11	>500	125
Kleb aerogenes A	125	<0.4
Serratia marcescens	>500	62
S. aureus Russell	500	<0.4

Figure 1.19

The Future

The future should see further advances in the chemotherapy of bacterial diseases along the following lines:

(1) more beta-lactam antibiotics with useful advantages over existing products;
(2) further pro-drug forms of beta-lactam antibiotics;
(3) combination products, using various ideas on synergism with the aim of overcoming the resistance problem;
(4) more and more attention being paid to the relationship between anti-bacterial treatment and the immune status of the host. The possibility of immunostimulants or inducers of non-specific immunity.

In this brief but broad view, it is hoped that your appetites have been sufficiently whetted for the feast of papers which follows.

2

ANTIBIOTICS BY THE THOUSAND: AN OVERVIEW FROM THE U.S.A.

D. PERLMAN
C.K.A. MARTIN*
School of Pharmacy, University of Wisconsin, U.S.A.

Examination of our accomplishments in antibiotic research in the past 30 years and study of the strategy used in directing this research leads to the formulation of several questions.

Do We Have a Sufficiency of Antibiotics?

We now have in the antibiotic literature descriptions of some 3800 microbial metabolites which are considered to have antibiotic properties. In many instances these represented, upon first description, new types of structures not previously investigated (or imagined) by the organic chemists of the day. Berdy (1974) has tentatively divided the 3800 into 15 major classes and 35 minor classes on the basis of chemical structure and other chemical features, and further subdivision will probably result when more of this group are subjected to x-ray analysis and their correct structures determined.

We also know that in many fermentations the antibiotic-producing organisms synthesize families of chemically related compounds, and in many instances only those produced in major amounts have been chemically characterized. (For example, one gentamicin-producing culture produces 17 antibiotics (Maehr and Schaffner, 1967).) It seems likely that for every antibiotic purified from a fermentation we have 'missed' or discarded three related compounds, and thus our 'real' inventory is closer to 12 000 than 3800.

In addition to the 3800 microbial metabolites described in the literature we have seen major research investments on the part of chemists in making antibiotic derivatives and analogues. Some 35 000 have already been prepared including about 20 000 penicillins, 10 000 cephalosporins, thousands of tetracyclines and rifamycins, and hundreds of aminoglycosides and lincomycins. The study of the structure/activity relationships of these thousands of antibiotic derivatives and analogues (Perlman, 1977) has led to some comprehension of the

*Current address: Gesellschaft für Molekularbiologische Forschung mbH, Stockheim über Braunschweig, West Germany.

portion of the molecule required for a specific type of antimicrobial activity and also for certain (perhaps unwanted) pharmacological and toxicological effects. This understanding in time will help the organic chemist in design of new derivatives and analogues with the desired biological activities. MK 641/MK 642 is the first example of the application of this approach (Kahan and Kropp, 1975).

Do We Need More Antibiotics?

With the current availability of the thousands of antibiotics mentioned above, is there a need for a continued search for a new compound? What will be the value of a new penicillin? A new cephalosporin? Another aminoglycoside? Or, another rifamycin? Can the medical profession utilize what is available now? Will another series of compounds be that much help to resolving therapeutic problems?

All of these questions have been repeatedly asked in the past 15 years, and the only conclusion that can be reached is that new derivatives and analogues have been accepted and even solicited to resolve therapeutic problems. Study

Table 2.1 Some semi-synthetic antibiotics and antibiotic derivatives used in clinical medicine

Class	*Number reported prepared*	*Some compounds now used in clinical medicine*	
Penicillins	~20 000	Ampicillin	Hetacillin
		Amoxicillin	Methicillin
		Azidocillin	Nafcillin
		Cloxacillin	Oxacillin
		Carbenicillin	Phenethicillin
		Cyclacillin	Propicillin
		Dicloxacillin	Pivampicillin
		Epicillin	Sulbenicillin
		Flucloxacillin	Tricarcillin
Cephalosporins	~7500	Cephalothin	Cephapirin
		Cephaloglycine	Cephacetrile
		Cephaloridine	Cefazolin
		Cephalexin	Cefoxitin
		Cephradine	Cefamandole
		Cephanone	Cefuroxime
Rifamycins	~1500	Rifamycin SV	Rifamide
		Rifampicin	Rifazin
Tetracyclines	~3000	Doxycycline	Minocycline
		Lymecycline	Methacycline
		Rollicycline	
Lincomycins	~750	Clindamycin	
Streptomycins	~300	Dihydrostreptomycin	
		Dihydrodeoxystreptomycin	
Kanamycins	~500	Amikacin (BB-K8)	

of the clinical acceptance of antibiotics suggests that about 1 of every 1000 studied eventually is accepted. This ratio may vary with the group of compounds involved; it is now more difficult to obtain acceptance of a new penicillin (since we have some 35 already in clinical use) (*see Table 2.1*) than a new cephalosporin (where only 10 are in clinical use).

Among the perennial problems that seem worthy of continued attention are developments of a penicillin which is non-allergenic, an aminoglycoside which is not ototoxic, an antifungal polyene which can be tolerated systematically, and a rifamycin which is likely to be effective against those organisms which now apparently develop resistance to rifampicin. Although it may require some education of the medical practitioners to best utilize these compounds, this is not an impossible situation.

In considering the question 'Whither the Cephalosporins?' Hamilton-Miller and Brumfitt (1974) have pointed out that an ultimate aim in chemotherapy could be to have two kinds of drugs; first, one would have a series of very broad-spectrum drugs, one of which would be used to initiate treatment of an infection before the pathogen had been identified. When the offending organism had been isolated, treatment would be changed at once to a 'secondary' drug, one with high activity against that specific organism, and little if any against other bacteria. In such a pattern of things, the cephalosporins have an obvious place at both levels. Such an approach is applicable to relatively few other antibiotics, and in any case prospects for success seem to be much less.

Do We Need New Types of Antibiotics?

Inspection of the dozens of types of chemical structures of microbial metabolites which have antimicrobial activity (Berdy, 1974) suggests that we still cannot predict with any degree of confidence the specific antimicrobial activity and pharmacology by inspection of the chemical structure of a candidate compound. Thus, it is possible that discovery of some additional structures will result in a whole new group of therapeutically useful compounds, or at least compounds which can help to better our understanding of useful mechanisms for inhibition of growth of infectious organisms.

Since most of the antibiotics utilized in 1976 were selected for initial study on a fairly random basis, it is not unlikely that many useful compounds still remain to be discovered, and one of the major decisions that has to be considered is the relative investment in searching for new microbial metabolites to that in preparing derivatives and analogues of compounds with demonstrated activities and deficiencies.

When is an Antibiotic Obsolete?

Obsolescence rates in pharmaceuticals have been as high as 10%, i.e. 1 out of 10 pharmaceutically useful compounds is replaced every year by another compound. This has not been the experience with antibiotics. Only three antibiotics have been withdrawn from the market: Ristocetin, a relative of the currently available vancomycin; Fumagillin, a chemically unstable compound with activity restricted to treatment of protozoal infections; and Stendomycin, an antifungal agent at one time used for agricultural purposes. Use of others has dropped as new compounds with more desirable properties have become available, e.g. phenethicillin has been replaced by ampicillin, carbenicillin, oxacillin etc., or toxicity and side-effects have been of such concern as to limit the use of the antibiotic to only a few situations, e.g. chloramphenicol and novobiocin.

It would appear that at the present time there is no positive evidence that we can expect all antibiotics eventually to become obsolete, and the need for replacement compounds cannot be programmed in the same fashion as was possible a few years ago in the research on organic compounds such as coccidiostats (where protozoal resistance in the field could almost be predicted as a function of length of use). Thus, the problem becomes one of determining the maximum numbers of antimicrobial agents that can serve a useful function, and the obsolescence problem is replaced by the economic competition problem. This latter is complicated by the vagaries of the market, in some instances the insistence of certain governments on having antibiotic-producing capabilities in their countries, and the complications of the patent protection systems.

Since it appears that there are advantages to continuing the search for new antibiotics, the strategy to be used should be discussed. Most of the antibiotics which have been found acceptable for clinical or agricultural use are listed in *Table 2.2*. As can be seen, these are mainly products obtained from streptomycete fermentations, and several workers have suggested (Porter, 1971; Routien, 1961) that the incidence of antibiotic-producing capacity in this group is over 50%. More than half the cultures examined will produce some antibiotic activity when grown in laboratory media. This is a much higher incidence of production than noted for fungi (15%), bacteria (3%) or yeasts (less than 1%), and has led many to focus their attention on streptomycetes in anticipation of at least finding some activity. The somewhat related *Micromonospora* have been studied rather extensively (Luedemann, 1969), and several hundred antibiotics have been detected from this group of filamentous organisms. In many instances the *Micromonospora* antibiotics which have been characterized are chemically related to streptomycete metabolites, but not always identical and these differences have been therapeutically significant. Similar intensive efforts have been made with *Actinoplanes* cultures (Thiemann *et al*., 1968) but fewer antibiotics apparently have been found than with the *Micromonospora*.

Thus, the problem in strategic terms can be defined as a choice between:

(1) examining metabolites from 'new' species of streptomycetes which may have unexpected metabolic potential and produce 'new' and hitherto untested compounds;
(2) studying *Micromonospora* or *Actinoplanes* cultures which might produce compounds somewhat related and still different from the *streptomycete*-produced antibiotics;
(3) searching other genera such as groups of bacteria, mycoplasma, yeasts, etc. for the possibilities of producing antibiotics.

A programme related to (1) is to examine more rigorously the producing capacity of previously studied antibiotic-producers in order to isolate the 'minor'

Table 2.2 Initial reports of antibiotics eventually found useful in clinical medicine or agriculture

Year of initial report	*Now used in clinical medicine*		*Now used in agriculture*
Before 1945	Actinomycin D	Penicillin G	
	Bacitracin	Penicillin V	
	Gramicidin D	Streptomycin	
	Griseofulvin	Tyrothricin	
1946–1950	Chloramphenicol	Neomycin	Antimycin A
	Chlortetracycline	Oxytetracycline	Cycloheximide
	Colistin	Polymyxin B	Nisin
	Fumagillin		
1951–1955	Actinomycin C	Nystatin	Staphylomycins
	Amphomycin	Oleandomycin	
	Candicidin B	Sarkomycin	
	Cycloserine	Spiramycin	
	Erythromycin	Staphylomycins	
	Gramicidin J	Tetracycline	
	Leucomycin	Trichomycin	
	Lucensomycin	Viomycin	
1956–1960	Aminosidin	Novobiocin	Blasticidin S
	Amphotericin B	Paromomycin	Cellocidin
	Chromomycin A3	Pentamycin	Hygromycin B
	Demethylchlor-tetracycline	Pimaricin	Mikamycin
		Pristinamycins	Stendomycin
	Hamycin	Rifamycin B	Thiostrepton
	Kanamycin	Ristocetin	Tylosin
	Mithramycin	Spectinomycin	
	Mitomycin	Vancomycin	
		Variotin	
1961–1965	Azalomycin	Gentamicin	Aureofungin
	Bleomycin	Lincomycin	Destomycin
	Capreomycin	Pyrrolnitrin	Kasugamycin
	Cephalosporin	Siccanin	Moenomycin
	Daunomycin		Polyoxin
	Fusidic Acid		Siomycin
1966–1970	Adriamycin	Ribostamycin	Monensin
	Enduracidin	Tobramycin	Validamycin
	Josamycin		
1971–1975	Maredamycin	Lividomycin	Lasalocid
	Bicyclomycin	Sisomicin	Macarbomycin
			Mocimycin
			Salinomycin
			Thiopeptin

constituents from the fermentation and to determine whether these might have activity comparable to the 'major' constituents. For example, perhaps one of the 14 minor components from the gentamicin-producing fermentation might have a therapeutic potential comparable to the very successful gentamicin C_1.

Among the limitations of each of these plans is the problem of obtaining sufficient amounts of the pure antibiotic for testing for therapeutic efficacy and initial pharmacology. The successes noted in production of the commercially important antibiotics (Thoma, 1971), give us some confidence that application of similar techniques will result in development of processes which will produce sufficient amounts for meeting the requirements for the laboratory evaluations and clinical trials.

The alternative to investing in programmes searching for new microbial metabolites with antibiotic properties, is to invest in a programme of preparation of semi-synthetic antibiotics. As mentioned earlier, we have already prepared thousands of penicillins, cephalosporins, tetracyclines, and rifamycins, and about 0.1% of those prepared have been found to be sufficient improvements on the older compounds to merit their successful introduction into clinical practice. A 0.1% yield for synthetic organic compounds is about the expected performance for pharmaceuticals with the expected 10-year obsolescence rate mentioned above. The practical limit on a programme focused on semi-synthetic antibiotics is the cost of evaluation of the compounds produced. In some laboratories the senior chemists are expected to synthesize about 40 compounds per year, and with a group of 10, it is relatively easy to generate nearly 500 compounds for testing. Both *in vitro* and *in vivo* testing are required, and all too often the testing techniques are not sufficiently sensitive to make the fine distinctions between competing compounds. The initial cost of evaluating these compounds may range from $200 for those with rather poor performance to over $5000 for those with some prospect of displacing several of the established compounds.

An alternative to the semi-synthetic antibiotic programme using the efforts of the organic chemist is to utilize bioconversion programmes similar to those used for bioconversions of steroids. In all antibiotics studied, at least one microorganism has been found which will convert a given antibiotic (Sebek, 1974). These range from the microorganism producing the antibiotic to the various organisms which are resistant to the antibiotic by virtue of being able to degrade it.

Examination of the reports suggests that with a few exceptions, the compounds produced by bioconversions are less potent than the starting materials. Of course, some of the transformation products (such as 6-aminopenicillanic acid) are very useful as building stones for making semi-synthetic antibiotics. But, in general, these transformation products do not have this utility. However, one of the by-products of these studies is a better understanding of mechanisms of biological degradation of the antibiotic and with this understanding it may be possible to reduce the rate of bioconversion by the antibiotic-producing microorganism (thus obtaining higher yields [Perlman, unpublished observations]) or by the resistant organisms.

Dowding and Davies (1975) have noted that the enzyme mechanisms for biotransformations frequently found in the antibiotic-producing organism are related to those found in the resistant organisms found in clinical situations. They suggest that the origin of these mechanisms is thus the producing organism and the occurrence in clinical organisms may be due to plasmid transfer. If this is indeed the origin, we can expect to find biotransformation mechanisms for all antibiotics.

The widespread use of antibiotic feed supplements has been of concern to those who are responsible for monitoring the antibiotic resistance patterns found in clinical infections and elsewhere. The Swann Committee's recommendations (Swann, 1969) which have been accepted in the United Kingdom include the requirements that the antibiotic:

(1) be of economic value in livestock production under U.K. farming conditions;
(2) have little or no application as therapeutic agents in man or animals;
(3) must not impair the efficacy of a prescribed therapeutic antibiotic or antibiotics through the development of resistant strains or organisms.

In their report they mention that zinc bacitracin, moenomycin, and virginiamycin met these objectives, and we can expect that in time these and perhaps others will replace penicillin, chlortetracycline, oxytetracycline, erythromycin, tylosin, and streptomycin now used in various countries as animal feed supplements. Some compounds which meet the Swann Committee objectives are thiopeptin, amphomycin, and chartreusin. These compounds are not well absorbed when fed to poultry or animals, and have some activity against a variety of organisms found in the intestinal tracts of these meat sources. If the use of penicillin, erythromycin, tetracyclines, and aminoglycoside antibiotics as animal feed supplements is eventually banned, it might be sufficient incentive to improve the production processes for these antibiotics to make them more economically attractive and competitive with zinc bacitracin.

Attempts to control plant diseases by the use of antibiotics have been made by plant pathologists all over the world after the discovery of penicillin. Those used in the U.S.A. and in Europe in practical situations have included streptomycin, tetracyclines, cycloheximide, and griseofulvin. Streptomycin is used in the U.S.A. for the control of 'fire blights', and a mixture of streptomycin and tetracycline has been useful in various bacterial plant diseases. Cycloheximide and griseofulvin have found some use for the control of fungal plant diseases. In surveying the antibiotic use for these purposes in the U.S.A. we find very small amounts are used in comparison with chemicals.

In Japan more intensive studies have been carried out on the use of antibiotics to control plant pathogens, and thousands of tons of material are now being used (Misato, Ko and Yamaguchi, 1976). The processes used to manufacture kasugamycin, validamycin, blasticidin S, and polyoxins, are now so efficient that the product cost is competitive with other pathogen control agents. The cost to the farming operation has been subsidized in some situations since food production in Japan is a very critical situation. The companies manufacturing the antibiotics for agriculture in some instances are not involved in manufacturing antibiotics for therapy of human diseases, and their economic considerations are perhaps a factor in the profit/loss calculations, e.g. profit margins in the pharmaceutical industry are usually larger than in the agricultural chemicals industry.

Conclusion

In reviewing the work that is being done in various laboratories we have come to the following conclusions concerning present and future antibiotic research.

(1) There are fewer laboratories screening for 'new' antibiotics in 1976 than there were in 1950. If we compare the effort in 1950 with that in 1975 we find that the number of industrial laboratories is down by a factor of nearly 2, and the academic laboratories by a factor of 5. (This latter situation may result from the 'easy money' currently available for research in molecular biology from various granting sources.)

(2) There are perhaps 30 laboratories involved in programmes on semi-synthetic antibiotics, with cephalosporins and penicillins being the most popular. In many instances the strategy involved in the semi-synthetic antibiotics may relate to the mode of action of the parent antibiotic, the pharmacology of the parent antibiotic, or the chemistry of the antibiotic group. The major determinant in the success of the programmes is the pharmacological supporting research.

(3) Fewer projects are currently operative in laboratories maintained by governmental organizations than 20 years ago. In spite of general concern about increasing food supplies for a larger population, many governments have severely cut back on research and development of antibiotics which might be very effective in increasing the amount of food available for consumption and reducing spoilage between the harvest area and the consumer. In some instances this reduction in support is the result of shifting budgetary priorities, and in others it may be the result of the appropriate governmental officer deciding the industry should be responsible for the research and development costs since they are making reasonably large profits.

(4) Consulting services are available (1976) to assist in antibiotic screening, antibiotic fermentation process development, and antibiotic evaluation. These services may be less costly in the short run than having the work done in the industrial organization's own laboratories. In the long run this deprives the company of technical expertise, but in the short run it does solve some problems quickly.

(5) There is some interest now in applying some of the information learned in molecular biological studies of mechanisms of antibiotic action to practical problems. The Merck Sharp and Dohme Research Laboratories research leading to MK 641/642 is a good example: this combination of deuterofluoroalanine and the sodium pentanedione conjugate of cycloserine is a synergistic combination with broad antibiotic spectrum.

The fluoroalanine irreversibly inactivates alanine racemase. At high concentrations it becomes incorporated into the cell wall peptide in place of D-alanine. The cycloserine eliminates self-reversal and potentiates the inhibitory activity of the fluoroalanine. Both actions result from sequential blockade of cell-wall biosynthesis first by fluoroalanine of D-alanine formation, and then by cycloserine of further assimilation of residual D-alanine or of fluoroalanine itself (Kahan and Kropp, 1975).

The success of this combination in treatment of infections will no doubt lead to other combinations and thus finally justify the work done over the past 20 years on the mechanism of action of antibiotics inhibiting cell-wall synthesis in Gram-positive bacteria.

References

BERDY, J. (1974). *Adv. Appl. Microbiol.*, **18**, 309

DOWDING, J. and DAVIES, J., (1975). In *Microbiology – 1974*, pp. 179–186. Ed. Schlessinger, D., American Society for Microbiology, Washington, D.C.

HAMILTON-MILLER, J.H.M. and BRUMFITT, J. (1974). *J. Inf. Dis.*, **130**, 81

KAHAN, F.M. and KROPP, H. (1975). Abst. 15th Interscience Conf. *Antimicrobial Agents and Chemotherapy*, p. 99. American Society for Microbiology, Washington, D.C.

LUEDEMANN, G. (1969). *Adv. Appl. Microbiol.*, **11**, 101

MAEHR, H. and SCHAFFNER, C.P. (1967). *J. Chromatog.*, **30**, 572

MISATO, T., KO, K. and YAMAGUCHI, I. (1977). *Adv. Appl. Microbiol.*, **21**, 53–88

PERLMAN, D. (Ed.) (1976). *Structure/Activity Relationships in the Semi-synthetic Antibiotics.* Academic Press, New York

PORTER, J.N. (1971). *Adv. Appl. Microbiol.*, **14**, 73

ROUTIEN, J.B. (1961). *J. Bact.*, **81**, 218

SEBEK, O.K. (1974). *Lloydia*, **37**, 115

SWANN, M.M. (1969). Report of Joint Committee on the Use of Antibiotics in Animal Husbandry and Veterinary Medicine. H.M.S.O., London

THIEMANN, J.E., CORONELLI, C., PAGANI, H., BERETTA, G., TAMONI, G. and ARIOLI, V. (1968). *J. Antibiot.*, **21**, 525

THOMA, R.W. (1971). *Folia Microbiol.*, **16**, 197

II

THE CONTEXT OF SYNERGISM

3

A SYNERGIC PERSPECTIVE

M. WOODBINE
Department of Applied Biochemistry and Nutrition, University of Nottingham, Sutton Bonington

Introduction – Delineation

Shakespeare, Homer or the Bible, are often attributed with the ideal quotation for any given situation. Consider, for example, how apposite for the present discussion may be:

Romeo and Juliet III; i, 112: 'A plague o' both your houses!
They have made worms' meat of me.'

or V; iii, 119: 'O true apothecary! Thy drugs are quick.'

The Odyssey, bk 1, 1.7: 'By their own follies they perished, the fools.'

Some decades ago, in the early days of the B.B.C.'s *Any Questions*, Professor C.E.M. Joad would very often begin a contribution with some such phrase as 'it all depends on what you mean by –'. This situation has to be faced in respect of the title selected for this particular Easter School. We need to have some working basis of what is meant by:

agriculture, antibiosis, antibiotic and *synergism.*

In the Faculty of Agricultural Science in the University of Nottingham, the farm gate has never been a bar and Soil Science, Plant Science and Animal Science (behind the gate) have all been regarded as precursors to e.g. Food Science (before the gate). Along with Environmental Science, which relates to all, the whole of Science then becomes relevant to Agricultural Science and, therefore, to Agriculture.

The terms *antibiosis* and *antibiotic* have been attributed to Vuillemin (1889) as antibiose and l'antibiotic in about 1889. The word *antibiotic* should now be used perhaps on the basis of the Waksman (1954) notation, which he, in his fascinating autobiography, first suggested in 1941 'to designate the group of compounds produced by micro-organisms and having a growth-inhibiting effect upon other microbes'.

However, with the consideration of *synergism*, deeper waters are entered. Jawetz (1968, p. 161) uses the definition of *Webster's Dictionary*. But a comparison of Webster with e.g. *Shorter Oxford English Dictionary* for the words associated with *synergism* throws up some intriguing points (my italics).

O.E.D.	*Webster*
1682 G. – (rare) *Synergetic* working together, co-operate	Working together, co-operating, co-operative
1859 *Synergic* physiol: Working together, co-operating, as a group of muscles	
1744 *Synergism* theol: *The doctrine that the human will co-operates with the Divine grace in the work of regeneration*	(1) Physiol: *Co-operative action of discrete agencies such that the total effect is greater than the sum of the two effects taken independently – the opposite of antagonism,* as in *the action of the mixtures of certain salts or drugs* Theol: The semi-Pelagian doctrine that in regeneration there is a *co-operation of divine grace and human activity.* One form held by followers of Melanchton, specified that in conversion, *three agencies* (the Holy Spirit, the Word and the human will) co-operate
1657 *Synergist* med and physiol: A medicine etc. or a bodily organ (e.g. a muscle) that co-operates with another *or others*	(2) Med: A remedy *acting similarly to another and increasing its efficiency when combined with it*
1847 *Synergy:* Combined or correlated action of a group of bodily organs (as nerve centres, muscles etc.); hence of mental faculties, of remedies (etc.)	*The combined effective action of two or more drugs*
Synergise: –	*To co-operate or co-ordinate*
Synergistic: –	Serving as a synergist; co-operating; co-operative.

Within these statements any shade of opinion may be encompassed e.g. 'the combined effective action of two *or more* . . .' which I would adumbrate being based on the 'total effect greater than the sum of the "two" taken independently' or 'increasing the efficiency when combined'. But the most piquant point is that of 'the human will co-operates with the Divine' or 'co-operation of divine grace and human activity', which might have some extra appeal to those with religious affiliations. The more so, within the present context, perhaps, if three agencies co-operate!

Personal Associations: 1943–1976

The association with synergism began in the early 1940s with work on anti-tubercular compounds; an interest in intestinal antisepsis, and in the responsibility for the veterinary chemotherapeutic area within the Chemotherapy Division of the Wellcome Research Laboratories, Beckenham – under the direction of Brownlee and Bushby. The tubercle work (Brownlee, Green and Woodbine, 1948) was extended to experimental guinea-pig studies in which Brownlee and Kennedy (1948) demonstrated synergism with streptomycin and a sulphone (Sulphetrone). Some work was also done on streptomycin and lowly-soluble sulphonamides in relation to Shigellosis, but this was not published in the light of events (sulphadiazine, broad-spectrum antibiotics).

The work on the Erysipeloid (of man) or Rotlauf (diamond back disease in pigs) organism *Erysipelothrix rhusiopathiae* started with an accident in the veterinary vaccine department. This early work on penicillin was followed by some studies on streptomycin (Woodbine, 1946; 1947). In this latter paper some work on combined penicillin-streptomycin – using mice infected with *E. rhusiopathiae* in 5% mucin using percentage survival-days – was done (*see Table 3.1*), which illustrates what I mean by synergism. The bacteriology and chemotherapy of the organism was reviewed (Woodbine, 1950) and formed the basis

Table 3.1 Synergism between penicillin and streptomycin administered intraperitoneally twice daily for 10 days, and then once daily for 5 days, in groups of 20 mice infected with a number of lethal doses of *E. rhusiopathiae,* 353. The numbers surviving are shown, for convenience, as percentage survival-days (from Woodbine, 1947)

Antibiotics	*Dose (I.P.)*	*At 10 days*	*At 15 days*	*At 20 days*
Streptomycin (μg base)	1000	94.5	80.0	64.5
	500	59.0	44.3	37.0
	250	35.0	23.3	17.5
	100	27.5	18.3	13.7
	50	25.5	17.0	12.7
Penicillin (units)	1000	100.0	100.0	98.2
	500	100.0	97.7	93.7
	250	84.0	71.8	64.2
	100	55.5	33.7	25.2
	50	36.0	24.0	18.0
Penicillin (units) + streptomycin (μg base)	500	100.0	100.0	100.0
	250	100.0	99.0	98.0
	50	61.0	44.7	36.0
Controls		16.0	10.7	8.0
Mucin controls		100.0	100.0	100.0

of further work. Through the 1950s, production of antibiotics proceeded apace and a comparative *in vitro* study of magnamycin (or carbomycin) also indicated (*Table 3.2*) potential synergism (Wix and Woodbine, 1955). An interesting example of simultaneous work was that of Klein and Kimmelman (1947) who also used penicillin and streptomycin on *E. rhusiopathiae*.

Some preliminary work was also done on *Listeria monocytogenes* (Jones and Woodbine, 1961) and this was later extended (*Table 3.3*) to a synergic approach (Khan, Seaman and Woodbine, 1972).

Table 3.2 The minimum inhibitory concentrations of magnamycin and penicillin (after 7 days) with *E. rhusiopathiae* (from Wix and Woodbine, 1955)

Number of strains	*Magnamycin* (μg ml^{-1})	+	*Penicillin* (units ml^{-1})
2	0.50		0.10
2	0.50		0.06
1	0.50		0.03
9	0.25		0.10
6	0.25		0.06
15	0.25		0.03
2	0.10		0.10
1	0.10		0.03

Table 3.3 *In vivo* activity of synergic mixtures of ampicillin-trimethoprim and tetracycline-trimethoprim against artificial injection of mice with *L. monocytogenes* (SB-611) (from Khan, Seaman and Woodbine, 1975)

	Percent survival days	
(mg kg^{-1}) *Body weight*	*Ampicillin-Trimethoprim**	*Tetracycline-Trimethoprim***
2.5 + 2.5	63.4	46.6
5.0 + 2.5	46.6	70.0
5.0 + 5.0	70.2	50.0
10.0 + 1.25	53.4	76.8
10.0 + 2.5	56.8	96.6
10.0 + 5.0	56.8	93.4
15.0 + 2.5	30.0	50.2
20.0 + 2.5	30.0	80.0
25.0 + 2.5	43.4	47.34
30.0 + 2.5	30.0	83.4
15.0 + 5.0	30.0	70.0
20.0 + 5.0	40.0	80.0
25.0 + 5.0	36.6	83.4

* Correlation coefficient – 1.1325
** Correlation coefficient – 0.5033

Synergism/Combinations

(a) DAIRY AND FOOD ASPECTS

Within the food industry, the dairy component has always exhibited some technological prowess. This may be illustrated (*Table 3.4*) with the kind of teaching aid produced here in the early 1950s. This illustrates the variety of

Table 3.4 Outline of the major principles of food preservation and prevention of microbial spoilage associated with milk and dairy products, illustrating two, three and four combined effects

Product	*High (time)*	*Low (+ 'frig')*	*Drying*	*Sugar*	*Salt*	*pH*	*Chemical disinfection*
Raw milk		+					
Pasteurized milk	+	+					
Sterilized milk	+	+					
Evaporated milk	+	+					
Sweetened condensed	(+)	(+)		+			
Roller dried	+	(+)	+				
Spray dried	+	(+)	+				
Ice cream	+	+					
Butter	+	+			+	(+) (ripened cream)	
Cheese	+	+			+	+	
Fermented milk	+	+				+	
Plant and utensils	+					+ (caustic for bottles etc.)	+
cf. Eggs	(+)	(+)	(+)				

multiple effects, or combinations, which were developed (cf. Swartling and Lindgren [1968] for the fundamental sort of approach needed for Tetrapak, long-life milk and cream: heat; H_2O_2:sterilized container). Further aspects are referred to by Witter and Ordal (this volume, ch. 9).

A similar kind – and no doubt much more extensive – compilation could be produced for other foods or commodities, along the lines, for example, of the egg addendum.

(b)

Within this overall approach there is the associated problem of how to assess the efficacy of the process. For quality control, resuscitation procedures may be involved. Some attempt (Woodbine, 1968) to survey these was made for the 4th International Symposium on Food Hygiene in *The Microbiology of Dried Foods* (1969) which referred *inter alia* to ageing, diluent, temperature, pH and CO_2.

(c) SYNERGISM/COMBINATIONS IN MICROBIOLOGICAL MEDIA

Some media – about 50 – are illustrated in *Table 3.5*, which indicates the very diverse combinations that have been evolved, based on chemicals, anti-metabolites, antibiotics, and especially (and no doubt for historical reasons) dyes with a variety of physical conditions included.

Table 3.5 Synergism: combinations in microbiological media

Organisms	*Agents*	*References*
Staphylococcus aureus	Mannitol NaCl	Chapman 1944; 1946
	K tellurite Glycine Mannitol Egg yolk	Zebovitz, Evans and Niven (1955) Nelson and Moore (1960) Innes (1960)
	K tellurite Na pyruvate Egg yolk LiCl	Baird-Parker (1962, 1969)
	K tellurite Polymyxin Egg yolk	Crisley, Peeler and Angelotti (1965)
	Mannitol NaCl Ascorbic acid	Jay (1963)
Micrococcus luteus	P bacitracin Novobiocin Paromomycin	Lacey and Boswell (1968)
Cl. perfringens	Sulphite Polymyxin B Sulphadiazine (SPS)	Southworth and Strong (1964)
	Tryptone Sulphite Neomycin (TSN)	Angelotti *et al.* (1962)
	Tryptose Sulphite Cycloserine	Harmon, Kautter and Peeler (1971)
	Oleandomycin Polymyxin B Sulphadiazine	Handford (1974)
	Metabisulphite Polymyxin B Kanamycin SO_4	Shahidi and Ferguson (1971)
	Oleandomycin Polymyxin Sulphadiazine	Hauschild and Hilsheimer (1974)
	Neomycin Polymyxin Heat	Barach, Flowers and Adams (1975)

Organisms	*Agents*	*References*
Streptococcus pyogenes	Polymyxin B SO_4 Neomycin SO_4 Fusidic acid (Horse blood agar)	Lowbury, Kidson and Lilly (1964)
Str. faecalis *faecium* *thermophilus* *pyogenes* *uberis* *lactis* *cremoris*	Crystal violet NaN_3 Thallous acetate	Richards, Soulides and Soulides (1945) (*see also* Hartman, Reinbold and Saraswat [1966])
Str. faecalis	NaN_3 Triphenyl tetrazolium Cl	Burman, Oliver and Stevens (1969)
	Sorbitol Thallous acetate	
Str. agalactiae	Crystal violet Thallous acetate	Edwards (1933)
Listeria monocytogenes	Trypaflavine Naladixic acid	Ralovich *et al.* (1971)
	Thallous acetate Naladixic acid	Kramer and Jones (1969)
	K tellurite Naladixic acid	Khan, Seaman and Woodbine (1972)
	Polymyxin B Naladixic acid Methylene blue	Despierres (1971)
	Acridin K thiocyanate	Bockemühl *et al.* (1974)
	K thiocyanate Naladixic acid	Durst (1973)
Proteus spp	Baird-Parker + Sulphamezathine	Smith and Baird-Parker (1964)
E. coli *E. aerogenes*	Eosin Methylene blue	Levine (1918) Oxoid Manual (1972)
Salmonella spp	Tetrathionate Novobiocin	Jefferies (1959)
	Bismuth citrate Ferric citrate Sodium sulphite Brilliant green	Cruikshank *et al.* (1975)
	Na thiosulphate Brilliant green	Cruikshank *et al.* (1975)
	Selenite Brilliant green	Osborne and Stokes (1955) Stokes and Osborne (1955)
Bacteroides spp	Phanamycin Vancomycin	Finegold, Sugihara and Sutter (1969)
	Neomycin Vancomycin	Finegold, Sugihara and Sutter (1969)

Table 3.5 (continued)

Organisms	*Agents*	*References*
	Ethyl violet NaN_3	Barnes and Impey (1969)
B. fragilis	Kanamycin Colistin	Sutter and Finegold (1969)
Pseudomonas aeruginosa	Cetrimide Naladixic acid	Lilly and Lowbury (1972)
Erysipelothrix	NaN_3 Crystal violet	Packer (1943) (*see also* Harrington and Hulse [1971])
	K tellurite Crystal violet	Miles and Wilson (in Topley and Wilson) (1955)
	Kanamycin Neomycin Vancomycin (Novobiocin)	Wood (1965)
Brucella spp (Taxonomy)	Basic fuchsin Thionin	Cruikshank *et al.* (1975)
	Bacitracin Polymyxin B Cycloheximide	Jones and Morgan (1958) (*see* Cruikshank *et al.* [1975])
Mycoplasma spp	Thallous acetate Penicillin (Methylene blue)	Hayflick (1965) Cruikshank *et al.* (1975) Fallon (1969) Whittlestone (1969)
M. suispneumoniae	Penicillin Thallous acetate Serum and salts	
Microbacterium thermosphactum	Streptomycin Actidione Thallous acetate	Gardner (1966)
Vibrio costicolus (bacon)	Crystal violet Kanamycin	Gardner (1973)
Rhizobium spp	Cycloheximide Pentachlorobenzene Na benzylpenicillin Chloromycetin Sulphathiazole Neomycin	Graham (1969)
Cytophaga spp	Penicillin Chloramphenicol Bile salt	Warke and Dhala (1968)
Soil bacteria	Rose bengal Streptomycin	Martin (1950)
(taxonomy)	Tetracycline Streptomycin Penicillin G Oleandomycin Novobiocin Erythromycin Chloramphenicol	Harris and Woodbine (1967)

Table 3.5 (continued)

Organisms	*Agents*	*References*
Agrobacterium radiobacter	Cycloheximide Bacitracin Tyrothricin Na selenite (Erythritol)	New and Kerr (1971)
Candida spp	Neomycin Polymyxin B	Cohen (1969)
	Chloramphenicol Cycloheximide	Buckley, Campbell and Thompson (1969)
	Penicillin Streptomycin (Cycloheximide)	
General	Rose bengal Chlortetracycline	Cooke (1954) Skidmore and Koburger (1966) Mace and Koburger (1967) Nelson (1972) Jarvis (1973)

A Selection of Diverse Dual Combinations

The amassing of information of general interest over three decades on a particular theme – such as synergism – can lead to a bewildering variety. An attempt has been made to put these on a thematic sectional basis (*Table 3.6*).

Table 3.6 A selection of diverse dual combinations

Organism	*Agent*	*Reference*
(a) Physical (two agents)		
(Fruit juice)	Mild heat (50°C) Irradiation	Kaindl (1968)
General (fresh food)	Mild heat Irradiation	Goresline (1973)
Thermophiles (pH 2–3; 75–80°C)	Temperature pH	Brock and Darland (1970)
B. subtilis *B. pumilis* *Str. faecium*	Heat Radiation	Anon (1969b)
Viruses Bacteria Yeasts	High and low temperatures	Wood (1956)
Yeast ascopores	Freezing and thawing	Chudyk (1971)
Pythium irregulare *P. vexans*	Temperature pH	Cantrell and Camper (1969)
Rhizopus nigricans (enzymes)	Heat pH	Harper (1971)

Table 3.6 (continued)

Organism	*Agent*	*Reference*
Bacterial spores	Heat or radiation Pressure	Anon (1974)
Coliforms	U.V. Ultrasonics	Elhamy and Munkácsi (1973)
Sewage Sterilization	Heat Radiation	Anon (1975)
(b) Physical + chemical		
B. cereus	H_2O_2 Heat	Curran, Evans and Leviton (1940)
S. cerevisiae *Z. soya* *E. coli*	NaCl Radiation	Okazawa, Namiki and Matsuyama (1960)
E. coli	Acriflavine Radiation	Alper (1963)
B. subtilis v. *niger*	Ethylene/propylene oxides Ultrasonics	Boucher *et al.* (1967)
B. subtilis (spores)	H_2O_2 Heat (Irradiation)	Swartling and Lindgren (1968)
B. subtilis	Ultrasonics Glutaraldehyde	Sierra and Boucher (1971)
Fusobacterium nucleatum *Veillonella parvula* *Str. sanguis*	H_2O_2 Ultrasonics	Ahmed and Russell (1975)
Bacillus (spores)	Benzylalkonium Cl^- *m*-Chlorocresol Heat	Briggs and Yazdany (1974)
Shigella flexneri	{Redox pH (Acetic and formic)	Hentges (1969)
Serratia marcescens	{Dehydration Salt	Zimmerman (1969)
E. coli	2-Fluoroadenosine Radiation	Pittillo and Lucas (1965)
E. coli	Chloral hydrate Radiation	Pittillo and Lucas (1965)
S. typhimurium *Ps. aeroginosa* *S. marcescens* *Sarcina lutea* *Str. faecalis*	(Iodoacetamide Bromodeoxyuridine)	Burns (1965)
Psychrophiles	Cold (−1.1°C) NaCl (6%) (pH)	Elliott and Michener (1965)
Cl. sporogenes (spores)	Heat Glucose	Mälkki (1965)
Cl. botulinum E	NaCl pH	Segner, Schmidt and Bultz (1966)
Spores	Heat Phenolics	Deasy, Küster and Timoney (1970)

Table 3.6 (continued)

Organism	*Agent*	*Reference*
B. anitratum	Temp (37°C) pH (6.1–7.2)	Brzin (1973)
Lung irritation	RH SO_2	McIlton, Frank and Charlson (1973)
S. cerevisiae	Radio-frequency Ethanol	Carroll and Lopez (1969)
(c) Physical + antibiotic		
B. stearothermophilus	Mild heat Penicillin	Curran and Evans (1945)
B. stearothermophilus *Cl. botulinum* *B. subtilis*	Mild heat Subtilin	Anderson and Michener (1950)
E. coli	Radiation Hadacidin	Pittillo and Moncrief (1965)
E. coli	Radiation Tetracyclines	Pittillo and Lucas (1967)
S. arizona (turtle eggs)	Chilling + Terramycin or Chloromycetin	Siebeling, Neal and Granberry (1975)
(d) Chemical + chemical		
E. aerogenes	Formamide Formic or acetic	Cooper and Goddard (1952a, b)
General	Benzoic SO_2	Rehm (1960)
General (spores)	Aldehydes and salts	Boucher (1975)
Staphylococcus aureus *Trichophyton mentagrophytes*	Undecylenic acid Quaternary ammonium compounds	Kull *et al.* (1961)
Ps. acidovorans (tryptophan oxidase)	L-Tryptophan 7-Azatryptophan	Rosenfeld and Feigelson (1969)
Ps. aeruginosa	Organic mercury Chlorine	Fitzgerald and Der Vartanian (1969)
Ps. aeruginosa	Polymyxin Polysorbate 80	Brown and Winsley (1971)
Ps. aeruginosa	Phenylethanol and benzalkonium Cl or chlorocresol	Richards (1975)
	Phenylethanol and chlorbutol or benzylalcohol	
	2-Phenylethanol and Ph $HgNO_3$ or acriflavine	
Ps. aeruginosa *Cladosporium* spp	Tetraethylthiuram and Na or Zn-omadine	Cooney (1969)

Table 3.6 (continued)

Organism	*Agent*	*Reference*
Malaria parasite	Chloroquine and pyrimethamine or chloroquanine or proguanil	Pinder (1975)
E. aerogenes (Enzyme [s])	Glucose NO_3	Turner and Eisenthal (1976)
Cocarcinogens	Alcohol and tobacco	Bross and Combs (1976)
(e) Chemical + antibiotic		
Staph. aureus	Fucidin Penicillin or erythromycin Methicillin Novobiocin Tetracycline	Robson and Stacey (1962)
Staphylococci	Neomycin Chlorhexidine	Alder and Gillespie (1967)
Ps. aeruginosa	EDTA and penicillin G Ampicillin Tetracycline or chloramphenicol	Weiser, Wimpenny and Asscher (1969)
Ps. aeruginosa	EDTA and benzalkonium Cl^- or chlorhexidine or polymyxin	Richards (1975)
Ps. aeruginosa	2-Deutero-3 fluoro-D-alanine Cycloserine derivative	Anon (1975b)
Shigella	Naladixic acid and kanamycin Gentamycin or colistin	Michel, Luboshitzky and Sachs (1973)
M. tuberculosis (mice)	Ethambutol and isoniazid	Grumbach (1966)
S. pastorianus (maltose)	Glucose Cycloheximide	Bradley (1962)
T. pallidum (rabbit orchitis)	Mapharsen Bi-salicylate Terramycin	Kolmer (1952)
	KI Mercury succinimide Penicillin	Kolmer (1953)
Vaccines	Neomycin, streptomycin and phenoxyethanol	Cameron (1974)
(f) Antibiotic + antibiotic		
Streptococci (endocarditis)	Penicillin G Bacitracin	Schwarz and Lazarus (1950)
Resistant streptococci	Penicillin Bacitracin	Goldin and Auerbach (1950)
Str. faecalis	Erythromycin Demethyl-chlortetracycline	Gori, Sangiovanni and Floris (1964) Gori *et al.* (1965)

Table 3.6 (continued)

Organism	*Agent*	*Reference*
Sarcina lutea *Staph. aureus* *Str. faecalis* *C. diphtheriae*	Demethylchlortetracycline Oleandomycin	Gori (1967)
S. lutea *Staph. aureus* *Str. faecalis* *B. bronchiseptica*	Demethylchlortetracycline Erythromycin	Gori (1967)
S. lutea	Oleandomycin Chloramphenicol Demethylchloretetracycline	Gori (1967)
Infantile gastroenteritis (0111,055)	Neomycin Bacitracin	Kadison and Borovsky (1951)
Enteropathogenic *E. coli* (0111,055)	Neomycin Polymyxin B	Barr (1956)
Enterococci	Penicillin Kanamycin (or streptomycin)	Hewitt and Deigh (1965)
Streptococci	Cephalosporin Streptomycin Penicillin Streptomycin	Mouton (1967)
Ps. aeruginosa	Penicillins Cephalosporins	Sabath and Abraham (1964)
Ps. aeruginosa	Carbenicillin with colistin Polymyxin B or gentamicin	Beechams (1967)
Ps. aeruginosa	Gentamicin Carbenicillin	Mouton and Holtrigter (1969)
Ps. aeruginosa	Polymyxin + neomycin, bacitracin tetracycline or kanamycin	Lowbury and Jones (1975)
G-range	Methicillin Benzylpenicillin Benzylpenicillin Cloxacillin	Sutherland and Batchelor (1964)
G-range	Ampicillin Cloxacillin	Russell and Sutherland (1974)
E. coli *Shigella* *E. aerogenes*	Polymyxin B Chlortetracycline or chloramphenicol or streptomycin	Jawetz, Coleman and Gunnison (1954)
E. coli	Polymyxin B Streptomycin	Jawetz, Coleman and Gunnison (1954)
S. paratyphi B	Polymyxin Chloramphenicol	Beeuwkes, Mouton and Durlinger (1960)
Enterococci Coliforms	Chloromycetin Tetracycline	Portolés (1958)

Table 3.6 (continued)

Organism	*Agent*	*Reference*
Diphtheroids Enterococci	Streptomycin Chloromycetin	
Staph. aureus *Str. pyogenes* *E. coli*	Penicillin + aureomycin Penicillin + chloramphenicol Streptomycin + chloramphenicol	Elek, Hilson and Jewell (1953)
Staph. aureus	Ostreogrycin A (Staephylomycin M1) or ostreogrycin G (Mikamycin A) + ostreogrycin B (Mikamycin B)	Lester-Smith (1963)
E. coli	Lincomycin Spectinomycin	Hamdy and Blanchard (1969)
Entamoeba histolytica	Carbomycin and tetracycline	Herrell (1955)
Vaccines	Neomycin and streptomycin	Cameron (1974)
(g) Antibiotic + antimetabolite		
Mycobacteria	Cycloserine Isoniazid	Gialdroni-Grassi and Grassi (1966)
M. tuberculosis	Streptomycin Sulphetrone (a soluble sulphone) Streptomycin Promin (a sulphone)	Brownlee and Kennedy (1948)
Staph. aureus	Penicillin Sulphonamide	Bonet-Maury and Perault (1946)
Staph. aureus	Tetracycline or fucidic acid + erythromycin or rifamycin	Mouton and Koelman (1965)
Staph. aureus	Fucidin Methicillin	Garrod (1968)
E. coli *Str. faecalis* *Ps. aeruginosa*	Streptomycin Chloramphenicol or tetracyclines Tetracycline Neomycin Tetracycline Chloramphenicol Polymyxin B Chloramphenicol or streptomycin or tetracyclines Tetracycline Sulphonamide	Rhoads, Billings and Adair (1953)
Ps. aeruginosa	Colistin Sulphamethoxazole	Lowbury and Jones (1975)
Nocadia asteroides	Ampicillin Sulphonamide	Orfanakis, Wilcox and Smith (1971)

Table 3.6 (continued)

Organism	*Agent*	*Reference*
Mouse tumour	Cycloserine 6-Mercaptopurine	Stock and Clarke (1954)
(h) Antimetabolite + antimetabolite		
Ps. aeruginosa	Trimethoprim Sulphamethoxazole	Lowbury and Jones (1975)
Wide range of bacteria (including *Proteus, Bordetella*)	Trimethoprim Sulphonamide	Bushby and Hitchings (1968) Anon (1969a) Finland and Kass (1973)
(i) Synergism/Combinations in food		
Animal feed Rainbow trout	(*a*) Mycotoxin + mycotoxin (*b*) Mycotoxin + Cyclopropenoid F.A.	Lillehoj and Ciegler (1975)
Vinegar products	Sorbic acid Acetic acid	Dakin and Crawford (1966)
Dill pickles	Temp. (120–200°F) pH (acetic)	Monroe *et al.* (1969)
Animal feed	K sorbate Heat (190°F) (Garlic)	Schara and Stocker (1968)
Meat	Cold (5°C) CO_2	Baran, Kraft and Walker (1970)
Cod Plaice Haddock	Cold (ice) Oxytetracycline	Wright (1962)
Shrimp (?)	Nitrofuran(s) Chlortetracycline	Waters and Hamdy (1969)
Foods in general	NaCl and benzoic acid or CO_2	Ingram and Kitchell (1967)
Apple cider	{U.V. K sorbate} {U.V. Cold storage}	Harrington and Hills (1966)
Apple juice (*Z. nadsonii*)	Aw (fructose) Radiation	Kiss and Farkas (1969)
Fruit (strawberries and pears) Vegetables (asparagus, spinach, beans, peas)	Heat Irradiation	Langerak and Brours (1973)
Green peas	{Tylosin lactate Irradiation}	Farkas and Andrassy (1967)
Peas	{Nisin Heat}	Kiss *et al.* (1967)
Cl. botulinum (Toxin)	NaCl Cold	Evans and Tanner (1934)

Table 3.6 (continued)

Organism	*Agents*	*Reference*
B. stearothermophilus *B. cereus* *Cl. thermosaccharolyticum* *Cl. nigrifaciens* *Cl. botulinum* *Cl. sporogenes*	Heat and subtilin, nisin, tylosin or chlortetracycline	*See* Hawley (1962)
Cl. botulinum	U.V. γ-rays	Durban and Grecz (1969)
Cl. sporogenes	(*a*) NO_2^- + cysteine (*b*) Heat + cysteine or ascorbic acid	Farkas and Incze (1974)
Bacillus cereus *Bacillus coagulans* *Bacillus pumilis* (spores)	Radiation pH	Farkas and Andrassy (1967)
E. coli (food)	Chilling (0°C) Fatty acids (C^{11}–C^{12})	Fay and Farkas (1976)
Staph. aureus (enterotoxin)	Temp. NaCl NO_3^- NO_2^-	McLean, Lilly and Alford (1968)
Staph. aureus (meat macerate)	NaCl $NaNO_2$(?) Heat	Bean and Roberts (1975)
Bacteria Yeasts Moulds	Aw pH PO_2	Mossel and Ingram (1955) Mossel (1971)
Pickles	pH Pasteurization Salt	Dakin (1960)
Meat with *Cl. botulinum* (A, B, F, E)	$NaNO_2$ NaCl Sorbic acid	Baird-Parker and Baillie (1974)
(j) Plants		
Bacterial wilt (sweet corn)	Tween 20 Terramycin	Williams and Lockwood (1957)
Agrobacterium radiobacter (selective medium)	Cycloheximide Bacitracin Tyrothricin Na selenite (with erythritol and Fe EDTA)	New and Kerr (1971)
Weed killers	β-Pinene 2, 4–D	Hurt and Templeton (1971)
Pollutants and vegetation	O_3, SO_2 NO_2, SO_2	Williams and Ricks (1975)

Table 3.6 (continued)

Organism	*Agent*	*Reference*
(k) Animals		
Calf scours (*E. coli*)	Chloramphenicol Phthalylsulphathiazole	Clara (1953)
Cald scour isolates	Polymyxin B Neomycin	Barr, Carmen and Clarkson (1955)
Anti-diarrhoeal	Bacitracin Streptomycin	Rossini and Hergott (1955)
	Neomycin Sulphaguanidine (Ivax)	Boots Co.
	Streptomycin Sulphaguanidine (Entavet)	Allen and Hanbury Ltd
C. renale	Penicillin Trypaflavine	Smrček (1957)
Toxoplasmosis (feed)	{Pyrimethamine Sulphonamide	Conney and Hitchings (1969)
Coccidiosis (feed)	Pyrimethamine or diaveridine Sulphonamide	Conney and Hitchings (1969)

Combinations of More than Two Agents

(*a*) *Antibiotic and antibiosis.*
(*b*) *Food aspects.*
A similar attempt (*Table 3.7*) has been made here under the two headings.

Table 3.7 (a) Combinations of more than two agents: antibiotics and antibiosis

Organism	*Agents*	*Host*	*Reference*
Pharmacological activity	Phenacetin Aspirin Codeine	Man	Loewe, Käer and Muischnek (1927)
Coliforms	Streptomycin Bacitracin Polymyxin	Man (Intestinal flora)	Welch, Randall and Price (1950)
S. typhosa *E. coli* *Staph. aureus* *Shigella* spp	Diphenylioclonium/Cl^- Terpineol Mustard oil soap	Broth (Skin?)	Ahmed, Siddiqui and Khan (1969)
E. coli *Proteus* spp Coliforms	Naladixic acid Nitrofurantoin Ampicillin	Man (Urinary infections)	Robertson (1968)
Proteus vulgaris	Nitrofurantoin Chloramphenicol Erythromycin	Urinary system (man)	Zwart Voorspuij and Bokma (1959)

Table 3.7 (a) (continued)

Organism	*Agents*	*Host*	*Reference*
Bacillus spp (spores)	Heat γ-Radiation Chemicals (lipids, sorbic acid, dipeptides, salt)		SIK Report (1967–68)
B. subtilis (spores)	Glutaraldehyde Heat (25–55°C) Ultrasonics (20–25 khz)	Peptone Water	Sierra and Boucher (1971)
Mastitis organisms	Penicillin Dihydrostreptomycin Neomycin Sulfisoxazole	Whole milk	Florestano and Bahler (1955)
M. tuberculosis	Isoniazid Streptomycin Rifampicin or pyrazinamide	Man	Anon (1974a)
M. tuberculosis	{Isoniazid Streptomycin *p*-Amino salicylic acid (PAS)} {Ethionamide PAS Cycloserine}	Man Man	*See* e.g. Radenbach (1965)
L. monocytogenes	{Sulphathiazole Sulphadiazine Sulphamerazine}	Chinchilla	Shalkop (1960)
C. renale	{Streptomycin Sulphonamide Urinary antiseptic}	Cow	Kwiatowski (1957)
Str. pyogenes	Polymyxin B sulphate Neomycin sulphate Fusidic acid	Blood agar	Lowbury, Kidson and Lilly (1964)
General use	Polymyxin Neomycin Bacitracin (Ointment)	Man (topical)	Rexall Drugs (U.S.A.) (1969)
General	Amphotericin B Benzylpenicillin Streptomycin	Tissue culture media	Hamilton-Miller (1973)
Enterobacteria	Trimethoprim Sulphamethoxazole Colistin	Broth	Simmons (1970)
Breast cancer	5-Fluorouracil Methotrexate Cyclophosphamide	Women	{Bonnadonna *et al.* (1976) Anon (1976)}
Testicular cancers	Includes:– Cyclophosphamide *cis*-platinum Chlorambucil Bleomycin	Men	Anon (1976)

Table 3.7 (a) (continued)

Organism	*Agents*	*Host*	*Reference*
	Vinblastine Actinomycin D Adriamycin		
Neuroblastoma (children-nerve)	Cyclophosphamide Vincristine Trifluorothymidine Papaverine	Children	Nelson (1976)

Table 3.7 (b) Combinations of more than two agents: food

Organism	*Agents*	*Host*	*Reference*
Cl. botulinum	Aw pH NaCl	Broth	Baird-Parker and Freame (1967)
Cl. botulinum	NaCl $NaNO_2$ Heat pH	Meat Broth	Jarvis *et al.* (1976)
Cl. botulinum (toxin production)	NaCl $NaNO_2$ Low temp. (15/17.5°C)	Meat Slurry	Roberts, Jarvis and Rhodes (1976)
Cl. botulinum E *Bacillus circulans* *cereus*	Heat Ionizing radiation NaCl Heat Irradiation Tylosin lactate or nisin	Seasoning Peas	Farkas (1967; 1970)
Cl. sporogenes	Na ascorbate $NaNO_2$ NaCl	Meat	Baldini, Ambelli and Casolari (1974)
Cl. sporogenes	(*a*) $NaNO_2$ NaCl Cysteine (*b*) Methionine NaCl $FeSO_4$	Broth Broth	Baldini (1974)
Bacillus subtilis *Clostridium sporogenes* *oedumatiens*	NaCl KNO_3 $NaNO_2$ Heat pH	Broth	Roberts and Ingram (1966)
Cl. perfringens	$NaNO_2$ Cysteine Fe^{++}/Fe^{+++} Heat	Broth	Asan and Solberg (1976)

 Table 3.7 (b) (continued)

Organism	*Agents*	*Host*	*Reference*
Cl. putrefaciens	Heat γ-Radiation NaCl $NaNO_2$ Temp. (1–25°C) pH (6.5–7.0)		Roberts and Derrick (1976)
Spoilage	K sorbate Diethylpyrocarbonate Temp. (3.3°C)	Apple cider	Harrington and Hills (1966)
Spoilage	K sorbate Diethylpyrocarbonate Heat	Prunes	Bolin and Boyle (1967)
Staph. aureus	K sorbate Na benzoate pH (4.5–5.0)	Synthetic cream pies	Schmidt, Gould and Weiser (1969)
Staph. aureus	$NaNO_2$ PO_2 pH (6.3+)	Broth	Buchanan and Solberg (1972)
Salmonella spp	NaCl pH (5.0) Temp. (4°C, 10°C)	Ground pork	Alford and Palumbo (1969)
E. coli *S. typhimurium* *Ps. aeruginosa*	Thiocyanate H_2O_2 Lactoperoxidase	Milk	Reiter and Marshall (1976)

COMMENT

The overall problems are:

(1) to delineate when we have had an additive versus synergic effect (*see* Zwart Voorspuij; Sutherland; Leaman, Fisher, Paulton, Seaman and Woodbine, this volume);

(2) to remember that having imposed a stress (combinations of two, three, or more, cf. Witter and Ordal, this volume, ch. 9), there is then a concomitant problem to confirm that effect by some method of recovery (cf. Corry, van Doorne and Mossel, this volume, ch. 12) – the absence of a positive response is then indicative that the effect(s) has indeed operated.

Attempts to check on the additive, synergic, or antagonistic responses within antibiotics and sulphonamides have been assayed by e.g. Mouton and Koelman (1966). A graphical presentation was produced by Jawetz and Gunnison (1953, p. 184). A sophisticated pattern of a quadripartite nature was earlier produced by Manten and Meyerman-Wisse (1962). This, in turn, was linked to the initial groupings evaluated by Jawetz (*see* eg. Jawetz, 1968):

I Penicillins, streptomycin, neomycin-kanamycin, bacitracin, polymyxins,
II Tetracyclines, chloramphenicol, erythromycins, novobiocin, sulphonamides,

in which synergism often occurred – often as enhanced bactericidal activity *in vitro* – among group I and hardly ever in group II (*see* e.g. Garrod, Lambert and O'Grady, 1973, pp. 282–286; 516). The effect of a combination of groups I and II was found to be proportional largely to the behaviour of the group I component (if rapidly killed by I, addition of II might be antagonistic; if relatively resistant to I then II might produce synergism). But how to account for the diverse dual, or multiple, sequences?

The rate of bactericidal action (if means exist for assessing non-resuscitation) could be examined as suggested by Jawetz, Coleman and Gunnison (1954). We could confirm that the three characteristics of Davis and Sevag (1955) hold:

(1) concentration of one – preferably both – must be *less* than the inhibitory concentration of either;
(2) concentration of either should never be greater than inhibitory level of either alone;
(3) growth survival showed promise – in presence of the combination – whether it gives, or does not give, a resistant population (and *not* within a *short* time).

Or should we look to the approaches suggested by Woods (1953) or the more complicated pattern of Conney and Hitchings (1969)? They lead to the concept of 'double blockade' (*see* Gale *et al.,* 1972, pp. 36–37; 432–433), and Goldberg (1959, p. 32) also gives a simple outline.

Stern and Elek (1955) argued that the chances of a variant arising which is simultaneously resistant to two antibiotics as opposed to one, are much reduced. A larger population may be necessary for such a doubly resistant variety to emerge with less chance of resistance developing. In addition the antibacterial spectrum may be widened. What then of: (*a*) more than two agents, or (*b*) a mix of an antibiotic plus some other chemical or physical agency?

Jawetz, Gunnison and Peck (1952) defined synergism as 'a marked increase in the rate of bactericidal action within the first 24 h of exposure as compared to the rate with either doing alone, and killing of greater numbers of bacteria than could be expected from simple summation of single drug effects'. This was criticized by Davis and Sevag (1955) who thought it to be restrictive in terms of a completely inhibiting concentration and limited incubation. The definition of Manten and Meyermann-Wisse (1961) was more explicit – synergism occurring when the effect of the combination exceeds the sum of the antibacterial effects of its components.

The combined effect may depend on the concentrations of the active substances, the inoculum size, the species, growth conditions, and susceptibility of the organism (Hobby and Dawson, 1946). The ratio of the concentrations is important (Weil and Kotsevalov, 1956; Zwart Voorspuij and Bokma, 1959) as is the growth medium (Davis and Sevag, 1955; Gunnison *et al.,* 1955) or the stage in the growth (Ter-Zakharyan, 1958) or time (Fogh, 1952).

More practical aspects arise from some of the suggestions of Williams-Smith (1958) that drug resistance could be minimized by: (*a*) new drugs, (*b*) combinations, (*c*) periodic use, (*d*) the minimal effective dose for the minimal time, (*e*) avoidance of prophylactic use for a long time, (*f*) support by surgical, immunological or sanitary measures. Succinct guidelines for combinations were presented by Kabins (1972), and Garrod, Lambert and O'Grady (1973) in their book *Antibiotic and Chemotherapy* deal with the types of combined effect (p. 282), tests for combined action (p. 512), and provide a table of combinations likely to show bacterial synergy (p. 516).

ANTI-COMBINATIONS

The contrasting arguments here may be highlighted by the older comments of Hobby and Lenert (1950) that the activity of Terramycin in combination with two *or more* agents is often far in excess of them alone, and Hobby (1953) who stated that synergism was introduced to microbiology in 1923 but in a slightly different manner than for pharmacology owing to the lack of precision in sensitivity determinations (which lead to synergism versus summation).

In contrast, McLachlan reviewing the book by Franklin and Snow (1975) says 'one is left wondering whether the old belief of changing drugs regularly is not the safest method of procedure instead of increasing the dosage . . .'. This view is strongly supported by Grindey (pers. comm. 1976; *see* also Grindey, Moran and Werkheiser, 1975), who says:

'Three basic concepts have been, for the most part, responsible for the widespread use of drug combinations in parasite chemotherapy. The first involves the fact that most of these agents are quite selective and have only moderate host toxicity. This allowed the utilization of combinations of agents with only a minimal increase in host toxicity. Secondly, most of these agents have a selective spectrum of activity and thus combinations were developed to assure effective therapy, should more than one organism be involved. Finally, the concept that the development of resistance was delayed in combination treatment also was considered an important aspect of drug combinations.'

'Unfortunately, the widespread use of drug combinations was responsible for the appearance of 'R Factors' in bacteria. These epigenic species are capable of conferring complete resistance to several drugs at once (*see* chapter by Reynard in *Drug Resistance and Selectivity*). Thus, in the presence of 'R Factors', resistance to a four- or five-drug combination can develop immediately and completely negate the proposed benefits from concurrent therapy. Thus, in retrospect, the use of sequential drugs to combat resistance and multiple organisms (or lack of ability or inclination to identify infectious organisms) would have been prudent rather than the concurrent combinations which were utilized . . .'

and by Falkow (pers. comm. 1976; *see* also Falkow, 1975), who says:

'Sequential or intermittent exposure to antibiotics can, of course, lead to selection for resistant microbial species. In most cases, however, the organisms are transient and lost after antibiotic selection is discontinued. Very simply put, it is a rare micro-organism which is adept at both maintaining an R plasmid and being proficient in bowel colonization. Given enough time and selective pressure such as that which occurs during continuous feeding such strains do arise however. Nevertheless, the finding by Richmond's group that fully one-third of all R-bearing strains of *E. coli* in both Man and his domestic animals belong to but 3 of the possible 160 0 antigenic types reveals that "special" strains are involved. We often see patients in our clinic who have received antibiotics and shed virtually 100% R^+ *E. coli* during treatment, but within a few months of recovery harbor only a few R^+ organisms. Yet, patients on continuous therapy for many months quite generally maintain a significant reservoir of R^+ species. It is the same in calves. Veal calves raised in an environment in which antibiotics are continuously employed will have from 40–60% of their *E. coli* R^+. Yet, range calves just 30 miles away which are treated only intermittently with antibiotics show less than 1% R^+ *E. coli.*'

'It seems clear that R plasmid-containing strains become permanently established in an individual as a result of long term selection with subtherapeutic and therapeutic levels of antibiotics, while intermittent use does not present a problem of the same magnitude. Certainly, the fact that R^+ bacteria are most commonly found in the hospital ward and on farms using medicated feed and only at a relatively low level in the community also argues for this view.'

In strong contrast to both these views, there is the very recent work of e.g. Bonadonna *et al.* (1976) who have put forward the benefits of multiple agents in breast cancer (with the use of cyclophosphamide, 5-fluorouracil, and methotrexate).

Peroration

The world undoubtedly faces a double demand: an improvement in the overall quality of life and a concurrent, allied insistence on the conservation and utilization of resources.

A critical and sustained appraisal of the value of combinations – and especially multiple ones (i.e. more than two) – for synergic potential, could well contribute to these aims, both on aesthetic and on economic grounds.

Acknowledgements

Very grateful thanks to colleagues throughout the world and over three decades who have helped in providing material and giving opinions. Among others, Ella Barnes, John Cavett, Alan Gardner and Richard Gilbert for the media aspect and to Gerald B. Grindey and Stanley Falkow for anti-combination comments.

References

AHMED, F.I.K. and RUSSELL, C. (1975). *J. appl. Bact.*, **39**, 31
AHMED, Z., SIDDIQUI, M.A. and KHAN, I. (1969). *Appl. Microbiol.*, **17**, 857
ALDER, V.G. and GILLESPIE, W.A. (1967). *Lancet*, **ii**, 1062
ALFORD, J.A. and PALUMBO, S.A. (1969). *Appl. Microbiol.*, **17**, 528
ALPER, T. (1963). *Nature, Lond.*, **200**, 534
ANDERSON, A.A. and MICHENER, H.D. (1950). *Food Tech., Champaign*, **4**, 188

ANGELOTTI, R., HALL, R.E., FOSTER, M.J. and LEWIS, K.H. (1962). *Appl. Microbiol.,* **10**, 193
ANON (1969a). The synergy of trimethoprim and sulphonamides. *Post-Grad. Med. J.,* **45**, Supplement
ANON (1969b). *Chem. Eng. News,* **29 Sept.**, 39
ANON (1974). *Chem. Eng. News,* **24 June**
ANON (1974a). *Med. Tech.,* **4**, July
ANON (1974b). *Chem. Eng. News,* **29 July**, 12
ANON (1975). *Chem. Eng. News,* **24 March**, 20
ANON (1975b). *Chem. Eng. News,* **6 Oct.**, 6
ANON (1976). *Chem. Eng. News,* **23 Feb.**, 6
ANON (1976). *Chem. Eng. News,* **17 May**, 23
ASAN, T. and SOLBERG, M. (1976). *Appl. envir. Microbiol.,* **31**, 49
BAIRD-PARKER, A.C. (1962). *J. appl. Bact.,* **25**, 12
BAIRD-PARKER, A.C. (1969). In *Isolation Methods for Microbiologists,* p. 1. Eds. Shapton, D.A. and Gould, G.W. Academic Press, London
BAIRD-PARKER, A.C. and BAILLIE, M. ANN (1974). *Proc. Int. Symp. Nitrite Meat Prod., Zeist.,* p. 77. Eds. Krol, B. and Tinbergen, B.J.
BAIRD-PARKER, A.C. and FREAME, BARBARA (1967). *J. appl. Bact.,* **30**, 420
BALDINI, P. (1974). *Industria Conserva,* **49**, 232
BALDINI, P., AMBANELLI, G. and CASOLARI, A. (1974). *Industria Conserva,* **49**, 155
BARACH, J.T., FLOWERS, R.S. and ADAMS, D.M. (1975). *Appl. Microbiol.,* **30**, 873
BARAN, W.L., KRAFT, A.A. and WALKER, H.W. (1970). *J. Milk Fd Tech.,* **33**, 77
BARNES, ELLA M. and IMPEY, C.S. (1969). In *Isolation of Anaerobes*, p. 115. Eds. Shapton, D.A. and Board, R.G. Academic Press, London
BARR, F.S. (1956). *Antibiotic Med.,* **2**, 324
BARR, F.S., CARMEN, P.E. and CLARKSON, J.B. (1955). *Am. J. vet. Res.,* **16**, 515
BEAN, P.G. and ROBERTS, T.A. (1975). *J. Food Tech.,* **10**, 327
BEECHAM RESEARCH LABORATORIES (1967). *Pyopen/carbenicillin,* p. 26
BEEUWKES, H., MOUTON, R.P. and DURLINGER, L. (1960). *Antonie van Leeuwenhoek,* **26**, 340
BOCKEMUHL, J., FEINDT, E., HOHNE, K. and SEELIGER, H.P.R. (1974). *Med. Mikrobiol. Immunol.,* **159**, 289
BOLIN, H.R. and BOYLE, F.P. (1967). *J. Sci. Fd Agric.,* **18**, 289
BONADONNA, G., BRASAMILINO, E., VALAGUSSA, P., ROSSI, ANNA, BRUGNATELLI, LUISE, BRAMBILLA, CRISTINA, DELENA, M., TANCINI, GABRIELLE, BAJETTA, E., MUSUMECI, R. and VERONESI, U. (1976). *New Engl. J. Med.,* **294**, 405, 440
BONET-MAURY, P. and PERAULT, R. (1946). *Nature, Lond.,* **157**, 131
BOUCHER, R.M.G. (1976). *Chem. Eng. News,* **24 May**, 12
BOUCHER, R.M.G., PISANO, M.A., TORTORA, G. and SAWICKI, E. (1967). *Appl. Microbiol.,* **15**, 1257
BRADLEY, S.G. (1962). *Nature, Lond.,* **194**, 315
BRIGGS, A. and YAZDANY, S. (1974). *J. appl. Bact.,* **37**, 623
BROCK, T.D. and DARLAND, G.K. (1970). *Science,* **169**, 1316
BROSS, I. and COOMBS, JEAN (1976). *Chem. Eng. News,* **20 May**, 19
BROWN, M.R.W. (Ed.) (1975). *Resistance of* Pseudomonas aeruginosa, Wiley, London
BROWN, M.R.W. and WINSLEY, B.E. (1971). *J. gen. Microbiol.,* **68**, 367

BROWNLEE, G., GREEN, A.F. and WOODBINE, M. (1948). *Brit. J. Pharmac. Chemother.*, **3**, 15

BROWNLEE, G. and KENNEDY, C.R. (1948). *Brit. J. Pharmac. Chemother.*, **3**, 37

BRZIN, BRONKA (1973). *Zentbl. Bakt. Parasit Kde.* (Abt I Orig. A.), **223**, 83

BUCHANAN, R.L. and SOLBERG, M. (1972). *J. Food Sci.*, **37**, 81

BUCKLEY, HELEN R., CAMPBELL, C.K. and THOMPSON, J.C. (1969). In *Isolation Methods for Microbiologists,* p. 113. Eds. Shapton, D.A. and Gould, G.W. Academic Press, London

BURMAN, N.P., OLIVER, C.W. and STEVENS, JANET K. (1969). In *Isolation Methods for Microbiologists,* p. 127. Eds. Shapton, D.A. and Gould, G.W. Academic Press, London

BURNS, J., GARCIA, J.P., LUCAS, MARY, MONCRIEF, F. CAROLYN and PITTILLO, R.F. (1965). *Radiat. Res.*, **25**, 460

BUSHBY, S.R.M. and HITCHINGS, G.H. (1968). *Br. J. Pharmac. Chemother.*, **33**, 72

CAMERON, J. (1974). *Int. Symp. Preservatives in Biological Products in Develop. Biol. Standard,* **24**, 155. (Karger, Basel)

CANTRELL, H.F. and CAMPER, N.D. (1969). *Bact. Proc.* (G118)

CARROLL, D.E. and LOPEZ. A. (1969). *J. Food Sci.*, **34**, 320

CHAPMAN, G.H. (1944). *J. Bact.*, **48**, 555

CHAPMAN, G.H. (1946). *J. Bact.*, **51**, 409

CHUDYK, R.V. (1971). Ph.D. Thesis, Nottingham

CLARA, I. (1953). *Atti Soc. ital. Sci. vet.*, **6**, 398

COHEN, S.N. (1969). *Appl. Microbiol.*, **17**, 486

CONNEY, A.H. and HITCHINGS, G.H. (1969). In *The Use of Drugs in Animals Feeds*, p. 180. N.A.S., N.R.C., Washington

COOKE, W.B. (1954). *Antibiot. Chemother.*, **4**, 657

COONEY, J.J. (1969). *Appl. Microbiol.*, **17**, 227

COOPER, E.A. and GODDARD, A.E. (1952a). *J. appl. Chem.*, **2**, 49

COOPER, E.A. and GODDARD, A.E. (1952b). *J. appl. Chem.*, **2**, 129

CRISLEY, F.D., PEELER, J.T. and ANGELOTTI, R. (1965). *Appl. Microbiol.*, **13**, 140

CRUICKSHANK, R., DUGUID, J.P., MARMION, B.P. and SWAIN, R.H.A. (1975). *Medical Microbiology,* 12th edn. Churchill Livingstone, London

CURRAN, H.R. and EVANS, F.R. (1945). *J. Bact.*, **34**, 179

CURRAN, H.R., EVANS, F.R. and LEVITON, A. (1940). *J. Bact.*, **40**, 423

DAKIN, J.C. (1960). In *Recent Advances in Food Science,* p. 128. Eds. Hawthorn, J. and Leitch, J.M. Butterworths, London

DAKIN, J.C. and CRAWFORD, D.C. (1966). *Tech. Circ.*, **166** (British Food Manufacturers' Industrial Research Association)

DAVIS, L. and SEVAG, M.G. (1955). *Antibiot. Chemother.*, **5**, 80

DEASY, P.B., KUSTER, E. and TIMONEY, R.F. (1970). *Appl. Microbiol.*, **20**, 455

DESPIERRES, M. (1971). *Ann. Inst. Pasteur.*, **121**, 493

DURBAN, E. and GRECZ, N. (1969). *Appl. Microbiol.*, **18**, 44

DURST, J. (1973). *Z. med. Labor. Tech.*, **14**, 111

EDWARDS, S.J. (1933). *J. comp. Path. Therap.*, **46**, 211

ELEK, S.D., HILSON, G.R.F. and JEWELL, PAMELA (1953). *Br. Med. J.*, **ii**, 1298

ELHAMY, M. and MUNKACSI, F. (1973). *Medicor News.* (Hungary), 25

ELLIOTT, R.P. and MICHENER, H.D. (1965). *USDA Tech. Bull.*, No. 1320

EVANS, FLORENCE L. and TANNER, F.W. (1934). *Zentl. Bakt. Parasit Kde.* (Abt. 2), **91**, 135

FALKOW, S. (1975). *Infectious Multiple Drug Resistance.* Pion Ltd, London

FALLON, R.J. (1969). In *Isolation Methods for Microbiologists*, p. 41. Eds. Shapton, D.A. and Gould, G.W. Academic Press, London

FARKAS, J. (1967). Microbiological problems in food preservation by irradiation. *Int. Atomic Energy Agency,* 123

FARKAS, J. (170). *Spore News Letter,* **Nov.**, 162

FARKAS, J. and ANDRASSY, EVA (1967a). *Elelmiszertudomany,* **2**, 59

FARKAS, J. and ANDRASSY, EVA (1967b). *Elelmiszertudomany* (Fd Sci.), **2**, 99

FARKAS, J. and INCZE, K. (1974). *Konzerves Paprikaipar* (Special issue), 50

FARKAS, J. and KISS, I. (1968). *Int. Atomic Energy Agency Report*

FAY, J.P. and FARKAS, R.N. (1976). *Appl. env. Microbiol.,* **31**, 153

FINEGOLD, S.M., SUGIHARA, P.T. and SUTTER, VERA L. (1969). In *Isolation of Anaerobes*, p. 99. Eds. Shapton, D.A. and Board, R.G. Academic Press, London

FINLAND, M. and KASS, E.H. (Eds) (1973). *Trimethoprim – sulfamethoxazole.* Univ. of Chicago Press, Chicago, U.S.A.

FITZGERALD, C.P. and DERVARTANIAN, M.E. (1969). *Appl. Microbiol.,* **17**, 415

FLORESTANO, H.J. and BAHLER, M.E. (1955). *Vet. Med.,* **50**, 441

FOGH, B. (1952). *Act. path. microbiol. scand.,* **31**, 481

FRANKLIN, T.J. and SNOW, G.A. (1975). *Biochemistry of Antimicrobial Action,* 2nd edn. Academic Press, London

GALE, E.F., CUNDLIFFE, E., REYNOLDS, P.E., RICHMOND, M.A. and WARING, M.J. (1972). *The Molecular Basis of Antibiotic Action.* Wiley, London

GARDNER, G.A. (1966). *J. appl. Bact.,* **29**, 455

GARDNER, G.A. (1973). *J. appl. Bact.,* **36**, 329

GARROD, L.P. (1968). *Lancet,* **ii**, 19 Oct

GARROD, C.P., LAMBERT, H.P. and O'GRADY, F. (1973). *Antibiotic and Chemotherapy,* 4th edn, pp. 282, 512, 516. Churchill Livingstone, London

GIALDRONI-GRASSI, G. and GRASSI, C. (1965). *Antimicrob. Ag. Chemother.,* – 1965, 1074

GOLDBERG, H.S. (1959). *Antibiotics: Their Chemistry and Non-medical Uses,* pp. 32, 24. Von Nostrand, New York

GOLDIN, M. and AUERBACH, HELEN (1950). *Bact. Proc.,* 119

GORESLINE, H.E. (1973). In *Food Irradiation Information.* International Project in the Field of Food Irradiation, Int. Atomic Energy Agency, Vienna

GORI, E. (1967). *Path. Biol., Paris,* **15**, 148

GORI, E., SANGIOVANNI, M. and FLORIS, M. (1964). *3rd Int. Congr. Chemother.,* 696. Georg Thieme, Stuttgart

GORI, E., SANGIOVANNI, E.P., FLORIS, E. and PAGAN, M. (1965). *Antimicrob. Ag. Chemother.* – 1965, 273

GRAHAM, P.H. (1969). *Appl. Microbiol.,* **17**, 769

GRINDEY, G.B., MORAN, R.G. and WERKHEISER, W.C. (1975). In *Drug Design,* p. 5. Ed. Ariens, E.J. Academic Press, New York

GRUMBACH, F. (1966). *Antimicrob. Ag. Chemother.* – 1966, 1058

GUNNISON, JANET B., KUNISHIGE, E., COLEMAN, VIRGINIA, R. and JAWETZ, E. (1955). *J. gen. Microbiol.,* **13**, 509

HAMDY, A.H. and BLANCHARD, C.J. (1969). *Poult. Sci.,* **48**, 1703

HAMILTON-MILLER, J.M.T. (1973). *Bact. Rev.,* **37**, 166

HANDFORD, P. MARION (1974). *J. appl. Bact.,* **37**, 559

HARMON, S.M., KAUTTER, D.A. and PEELER, J.I. (1971). *Appl. Microbiol.,* **22**, 688
HARPER, K.A. (1971). *Chem. Ind.,* 462
HARRINGTON, W.O. and HILLS, C.H. (1966). *Fd Technol., Champaign.,* **20**, 120
HARRINGTON, R. and HULSE, D.C. (1971). *Appl. Microbiol.,* **22**, 141
HARRIS, P.J. and WOODBINE, M. (1967). *Plant and Soil.,* **27**, 167
HARTMAN, P.A., REINBOLD, G.W. and SARASWAT, D.S. (1966). *Adv. appl. Microbiol.,* **8**, 253
HAUSCHILD, A.H.W. and HILSHEIMER, R. (1974). *Appl. Microbiol.,* **27**, 78
HAWLEY, H.B. (1962). In *Antibiotics in Agriculture*. Ed. Woodbine, M. Butterworths, London
HAYFLICK, L. (1965). *Tex. Rep. biol. Med.,* **23** (Suppl. 1), 285
HENTGES, D.J. (1969). *J. Bact.,* **97**, 513
HERRELL, W.E. (1955). *Int. Rec. Med. gen. Pract. Clinics.,* **168**, 463
HEWITT, W.L. and DEIGH, ROSALYN A. (1965). *Antimicrob. Ag. Chemother.* – 1966, 278
HOBBY, GLADYS L. (1953). *Int. Congr. Microbiol., Rome,* (Abstr.), p. 182
HOBBY, GLADYS L. and DAWSON, M.H. (1946). *J. Bact.,* **51**, 447
HOBBY, GLADYS L. and LENERT, TULITA F.(1950). *Bact. Proc.,* 99
HURT, W. and TEMPLETON, A.R. (1971). In *Chem. Eng. News,* **11 Jan.**, 25
INGRAM, M. and KITCHELL, A.G. (1967). *J. Food Tech.,* **2**, 1
INNES, A.G. (1960). *J. appl. Bact.,* **23**, 105
JARVIS, B. (1973). *J. appl. Bact.,* **36**, 723
JARVIS, B., RHODES, ANNETTE, C., KING, SUSAN E. and PATEL, M. (1976). *J. Food Tech.,* **11**, 41
JAWETZ, E. (1968). *A. Rev. Pharmac.,* **8**, 151
JAWETZ, E., COLEMAN, VIRGINIA and GUNNISON, JANET B. (1954). *Ann. intern. Med.,* **41**, 79
JAWETZ, E. and GUNNISON, JANET B. (1953). *Pharmac. Rev.,* **5**, 175
JAWETZ, E., GUNNISON, JANET B. and PECK, R.S. (1952). *Am. J. med. Sci.,* **222**, 404
JAY, J.M. (1963). *J. appl. Bact.,* **26**, 69
JEFFERIES, L. (1959). *J. clin. Path.,* **12**, 568
JONES, SUSAN M. and WOODBINE, M. (1961). *Vet. Revs Annot.,* **7**, 39
KABINS, S.A. (1972). *J. Am. Med. Ass.,* **219**, 206
KADISON, E.R. and BOROVSKY, M.P. (1951). *J. Pediat.,* **38**, 576
KAINDL, K. (1968). *Chemy Ind.,* (Abstr.) 254
KHAN, M.A., SEAMAN, A. and WOODBINE, M. (1972). *Acta microbiol. hung.,* **19**, 371
KHAN, M.A., SEAMAN, A. and WOODBINE, M. (1975). In *Problems in Listeriosis,* p. 52. Ed. Woodbine, M. Leicester University Press
KISS, I. and FARKAS, J. (1969). *Elelmiszestudomany,* **3**, 93
KISS, I., KISSNE, K. NATALIA, FARKAS, J., FABRI, ILONA and VAS, K. (1967). *Elelmiszestudomany,* **2**, 51
KLEIN, M. and KIMMELMAN, J.L. (1947). *J. Bact.,* **54**, 363
KOLMER, J.A. (1952). *Proc. Soc. exp. Biol. Med.,* **79**, 143
KOLMER, J.A. (1953). *Am. J. Syph. Gonorrhea vener. Dis.,* **37**, 77
KRAMER, PAMELA A. and JONES, DOROTHY (1969). *J. appl. Bact.,* **32**, 381
KULL, K.C., EISMAN, P.C., SYLWESTROWICZ, H.D. and MAYER, R.L. (1961). *Appl. Microbiol.,* **9**, 538

KWIATOWSKI, T. (1957). *Medycyna wet.*, **13**, 289
LACEY, R.W. and BOSWELL, P.A. (1968). *J. appl. Bact.*, **31**, 302
LANGERAK, D.I. and BROURS, M.F.J. (1973). *Acta Alimentaria*, **2**, 229
LESTER-SMITH, E. (1963). *J. gen. Microbiol.*, **33**, iii–iv
LEVINE, M. (1918). *J. infect. Dis.*, **23**, 43
LILLEHOJ, E.B. and CIEGLER, A. (1975). *Microbiology*, p. 344. Am. Soc. Microbiol., Washington
LILLY, H.A. and LOWBURY, E.J.L. (1972). *J. med. Microbiol.*, **5**, 151
LOEWE, S., KAER, E. and MUISCHNEK, H. (1927). *Arch. exp. Path. Pharmak.*, **120**, 25, 41
LOWBURY, E.J.L. and JONES, R.J. (1975). In *Resistance of* Pseudomonas aeruginosa, pp. 237–269. Ed. Brown, M.R.W. Wiley, London
LOWBURY, E.J.L., KIDSON, A. and LILLY, H.A. (1964). *J. clin. Path.*, **17**, 231
MACE, F.E. and KOBURGER, J.A. (1967). *Proc. W. Va. Acad. Sci.*, **39**, 102
MALKKI, Y. (1965). State Inst. Tech. Res., Helsinki, Finland. Publ. 96
MANTEN, A. and WISSE, M.J. (1962). *Antonie van Leeuwenhoek.*, **28**, 321
MANTEN, A. and WISSE, M.J. (1961). *Nature, Lond.*, **192**, 671
MARSHALL, R.S., STEENBERGEN, J.F. and McCLUNG, L.S. (1965). *Appl. Microbiol.*, **13**, 559
MARTIN, J.P. (1950). *Soil Sci.*, **69**, 215
McILTON, C., FRANK, R. and CHARLSON, R. (1973). *Science*, **182**, 503
MCLEAN, R.A., LILLEY, H.D. and ALFORD, J.A. (1968). *J. Bact.*, **95**, 1207
MICHEL, J., LUBOSHITZKY, R. and SACHS, T. (1973). *Antimicrob. Ag. Chemother.* – 1963, 201
MONROE, R.J., ETCHELLS, J.L., PACILIO, J.C., BORG, A.I.F., WALLACE, D.H., ROGERS, M.P., TURNEY, L.J. and SCHOENE, E.S. (1969). *Food Tech., Champaign.*, **23**, 71
MOSSEL, D.A.A. (1971). In *Microbes and Biological Productivity*, p. 117. Eds. Hughes, D.E. and Rose, A.H. Cambridge University Press
MOSSEL, D.A.A. and INGRAM, M. (1955). *J. appl. Bact.*, **18**, 232 (esp. 253–4)
MOUTON, R.P. (1967). *Int. Congr. Chthy, Vienna*, 735
MOUTON, R.P. and HOLTRIGTER, B. (1969). *Chemotherapy*, **14**, 371
MOUTON, R.P. and KOELMAN, A. (1965). *Antimicrob. Ag. Chemother.* – 1965, 261
MOUTON, R.P. and KOELMAN, E. (1966). *Chemotherapia*, **11**, 10
MOYNIHAN, I.W. and STOVELL, D.L. (1954). Amer. Vet. Med. Assoc., 91st Meeting, p. 327
NELSON, F.E. (1972). *Appl. Microbiol.*, **24**, 236
NELSON, F.E. and MOORE, T.D. (1960). *Bact. Proc.*, 45
NELSON, L. (1976). *Chem. Eng. News*, **17 May**, 73
NEW, P.B. and KERR, A. (1971). *J. appl. Bact.*, **34**, 233
OKAZAWA, Y., NAMIKI, M. and MATSUYAMA, A. (1960). *Bull. Agr. Chem. Soc., Japan*, **24**, 435
ORFANAKIS, M.G., WILCOX, H. and SMITH, C.B. (1971). *Antibiot. Chemother.*, No. 103
OSBORNE, W.W. and STOKES, J.L. (1955). *Appl. Microbiol.*, **3**, 295
PACKER, R.A. (1943). *J. Bact.*, **46**, 343
PINDER, R.M. (1975). *Progr. med. Chem.*, **8**, 231
PITTILLO, R.F. and LUCAS, MARY B. (1965). *Nature, Lond.*, **205**, 824

PITTILLO, R.F. and LUCAS, MARY B. (1967). *Radiat. Res.*, **31**, 36
PITTILLO, R.F. and MONCRIEF, F. CAROLYN (1965). *Proc. Soc. exp. Biol. Med.*, **118**, 525
PORTOLES, A. (1958). *Int. Congr. Microbiol., Stockholm.* (Abstr.), 340
RADENBACH, K.L. (1965). *Antimicrobial Agents and Chemotherapy – 1965*, 1065
RALOVICH, B., FORRAY, A., MERO, E., MALOVICS, HELEN and SZAZADUS, I. (1971). *Zentbl. Bakt. Parasit. Kde.* (Abtl orig.), **216**, 88
REHM, H.J. (1960). *Annls. Inst. Pasteur, Paris*, **11**, 217
REITER, B. and MARSHALL, VALERIE M. (1976). *Proc. Soc. gen. Microbiol.*, **4 (Jan.)**, pp. 108, 109
RHOADS, P.S., BILLINGS, C.E. and ADAIR, DORIS M. (1953). *Antibiot. Chemother.*, **3**, 721
RICHARDS, R.M.E. In *Resistance of* Pseudomonas aeruginosa. Ed. Brown. M.W.R. Wiley, London.
RICHARDS, T., SOULIDES, D.A. and SOULIDES, E. (1945). *Proc. Soc. appl. Bact.* (Abstr.), 44
ROBERTS, T.A. and DERRICK, CHRISTINE M. (1976). *J. appl. Bact.*, **38**, 33
ROBERTS, T.A. and INGRAM, M. (1966). *J. Food Tech.*, **1**, 147
ROBERTS, T.A., JARVIS, B. and RHODES, ANNETTE C. (1976). *J. Food Tech.*, **11**, 25
ROBERTSON, M.H. (1968). *Br. J. clin. Pract.*, **22**, 63
ROBSON, J.M. and STACEY, R.S. (1962). In *Recent Advances in Pharmacology*, p. 354. Churchill, London. (*See also* Leo Labs, Copenhagen, 1967)
ROSENELD, H. and FEIGELSON, P. (1969). *J. Bact.*, **97**, 697
ROSSINI, L.J. and HERGOTT, J.A. (1955). *N. Am. Vet.*, **35**, 384
RUSSELL, E.J. and SUTHERLAND, R. (1964). *Progr. Chthy., Athens*, 109
SABATH, L.D. and ABRAHAM, E.P. (1964). *Nature, Lond.*, **204**, 1066
SCHARA, R.E. and STOCKER, C.T. (1968). S.A. Patent 67,03647
SCHMIDT, E.W., GOULD, W.A. and WEISER, H.H. (1969). *Food Tech., Champaign.*, **23**, 1197
SCHWARZ, L.H. and LAZARUS, J.A. (1950). *Bact. Proc.*, p. 117
SEGNER, N.P., SCHMIDT, C.F. and BULTZ, J.K. (1966). *Appl. Microbiol.*, **14**, 49
SHAHIDI, S.A. and FERGUSON, A.R. (1969). *Bact. Proc.*, p. 1
SHAHIDI, S.A. and FERGUSON, A.R. (1971). *Appl. Microbiol.*, **21**, 500
SHALKOP, W.T. (1960). *J. Am. vet. med. Ass.*, **116**, 447
SIEBELING, R.J., NEAL, P.M. and GRANBERRY, W.D. (1975). *Appl. Microbiol.*, **30**, 791
SIERRA, G. and BOUCHER, R.M.G. (1971). *Appl. Microbiol.*, **22**, 160
SIK REPORT (1967–8). *Swedish Institute for Food Preservation Research*, Göteborg
SIMMONS, N.A. (1970). *J. clin. Path.*, **23**, 757
SKIDMORE, N.C. and KOBURGER, J.A. (1966). *Proc. W. Va. Acad. Sci.*, **38**, 63
SMITH, B.A. and BAIRD-PARKER, A.C. (1964). *J. appl. Bact.*, **27**, 78
SMRCEK, Z. (1957). *Vet. Glasn.*, **11**, 426
SONNE, M. and JAWETZ, E. (1969). *Appl. Microbiol.*, **17**, 893
SOUTHWORTH, JILL M.L. and STRONG, DOROTHY H. (1964). *J. Fd Sci.*, **27**, 205
STERN, H. and ELEK, S.D. (1955). *Brit. med. J.*, **ii**, 1304
STOCK, C.C. and CLARKE, D.A. (1954). *Chem. Eng. News*, **5 April**, 1321

STOKES, J.L. and OSBORNE, W.W. (1955). *Appl. Microbiol.*, **3**, 217
SUTTER, VERA L. and FINEGOLD, S.M. (1969). *Bact. Proc.*, p. 35
SUTHERLAND, R. and BATCHELOR, F.R. (1964). *Nature, Lond.*, **201**, 868
SWARTLING, P. and LINDGREN, B. (1968). *J. Dairy Res.*, **35**, 423
TER-ZAKHARYAN, YU Z. (1958). *See Biol. Abstr. 1958,* 12984
TOPLEY, S. and WILSON, G.S. (1955). *Topley and Wilson's Principles of Bacteriology and Immunity*, 4th edn. Eds. Wilson, G.S. and Miles, A.T. Arnold, London
TURNER, W.H. and EISENTHAL, R. (1975). *Proc. Soc. gen. Microbiol.*, **3 (Nov.)**, p. 59
VUILLEMIN, P. (1889). *Assoc. Franc. Avanc. Sci., Paris,* pt 2, 525
WAKSMAN, S.A. (1954). *My Life with the Microbes,* p. 207. Simon and Schuster, New York
WARKE, G.M. and DHALA, S.A. (1968). *J. gen. Microbiol.*, **51**, 43
WATERS, M.E. and HAMDY, M.K. (1969). *Appl. Microbiol.*, **17**, 21
WEBSTER'S NEW INTERNATIONAL DICTIONARY OF THE ENGLISH LANGUAGE (1958). 2nd edn. G. and C. Merrian, Springfield, Mass.; Bell, London
WEIL, A.J. and KOTSEVALOV, O. (1956). *Zentbl. Bakt. Parasit Kde.* (Abt. I. Orig.), **165**, 459
WEISER, R., WIMPENNY, J. and ASSCHER, A.W. (1969). *Lancet,* **ii**, 619
WELCH, H., RANDALL, W.A. and PRICE, C.W. (1950). *Bact. Proc.*, p. 96
WHITTLESTONE, P. (1969). In *Isolation Methods for Microbiologists,* p. 51 Eds. Shapton, D.A. and Gould, G.W. Academic Press, London
WILLIAMS, L.E. and LOCKWOOD, J.L. (1957). *Phytopathology,* **47**, 44
WILLIAMS, R.J.H. and RICKS, G.R. (1975). In *The Ecology of Resource Degradation and Renewal,* p. 127. 15th Symp. Ecological Soc. Blackwell, Oxford
WILLIAMS-SMITH, H. (1958). *Vet. Rec.*, **70**, 575
WILLIAMS-SMITH, H. and CRABB, W.E. (1955a). *J. comp. Path.*, **65**, 55
WILLIAMS-SMITH, H. and CRABB, W.E. (1955b). *Vet. Rec.*, **67**, 749
WILLIAMS-SMITH, H. and CRABB, W.E. (1957). *Vet. Rec.*, **69**, 24
WIX, P. and WOODBINE, M. (1955). *Brit. vet. J.*, **111**, 432
WOOD, R.L. (1965). *Amer. J. vet. Res.*, **26**, 1303
WOOD, T.H. (1956). *Adv. biol. med. Phys.*, **4**, 119
WOODBINE, M. (1946). *Vet. J.*, **102**, 88
WOODBINE, M. (1947). *Vet. J.*, **103**, 149
WOODBINE, M. (1950). *Bact. Rev.*, **12**, 161
WOODBINE, M. (Ed.) (1962). *Antibiotics in Agriculture.* Butterworths, London
WOODBINE, M. (1968–69). 6th Int. Symp. Fd Hyg. *Microbiology of dried foods.* Ed. Kampelmacher, E.H. Bilthoven, The Netherlands
WOODS, D.D. (1953). *J. gen. Microbiol.*, **9**, 151
WRIGHT, H.B. (1962). *Int. Congr. Microbiol., Montreal,* (Abstr.), p. 49
ZEBOVITZ, E., EVANS, J.B. and NIVEN, C.F. (1955). *J. Bact.*, **70**, 686
ZIMMERMAN, L. (1969). *J. Bact.*, **97**, 749
ZWART VOORSPUIJ, A.J. and BOKMA, L.H. (1959). *Antibiot. Chemother.*, **9**, 27

4

SYNERGY IN CHEMOTHERAPY

F. O'GRADY
Department of Microbiology, University of Nottingham, City Hospital, Nottingham

Before the introduction of co-trimoxazole, the use of synergic combinations of antimicrobial agents in clinical practice was virtually restricted to 'totally bactericidal' combinations for the treatment of difficult cases of bacterial endocarditis. In reviewing the current situation it is perhaps appropriate to deal very briefly with the use of pairs of agents, sometimes described as 'synergic' combinations which are really complementary pairs used for several different purposes.

Antibacterial Complementation

Simplest, and clearly least 'synergic', is the use of two antibiotics which act sufficiently similarly for half an MIC of one plus half and MIC of the other to act as though it were an inhibitory concentration of a single agent. An example of such a mixture, at least in its action on some strains of staphylococci, is the combination of novobiocin and tetracycline marketed in this country under the name of albamycin T. In a rather different way, a mixture of cloxacillin and polymyxin can be used to obtain a wide spectrum of antibacterial activity, the cloxacillin acting against Gram-positive organisms and the polymyxin against Gram-negative organisms. A special kind of complementation is the use of pairs, or even triplets, of agents to prevent the emergence of resistance – a use which has had notable success in the field of tuberculosis though much less obvious success when applied elsewhere.

Antibacterial Synergy

Truly 'synergic' combinations are those where the effect of the pair of agents is together greater than that obtainable by using either alone even in substantially increased concentrations. The outstandingly important example of this in therapeutic practice – certainly as judged by volume of usage – is, of course, the combination of trimethoprim and sulphamethoxazole in co-trimoxazole. A good deal of attention is to be paid to this in later papers and it is necessary in the present review only to say something about the clinical uses of the combination (O'Grady, 1973).

If we look at the antibacterial spectrum of the two agents, it is in each case remarkably broad and for the two agents broadly similar, but there are some differences in the ratios of activity: trimethoprim is generally the more active notably against *Streptococcus faecalis*, but the sulphonamide is the more active against the pathogenic Neisseria and neither agent shows much activity against *Pseudomonas.* Otherwise a very wide range of organisms including the common pyogenic Gram-positive cocci, *Haemophilus influenzae* and a wide range of enterobacteria are included in their joint spectrum. What is more, of course, not only are the two agents active in their own rights but when combined together they greatly potentiate one another's activity, so producing a genuine synergic interaction.

For this synergic interaction to be utilized in treatment it is of course essential for the two agents to be in the same place at the same time. A look at the plasma profiles of the two compounds shows that they approximate reasonably well so that the concentration ratio of the two agents is maintained through the inter-dose interval (Fowle, 1973). On this basis, the combination has been used for the treatment of a wide variety of infections: respiratory infections on the basis of activity against streptococci, pneumococci and Haemophilus, and meningitis on the basis of their activity against the pneumococcus, Haemophilus and *Neisseria meningitidis.* The combination has been particularly widely and successfully used in the treatment of urinary tract infection, the combination being active against far and away the great majority of *Escherichia coli,* much the commonest cause of acute urinary tract infection. The combination has also been successfully used in the treatment of enteric fever and in the uncommon but otherwise difficult to manage infections – brucellosis and nocardiasis. The success of co-trimoxazole in clinical practice has been recognized in a whole series of symposia held in various parts of the world, and a huge amount of clinical data now attests to the success of the combination (O'Grady, 1975). On the face of it, co-trimoxazole has provided a remarkable example of the way in which the two agents can be used together to therapeutic advantage. How much of its therapeutic success is due to interaction between the two components and how much to the high intrinsic activity of trimethoprim itself is now undergoing critical review (O'Grady, 1975).

Penetration Synergy

A situation where there is no doubt of the contribution of each component of the mixture is provided by the classical example of synergy between penicillin and aminoglycosides in the treatment of enterococcal endocarditis. Enterococci are slowly killed by penicillin and tend not to be affected by streptomycin except in high concentrations. The combination, on the other hand, is extremely successful in 'totally' or near-totally extinguishing the enterococcal population. The reason for this is that the streptococcus is potentially lethal to the organism but is prevented from exerting as much effect as it might by the fact that it is excluded from its site of action on the streptococcal ribosome by the relatively impermeable cell wall. When the organism is simultaneously exposed to penicillin the cell wall is damaged and the streptomycin is able to gain access and exert its lethal effect. It transpires that some enterococci owe their resistance to streptomycin not to the impermeability of the cell wall – a resistance which is amenable to modification by treatment with penicillin – but to a change in the ribosome itself whereby, as a result of mutation, a single protein in the ribosome – the one to which streptomycin clings – is replaced, streptomycin is no longer bound by the ribosome and the organism becomes totally indifferent to its action whether or not it is able to gain access to the cell. The existence of these two forms of resistance is apparent from the distribution of sensitivity to streptomycin among enterococci. The organisms fall into two groups (Standiford, de Main and Kirby, 1970): those sensitive to 250 μg streptomycin ml^{-1} or less and those resistant to 1000 or more μg streptomycin ml^{-1}. The less resistant organisms are those which are fundamentally sensitive to streptomycin and are susceptible to treatment with penicillin which allows streptomycin to enter the cell and exert a synergic effect. In contrast, the group which is much more resistant owes its resistance to changes in the ribosome which cannot be overcome by improvement in access and consequently shows no synergic effect on exposure to the combination of penicillin and streptomycin.

The interaction between penicillins or cephalosporins and aminoglycosides is clinically particularly important, not because of its use – like that of co-trimoxazole – in large numbers of patients, but because of the severity of the infections in which such combinations are indicated. Not only are such combinations the most likely to be effective in the management of difficult cases of endocarditis but they also find an important application in the treatment of generalized *Pseudomonas* infections, where the combination of carbenicillin with gentamicin or other aminoglycosides, active against the *Pseudomonas*, often shows a striking synergic effect with much more rapid and complete killing of the organism than can be achieved by either agent alone. As a result, such combinations are widely regarded as the optimum treatment for severe *Pseudomonas* infections, particularly in patients with impaired defences in whom such infections often occur.

Internal Synergy

There are two classes of agent that exhibit a very special kind of interaction which might be described as 'internal synergy'. The first example of this is cycloserine. This is an agent which has been used quite extensively for the treatment of tuberculosis and urinary tract infection, though its use for both these conditions has now largely been superseded by other compounds. The interest in cycloserine as a synergic compound is that it affects the synthesis of bacterial cell wall by inhibiting two successive reactions at the very earliest stage of the construction of cell wall units. In effect it produces by itself sequential blockade of successive steps in the same metabolic pathway, in much the same way as sulphonamide and trimethoprim sequentially block the pathway leading to folate synthesis.

The other example of 'internal synergy' is that of the depsipeptides. These are an extremely interesting large group of natural compounds which include substances with no detected biological activity, some which are extraordinarily toxic, and a large and complex group of antibiotics. The special interest of the antibiotics in the present connection is that they consist of pairs of agents which are separated with difficulty and which individually exert a relatively limited bacteristatic effect. The two components together, however, are substantially more active and commonly bactericidal. Some of these agents have been widely used in Europe, particularly virginiamycin and pristinamycin which can be given orally. These are extremely active against staphylococci and have been very successfully used for the management of such severe staphylococcal infections as osteomyelitis. Virginiamycin is also used as a feed supplement.

Potential Therapeutic Synergic Combinations

Having dealt with the varieties of synergy which have direct therapeutic applications, there remain a number of combinations which have been used for experimental therapy. The first example is potentially extremely important, though it has so far had little therapeutic use. This is the possibility of protecting antibiotics against their destruction by bacterial enzymes. Much clinically important resistance to aminoglycosides and to β-lactam antibiotics is due not to intrinsic resistance on the part of the organism, but to the capacity of the bacteria to generate enzymes which destroy the antibiotics before they can exert their effects. A good example is provided by the cephalosporins – an important group of antibiotics – of which the major defect is the susceptibility of many of the more active members of the group to degradation by enterobacterial enzymes. Protection of the agent against such degradation would, of course, preserve its intrinsic activity and greatly improve its therapeutic potential. One way of achieving such protection is to expose the bacteria simultaneously to other β-lactam antibiotics which have a much higher affinity for the degrading enzyme. An early example of the application of this principle was the exposure of *Pseudomonas* to higher concentrations of cloxacillin – itself inactive against the *Pseudomonas* – which has a very high affinity for the *Pseudomonas* β-lactamase which is pre-occupied thereby allowing a simultaneously administered penicillin or cephalosporin to act unhindered on the *Pseudomonas.* Some application has been made of this in the treatment of difficult urinary tract infections with highly resistant organisms. The restriction of the combination to the field of urinary infection depends upon the fact that very high concentrations of the inhibitory substance are required.

In our own work we have had the opportunity to look at the possibilities of such protective mechanisms by utilizing a mechanical model of the urinary tract in which various treatment regimens can be investigated (O'Grady *et al.,* 1973). When this mechanical patient empties its bladder at regular intervals, the concentration of bacteria in the infected bladder falls promptly and then settles, just as it does in many human patients, to a fluctuating concentration of around $10^6 – 10^7$ organisms ml^{-1}. Clearance of this infection cannot be achieved without treatment by antibiotics. If infection with a β-lactamase-producing organism is treated with a dose of a cephalosporin there is initially a very marked fall in the bacterial concentration due to rapid destruction of the infecting organism, but subsequently there is prompt regrowth of the survivors as the cephalosporin is degraded by the bacterial enzymes. If the cephalosporin treatment is supplemented by simultaneous administration of a potent β-lactamase inhibitor then very substantial enhancement of the antibacterial effect occurs (Greenwood and O'Grady, 1975). A number of agents have now been investigated as inhibitors of microbial β-lactamases. At the present time, for various reasons, these compounds are not in a state to be used therapeutically but this is an extremely promising area for further exploration, certainly as far as highly resistant urinary tract infection is concerned.

Spheroplast Generation and Inhibition

Still in the field of urinary tract infection, another ingenious use has been made of pairs of agents in an attempt to overcome another essential defect in the otherwise highly desirable group of β-lactam antibiotics. When enterobacteria – and proteus in particular – are exposed to penicillins, for example ampicillin, many of the bacteria are lysed, but a substantial number of them generate protoplasts which are supported by the relatively high osmolarity of the urine and, because they are devoid of cell wall, are no longer susceptible to the action of the penicillin. As a result, when the concentration of penicillin falls below inhibitory levels the spheroplasts are able to re-assemble their cell walls, resume growth and re-establish infection. In their natural state the organisms are not susceptible to agents like erythromycin because the way to their site of action on the bacterial ribosome is blocked by the enterobacterial cell wall in much the same way as streptomycin is excluded from the enterococcal ribosome by the streptococcal cell wall. Once the cell wall has been breached by the penicillin, however, erythromycin is able to cross the cell membrane and act on the ribosome. On this basis the combination of ampicillin plus erythromycin, or the sequential use of ampicillin and erythromycin, has found a place – though a limited place – in the treatment of relapsing proteus infections. The main defect in this form of therapy is that by no means all the survivors from penicillin action are in the form of spheroplasts. Some are apparently morphologically intact – and hence unresponsive to erythromycin – and the proportion of survivors in the spheroplast or intact forms differs from one bacterial species (and very likely one bacterial strain) to another (Greenwood and O'Grady, 1970).

Complexity of Antibiotic Interactions

The subject of therapeutic applications of antibiotic combinations for synergic or other reasons cannot be left without reference to the complicated nature of the interactions that may occur. Quite apart from the pharmacokinetic difficulties of achieving concentrations of the two agents at the same place at the same time, appropriate to the desired effect, not only the magnitude but the nature of the interaction between the two agents can differ in the laboratory on changing the relative concentrations, or the conditions of test or the strains tested. A good example is provided by a combination commonly used therapeutically: that of penicillin and sodium fusidate. It is easy the show in the laboratory that sodium fusidate and penicillins are commonly antagonistic. It is nevertheless widespread clinical practice to give penicillin together with sodium fusidate because resistant staphylococci very easily emerge on exposure of previously sensitive strains to fusidate, and it is well established that the presence of penicillin will prevent their emergence. In order to judge the clinical significance of the interaction between sodium fusidate and penicillins we examined the behaviour of a number of strains of *Staphylococcus aureus.* Among as few as ten strains we found no less than four ways in which the two compounds interacted with one another (O'Grady and Greenwood, 1973). Rather more than half the strains showed, as previously found, two-way antagonism: that is to say, the number of survivors from exposure to the two bactericidal agents in combination was greater than that from exposure to either alone. The remaining strains showed one-way antagonism (that is to say the number of survivors was more than that which resulted from exposure to the more active agent alone but less than that which resulted from exposure to the less active agent) or indifference, or synergy; in the presence of the two agents, therefore, there were fewer survivors than in the presence of either of the agents alone. What emerges from the therapeutic standpoint is firstly that the nature of the interaction cannot be prophesied without some fairly elaborate laboratory investigations; secondly, two-way antagonism is the common response but one-way antagonism or synergy may occur; thirdly, that even where two-way antagonism is found the number of survivors is extremely small so that the combination still exerts a bactericidal effect to a degree which would be regarded as adequate in the management of endocarditis; and fourthly, that even where two-way antagonism occurs, the presence of penicillin is still highly effective in preventing the emergence of mutants resistant to fusidate.

Future of Therapeutic Synergic Combinations

It is easy to see several ways in which synergic interactions might be exploited therapeutically. The simultaneous administration of potent but enzyme-labile β-lactam antibiotics together with a wide-spectrum β-lactamase inhibitor is an obvious one. Another is the possibility of administering with tetracycline an agent capable of breaching the cellular barrier on which bacterial resistance to tetracycline depends.

If such developments are to be successful, it will be necessary not only to develop compounds which possess the necessary biochemical properties – a daunting enough task in itself – but to overcome three major difficulties: the need for near identity in the pharmacokinetics of the paired agents, the inevitably increased toxic hazard of administering two agents instead of one, and the sceptical view of combination therapy taken by a number of regulatory bodies around the world.

Intriguing possibilities of fundamental microbiological interest exist. Certainly no less interesting will be the extent to which they can be put to therapeutic use.

References

FOWLE, A.S.E. (1973). In *Trimethoprim/Sulphanethoxazole in Bacterial Infections*, p. 63. Eds. Bernstein, L.S. and Salter, A.J. Churchill Livingstone, London

GREENWOOD, D. and O'GRADY, F. (1970). *Nature,* 228, 457

GREENWOOD, D. and O'GRADY, F. (1975). *Chemother.,* **21**, 330
O'GRADY, F. (1973). *Med. J. Aust.,* Special Suppl., **1**, 19
O'GRADY, F. (1975). *Canad. med. J.,* **112**, 5
O'GRADY, F. and GREENWOOD, D. (1973). *J. med. Microbiol.,* **6**, 441
O'GRADY, F., MACKINTOSH, I.P., GREENWOOD, D. and WATSON, B.W. (1973). *Brit. J. exp. Path.,* **54**, 283
STANDIFORD, H.D., DE MAINE, J.B. and KIRBY, W.M.M. (1970). *Arch. Int. Med.,* **126**, 255

5

SYNERGY OF TRIMETHOPRIM AND SULPHONAMIDES: HISTORY AND CURRENT STATUS

S.R.M. BUSHBY
Wellcome Research Laboratories, Research Triangle Park, U.S.A.

Trimethoprim (TMP), the antibacterial which is now widely used in conjunction with a sulphonamide for the treatment of many infections, is 2,4-diamino-5-(3,4,5-trimethoxybenzyl)pyrimidine.

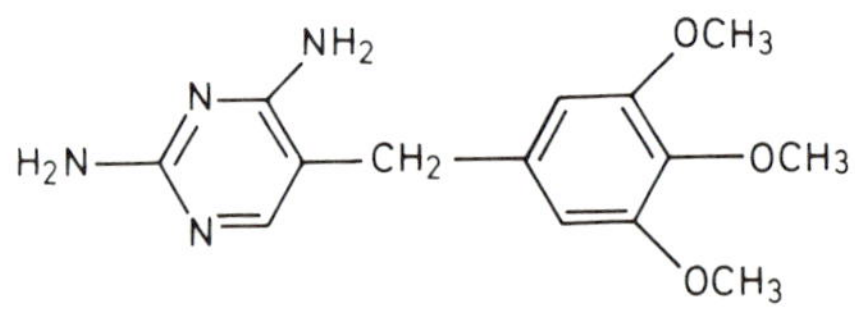

Development of TMP

TMP arose from an extensive study initiated by Hitchings in 1942 (*see* Hitchings *et al.*, 1950). The purpose of the study was to determine the effects of analogues of the natural purines and pyrimidines on the biosynthesis of nucleic acid, especially in relation to the chemotherapy of cancer but with the full appreciation that success could apply in other medical fields. Initially, emphasis was on the purine analogues and this led to the development of the antileukaemic drug, 6-mercaptopurine, and later to the immunosuppressive drug, azathioprine, and the antiuricaemic (especially gout) drug, allopurinol.

At an early stage of this study, the inhibition of the growth of *Lactobacillus casei* was chosen as the screening test for the antagonists (Hitchings *et al.*, 1949). The test was chosen because Snell and his colleagues and Stokstad (Snell and Peterson, 1940; Mitchell, Snell and Williams, 1941; Snell and Mitchell, 1941; Stokstad, 1941) had shown that the needs of *L. casei* for a then unidentified vitamin were closely related to thymine and purine syntheses. The needs for this vitamin were known to be replaceable by these substances and so the test allowed potential antimetabolites to be studied. The choice of this screening test proved especially fortunate when the chemical structure of the unidentified vitamin, folic acid, was elucidated and shown to contain a pyrimidine moiety (Angier *et al.*, 1946; Mowat *et al.*, 1948), for it then became apparent that the antagonists could be competing directly with the vitamin rather than with the end-products. This possibility proved to be correct and the 2,4-diaminopyrimidines as a class were identified as antifolates (Hitchings *et al.,* 1948).

During the early stages of studies by Hitchings and his colleagues, an independent search for new antibacterial drugs was being made by Rose and his colleagues in collaboration with chemists at the University of Manchester, England (Curd, Davey and Rose, 1945; Hull *et al.,* 1946; Basford *et al.,* 1947). In this search, pyrimidines were selected because of their structural relationship with certain antimalarial drugs and with some of the more active sulphonamides. The selected pyrimidines were mainly substituted aminopyrimidines and, although the more active ones appeared to act through direct interference with nucleoside biosynthesis, the study led to the development of proguanil (chlorguanide hydrochloride) which was later shown to act, after metabolism by the host, as an antifolate (Hawking and Perry, 1948; Carrington *et al.,* 1951); the active metabolite is 4,6-diamino-1-*p*-chlorophenyl-2,2-dimethyl-(1,2-dihydro-1,3,5-triazine).

Although, as a class, the 2,4-diaminopyrimidines are antifolates, their behaviour varied in different biological systems depending on the substitutions in the 5- and 6-positions (Hitchings *et al.,* 1952). High antibacterial activity was associated with 5-benzyl substitutions and high antimalarial activity with 5-phenyl substitutions especially if combined with 6-alkylation; high mammalian toxicity was also associated with these latter substitutions. Alkoxyl-substitutions on the benzene nucleus greatly increased antibacterial activity and peaked with trimethoxy substitution, as in TMP, with the 6-position remaining unsubstituted (Roth *et al.,* 1962).

Synergy between the sulphonamides and the 2,4-diamino-pyrimidines was first reported by Greenberg and Richeson (1950); it was observed in chicks infected with *Plasmodium gallinaceum* and treated with sulphadiazine and 2,4-diamino-5-(*p*-chlorophenoxy)pyrimidine. Earlier Greenberg, Boyd and Josephson (1948) had observed similar synergy with proguanil and, although at that time it was not realized that proguanil is, through metabolism, an antifolate, these investigators suggested that the potentiating effect may extend to bacterial infections, including those in which sulphonamides are only partially effective. A little later, Greenberg (1949) did, in fact, suggest that proguanil interfered with either the synthesis of the utilization of pteroylglutamic acid; this suggestion was based on the knowledge that certain proguanil-resistant strains of *Pl. gallinaceum* were cross-resistant to sulphadiazine and vice versa (Bishop and McConnachie, 1948), that one of the end-products of *p*-aminobenzoic metabolism is pteroylglutamic acid (Lampen and Jones, 1946) and that the activity of proguanil is not reversed by *p*-aminobenzoic acid.

Encouraged by these observations of synergy, Eyles and Coleman (1953 and 1955) sought and successfully demonstrated synergy between pyrimethamine and sulphadiazine in experimental toxoplasmosis of mice. Pyrimethamine is 2,4-diamino-5-*p*-chlorophenyl-6-ethylpyrimidine and it was chosen because Falco *et al.* (1951) had shown that, of a large series of 2,4-diaminopyrimidines, it and some closely related analogues had the highest antimalarial activity in chicks and mice infected with *Pl. gallinaceum* and *Pl. berghei*. Potentiation between the 2,4-diaminopyrimidines and the sulphonamides was also demonstrated by Lux (1954) in coccidiosis in poultry; the causal agent was *Eimeria tenella* and the potentiation was between pyrimethamine and sulphaquinoxaline or sulphanilamide.

Although synergy against bacteria had previously been shown to occur *in vitro* between sulphathiazole and some synthetic pterins, 2,4-diaminopyrimido-pyrazines (Daniel and Norris, 1947), it was not reported for the 2,4-diamino-pyrimidines until 1955 when Hitchings (1955), described increased *in vitro* activity against *Proteus vulgaris* with the combination of sulphadiazine and 2,4-diamino-5-(3,4-dimethoxybenzyl)pyrimidine, which is a close analogue of TMP. That the synergy of members of this series applies to a wide range of bacterial species and also occurs *in vivo* was shown by Hitchings and Bushby (1961). Especially important was the demonstration of synergy *in vivo* for the degree of *in vitro* activity of these antibacterials was known to depend upon the nature of the test medium, and there was no certainty that the *in vitro* conditions in which it occurred simulated those present *in vivo*.

Mode of Action of 2,4-Diaminopyrimidines

By the time 2,4-diaminopyrimidines were being seriously considered as potential antibacterial chemotherapeutic agents, their site of action had been determined.

From earlier evidence, Hitchings *et al.* (1952) had suggested that the 2,4-diaminopyrimidines may be regarded as structural analogues of folinic acid but, because they resemble it less closely than do the structurally close analogues of folic acid (e.g. aminopterin), minor changes in their fine chemical structure might enable them to be more selective in toxicity than are the close analogues, presumably due to their having fewer essential binding sites. At that point in time, however, the precise relationship and roles of folic acid and of folinic acid were not known.

The first indications of the relationship between folic and folinic acid came from the studies by Sauberlich (1949) which showed that the excretion of folinic acid was increased after administration of folic acid. Nichol and Welch (1950a), from the studies with rat liver slices, concluded that a reductive step was involved and their later studies (Nichol and Welch, 1950b) showed that aminopterin interferes both *in vivo* and *in vitro* with the conversion. That interference at this point was the probable site of action of the 2,4-diaminopyrimidines, was suggested by the observation that, whereas *Streptococcus faecalis* grew equally as well in the presence of folinic acid or folic acid, pyrimethamine was 3000 times more inhibitory in the presence of folic than in the presence of folinic acid and, in rats, the toxic effects of pyrimethamine were alleviated by folinic but not by folic acid (Hitchings, 1952). The identification of the precise sites of action of these drugs had to await the isolation from chicken liver of the enzyme responsible for the conversion of folic acid and the inhibition of its action, non-competitively, by aminopterin and amethopterin (Osborn, Freeman and Huennekens, 1956; Osborn and Huennekens, 1958) and for Wood and Hitchings (1959a) to show with whole cells and cell-free extracts of *Strep. faecalis*, that pyrimethamine is a potent inhibitor of this reaction.

Although these studies showed that both the close analogues of folic acid and the small molecular inhibitors act by the same mechanism, they did not explain why the close analogues affected mammalian cells but not bacteria (except for the few species that could use exogenous folates), whereas the small molecular inhibitors were inhibitory for mammalian and almost all bacterial cells. These differences were usually attributed to differences in transport and this explanation was confirmed by Wood and Hitchings (1959b) and by Wood, Ferone and Hitchings (1961). Similarly, the variations in the activities of the 2,4-diaminopyrimidines for different biological systems could be explained in terms of transport, but structure–activity relationships suggested that differences in affinities for the various dihydrofolate reductases were a more likely explanation. The latter explanation was shown to be true when Baker and Beng-Thong Ho (1964) and Burchall and Hitchings (1965) showed that the degree of binding of the various antifolates to isolated dihydrofolate reductases from bacteria and mammalian tissues varied directly with their spectra of biological activities. Thus, as chemotherapeutic agents, the selective toxicities of antifolates reflect selective binding at the same locus, a conclusion which is important for its implications extend beyond the antifolates. It shows that, although in general biosynthetic pathways are common to all species, the enzymes involved can differ slightly and such differences can be exploited chemotherapeutically.

Effects of Inhibition of Dihydrofolate Reductase

The consequences of the specific inhibition of dihydrofolate reductase by antifolates have been extensively studied. After reduction to the tetrahydroform, the folates are converted into a series of coenzymes the functions of which are to act solely, except for one, as donors of certain 1-carbon fragments in the biosynthesis of proteins and nucleic acids. The exception is 5,10-methylene tetrahydrofolate, which is concerned with the synthesis of thymidylate from deoxyuridylate, for it also acts as a donor of two hydrogen atoms; thus, this coenzyme is oxidized back to dihydrofolic acid. Therefore, in the presence of an antagonist of dihydrofolate reductase, depletion of the tetrahydrofolate pool occurs through the trapping of a molecule of the acid in the oxidized state on each occasion that a molecule of thymidylate is synthesized.

The 2,4-diaminopyrimidines therefore affect not only *de novo* synthesis but also its recycling.

Biochemistry of TMP-Sulphonamides

TMP was chosen from some 50 analogues because of its wide and high antibacterial activity (Roth *et al.*, 1962) and, although in general it is more active on a weight basis than are the sulphonamides, clinically it has almost been exclusively used in combination with a sulphonamide in order to take advantage of the synergy which occurs. This synergy, which is well documented (Hitchings, 1971) is attributed to sequential blockade as defined by Potter (1951), i.e. due to the effects of the two inhibitors acting in the same metabolic pathway but on different enzymes within a limited portion of the pathway. The biochemical steps involved and the double blockade are depicted in *Figure 5.1.*

In the blockade the sulphonamide acts as a competitor for *p*-aminobenzoic acid in the formation of dihydropteroic acid by dihydropteroate synthetase, which is condensed with glutamic acid to form dihydrofolic acid (Brown, 1962).

TMP then acts through binding with dihydrofolate reductase, thus interfering with the reduction to tetrahydrofolate.

The blocking of the enzyme dihydropteroate synthetase by sulphonamides and of dihydrofolate reductase by TMP is competitive, and the amount of inhibitor needed to reduce the biosynthesis of dihydropteroic acid or tetrahydrofolic acid to levels below those essential for growth depends on the amount of substrate present. Because the sulphonamide acts before TMP in these biosyntheses, its role in the dual action is to reduce the amount of dihydrofolic acid

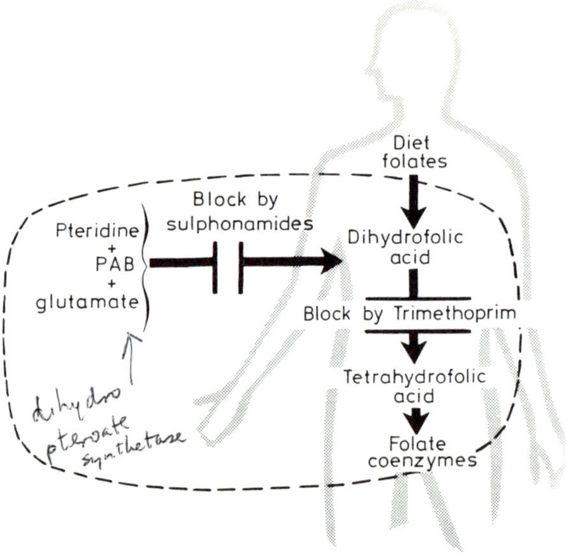

Figure 5.1 Sequential blockade of TMP and SMX in bacteria and animals

against which TMP competes. If the competition between TMP and dihydrofolic acid were linear then the effects of the dual action would not be expected to be more than additive, but the synergy becomes explicable if the competition by TMP increases relatively with decreases in dihydrofolic acid.

Both inhibitors are antifolates and could be expected to interfere in the folate metabolism of both host and parasite. The sulphonamides satisfy the ideal criterion for chemotherapeutic agents for their role in the sequential blockade is not involved in the metabolism of animals. The sulphonamides interfere with the biosynthesis of dihydrofolic acid and, during the course of evolution, animals have lost the ability to perform this synthesis so that they depend on dietary sources from which they obtain them either in the fully oxidized form, folic acid or as dihydrofolic acid. The next biosynthetic step, i.e. the reduction to the tetrahydro-form, is common to both animals and bacteria and is accomplished by dihydrofolate reductase. Sulphonamides are therefore antifolates for bacteria but not for animals while TMP is an antifolate for both. In practice, however, TMP shows selective toxicity for the bacterial parasite depending, as shown by Burchall and Hitchings (1965), on its greater affinity for the dihydrofolate reductase of bacteria than for that of mammals. These investigators demonstrated this greater affinity by measuring the effects of TMP on the decrease in absorbance when dihydrofolate is reduced to tetrahydrofolate by the semi-purified enzymes in the presence of the reductant, nicotinamide-adenine dinucleotide phosphate. For example, TMP produced 50% inhibition of the enzyme from *P. vulgaris* at a concentration of 4×10^{-9} M whilst a similar inhibition of the enzyme from rat liver occurred only when the concentration reached 3.6×10^{-4} M.

The Effects of Synergy

The advantages claimed for the use of the combination TMP–sulphonamide are (*a*) reduction in minimum inhibitory concentration (MIC), (*b*) increased bactericidal activity and (*c*) lessening of the risk of emergence of resistant mutants.

REDUCTION IN MIC

That the MICs of the sulphonamides depend upon the medium in which they are measured was recognized soon after their introduction as chemotherapeutic agents, and the same dependence applies to TMP and to its synergy with sulphonamides (Bushby and Hitchings, 1968; Darrell, Garrod and Waterworth, 1968). The differences in activities obtained in the different media were attributed to variable concentrations of reversing substances in the media and, in the case of the sulphonamides, these were assumed to be *p*-aminobenzoic acid and peptones. Harper and Cawston (1945) showed that the presence of lysed horse red cells in the medium increased the activity of the sulphonamides, and Bushby and Barnett (1967) and Darrell, Garrod and Waterworth (1968) reported similar effects on the activity of TMP. The factor in horse red cells responsible for this effect has been identified as thymidine phosphorylase (Ferone *et al.*, 1975) and the increase in activity is due to its converting thymidine to thymine which is some 30 times less effective as a reversing agent than is the nucleoside. Koch and Burchall (1971) showed that the activity of TMP in 13 different media correlated inversely with the thymidine content.

For most organisms TMP is, on a weight basis, more active than are the sulphonamides. *Table 5.1* compares, in a medium containing low concentrations of inhibitory substances, the MICs of TMP and sulphamethoxazole (SMX) for representative strains of the major pathogenic species (Bushby, 1973a).

Constituents of the culture medium also affect the degree of synergy. In two-dimensional titrations, Then (1973) found that the most impressive synergy occurred in the presence of all of the known antagonists of the inhibition, i.e. methionine, glycine, inosine as a purine and thymine, but under these conditions the required concentrations of SMX and TMP to inhibit growth of *E. coli* were 2.3 and 36 times higher, respectively, than those needed when omitting thymine. The effects of the presence of all the antagonists were interpreted as indicating that, although the synergy depends on the induction of a general tetrahydrofolate deficiency rather than deprivation of a single metabolite, the marked synergy that occurs in the presence of all the known available antagonists is due

Table 5.1 Antibacterial activity *in vitro.* The activities of TMP and SMX were compared in Wellcotest Sensitivity Test Agar containing 7.5% lysed horse blood. For the *Haemophilus* and *Neisseria* the medium was heated at 80°C for 5 min, and in the case of *Mycobacterium tuberculosis,* Peizer and Schector medium was used. One-third dilutions were used

	Minimum inhibitory concentration (μg ml^{-1})	
Organism	*Trimethoprim*	*Sulphamethoxazole*
Streptococcus pyogenes	0.5	95
Streptococcus pneumoniae Type II	1.5	28.5
Viridans streptococci	0.15	9.5
Streptococcus faecalis	0.5	95
Streptococcus agalactiae	5.0	28.5
Staphylococcus aureus	0.15	2.85
Erysipelothrix rhusiopathiae	5.0	>95
Corynebacterium pyogenes	0.5	>95
Corynebacterium diphtheriae	0.5	>95
Clostridium perfringens	50	28.5
Mycobacterium tuberculosis	150	>950
Nocardia asteroides	15	2.85
Escherichia coli	0.15	9.5
Citrobacter freundii	0.15	2.85
Klebsiella pneumoniae	0.5	28.5
Enterobacter aerogenes	5.0	>95
Salmonella typhi	0.5	2.85
Salmonella typhimurium	0.5	9.5
Shigella spp.	0.5	2.85
Vibrio comma	1.5	28.5
Pasteurella septica	0.15	9.5
Haemophilus influenzae	0.5	9.5
Moraxella lacunata	5.0	9.5
Proteus spp.	1.5	28.5
Providence B	1.5	28.5
Pseudomonas aeruginosa	150	28.5
Neisseria gonorrhoeae	15	0.95
Neisseria meningitidis	5.0	0.285
Brucella abortus	15	2.85

to selective inhibition of the formylation of methionyl-tRNA by 10-formyltetrahydrofolate, the product of which is essential for the initiation of protein translation; however, according to Harvey (1973) protein synthesis can proceed although less rapidly without this formylation, and so this explanation is unlikely to be that simple.

The degree of synergy is also dependent to some extent on the particular sulphonamide; it is less with the weaker ones and for obtaining maximum effects there is probably little to choose between the more active members. The early studies (Hitchings and Bushby, 1961; Bushby and Hitchings, 1968) were made mainly with sulphadiazine but most of the later ones have been made with SMX because it is the sulphonamide that is generally used with TMP in human medicine, in the ratio of 5:1. This sulphonamide was chosen because its plasma half-life after oral administration in man is similar to that of TMP; matching half-lives simplifies dosing but it is not essential. In veterinary medicine, matching of half-lives cannot be conveniently achieved because the pharmacokinetics vary greatly in different animal species; the sulphonamides in current veterinary use are sulphadiazine and sulphadoxine with TMP and sulphadimethoxine with the close analogue of TMP, ormetoprim (2,4-diamino-5-[2-methyl-4,5-dimethoxy-benzyl] pyrimidine).

In practice, the decrease in the MIC varies with the ratio of the drugs present, therefore maximal potentiation can be determined only by measuring activity with the drugs present in multiple ratios as in the two-dimensional, serial dilution procedure (Bushby and Hitchings, 1968). In order that the results obtained by this method with strains of bacteria of differing sensitivities to TMP and the sulphonamides may readily be compared, the MIC of each of the drugs in the various ratios can be expressed as a decimal fraction of the MIC of the respective drug when acting alone. This fraction was termed the 'fractional inhibitory concentration' (FIC) by Elion, Singer and Hitchings (1954) and when the sum of the FIC for each of the drugs, the FIC index, is less than unity, synergy is indicated; the lower this sum, the greater is the synergy. The indices for the various strains of the 14 species examined by Bushby and Hitchings (1968) ranged from 0.02 to 0.56. The results of such studies can also be presented graphically as isobolograms, in which curves falling below the diagonal indicate synergy. With TMP and SMX, the curves are symmetrical (*Figure 5.2*)

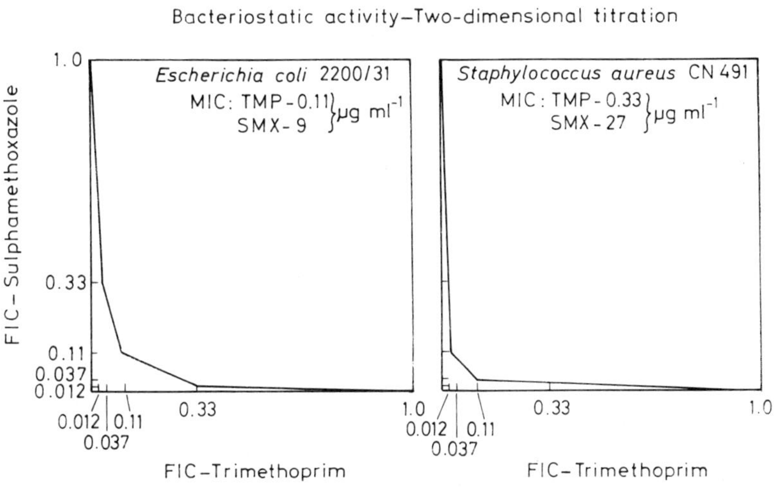

Figure 5.2 Synergism of TMP and SMX. FIC = (MIC in combination)/(MIC singly)

indicating that the optimum ratio, as measured by maximal reduction in the MICs of both drugs, is that in which the drugs are present in proportions corresponding to their respective MIC when acting singly (Acar, Goldstein and Chabbert, 1973; Bushby, 1973b). For example, if the MIC for TMP is 1 μg ml^{-1} and that for SMX is 20 μg ml^{-1}, the optimum ratio is 1:20 but, because of the wide variation in sensitivities of organisms to TMP and SMX, the optimum ratio is also variable. The use of this term 'optimum ratio', for this ratio has created the false impression that for each organism there is a ratio with which maximum antibacterial activity occurs, it cannot be stressed too strongly that the effect on the organism is the same over a wide range of ratios and that the 'optimum ratio' is merely the one with which the effect is produced by the lowest concentration of each drug. With other ratios, the minimum effective concentration of one of the components will be less than with the 'optimum ratio' but the concentration of the other component will be greater. The need for attaining the 'optimum ratio' arises only when there is a problem in reaching adequate concentrations of both drugs at an infection site.

In the main, TMP is 10 to 100 times more active than is SMX; therefore demonstration of enhanced susceptibility to the combination has most usually been done with TMP and SMX in the ratio of 1:20 which is not only near the modal optimal mean but is also the ratio at which the drugs are present in the blood of patients treated with standard doses of the combination. Examples of the increase in activity with this ratio are shown in *Table 5.2.*

Table 5.2 Effect on MIC of combining one part trimethoprim with 20 parts sulphamethoxazole. Medium: Wellcotest Sensitivity Test Agar + 7% lysed horse blood. For the *Haemophilus* the medium was heated at 80°C for 5 min

	MIC (μg ml^{-1})			
Organism	*Sulphamethoxazole*		*Trimethoprim*	
	Alone	*Mixture*	*Alone*	*Mixture*
Streptococcus pyogenes	285	2.85	1.5	0.15
Streptococcus pneumoniae	28.5	0.95	1.5	0.05
Staphylococcus aureus	9.5	0.95	0.5	0.05
Haemophilus influenzae	9.5	0.95	1.5	0.05
Klebsiella pneumoniae	9.5	0.95	0.5	0.05
Klebsiella aerogenes	9.5	0.95	0.5	0.05
Escherichia coli	2.85	0.285	0.15	0.015
Salmonella typhimurium	9.5	0.95	0.5	0.05
Shigella sonnei	2.85	0.285	0.15	0.015
Proteus vulgaris	28.5	0.95	0.5	0.05

The decrease in the minimum effective concentration is also demonstrated by the diffusion method. Grace, Bushby and Sigel (1975) have shown that the two drugs diffuse at the same rate, therefore, a larger zone of inhibition produced by a disc containing TMP and SMX, together, than that produced by discs containing the same quantity of TMP and SMX, singly, is indicative of enhanced susceptibility. This method has been widely used.

INCREASED BACTERICIDAL ACTIVITY

Both TMP and the sulphonamides are bactericidal *in vitro* but the conditions necessary for demonstrating this activity are critical. Increased bactericidal activities by the drugs in combination were reported by Bushby and Hitchings (1968), Darrell, Garrod and Waterworth (1968), Garrod and Waterworth (1968), Böhni (1969a), Bushby and Barnett (1969), Bushby (1973a), and Seydel *et al.*, (1972).

Death caused by the drugs, either singly or in combination, is due to the abnormal growth that occurs when the organism is deprived of thymidine and when the conditions permit continuation of protein synthesis (Angehrn and Then, 1973; Then, 1973). Therefore, for death to occur, it is essential for exogenous methionine, glycine and purines to be present in order that the effects of the drugs on the biosynthesis of ribonucleic acid and protein may be by-passed. These metabolites are, in fact, present in adequate quantities in most bacteriological media, but of equal importance is the need for the medium to be free from metabolites that would enable the organism to escape the effects of thymine deprivation. Thymidine is such a metabolite and it is present in many media. Concentrations as low as 0.01 $\mu g\ ml^{-1}$ will convert the bactericidal action of the drugs to bacteriostasis, and concentrations of around 0.1 $\mu g\ ml^{-1}$ will permit the partial growth within the zone of inhibition that has caused much confusion in susceptibility testing by the disc diffusion method (Bushby, 1973b).

Further evidence that killing by these agents is due to 'thymineless death' are the morphological changes which occur in organisms exposed to lethal concentrations of TMP. For example, under these conditions, *Haemophilus influenzae* assumes long, broad, filamentous forms (Bushby, 1973c; Bushby and Bushby, 1973) similar to those described by Cummings and Mondale (1967) for thymine-dependent *E. coli* deprived of thymine. *Escherichia coli* and *Staph. aureus* exposed to TMP assume large, vacuolated involute forms.

Whether the combination is, in fact, bactericidal under *in vivo* conditions is not known. Undoubtedly, the combination is highly effective in the treatment of many infections but, of course, it is not essential for an antibacterial drug to be bactericidal for it to be curative. Although elimination of an infection implies death of the invading organism, in practice, it is rarely possible to separate the role played by the antibacterial agent in the killing from that played by the natural defence mechanisms of the host. However, Then and Angehrn (1974), have shown that in blood *in vitro* the conditions are suitable for the effects of the combination to be bactericidal and that the conditions can be rendered unsuitable by adding thymine or, preferably thymidine. Because the conditions are not improved by adding glycine, methionine, and either adenine or inosine as a source of purine, these investigators concluded that the conditions in blood are optimal. By conducting similar experiments in urine they reached, for this fluid, the same conclusion which conflicts, however, with that of Anderson *et al.* (1974). These latter workers maintain from their experiences that the combination of TMP and SMX is rarely bactericidal *in vitro* in urine during a 6-hour observation period at 37°C, and that, in the instances in which it is lethal, the effects are due solely to the action of TMP; in fact, they maintain that SMX in urine interferes with the action of TMP. The difference between the results of these two groups of workers may be due to their use of different concentrations of the drugs for although apparently paradoxically, Anderson *et al.*, who found less activity, used concentrations some 10 times higher than those used by Then and Angehrn. The concentrations used by Anderson *et al.* were similar to those present in the urine of patients undergoing treatment with standard doses of the combination, i.e. 50–100 μg of TMP and 250–500 μg of SMX per ml, and so their conditions resembled more closely the *in vivo* conditions than did those of Then and Angehrn. Bushby (1975) has conducted experiments similar to those of Anderson *et al.* on urine from five patients undergoing treatment with the combination. The viability of six strains of urinary pathogens in each of the urine samples was determined during an observation time of 24 hours at 37°C, and although with none of the strains was viability affected during the first 6 hours, most of the organisms were dead by the 24th hour. The relatively slow killing in urine with high concentrations of the drug may be due, under these circumstances, to stronger inhibition affecting protein synthesis, which would counteract killing from unbalanced growth, the stronger inhibition affecting the synthesis of formylmethionyl-tRNA (Then and Angehrn, 1973).

Effects of Synergy *In Vivo*

The combination was shown to be more active in experimental infections of mice than either of the single components and was first reported by Hitchings and Bushby (1961) and later by Grunberg and DeLorenzo (1967) and by Böhni (1969b). As is predictable, the protection is not affected by administration of folinic acid (Böhni, 1969c; Grunberg, Prince and DeLorenzo, 1970) or by the administration of thymidine (Bushby, 1973b) because, of the common pathogens, only *Strep. faecalis* can use preformed folates and thymidine is very rapidly excreted, its concentrations in blood and urine being, according to Then and Angehrn (1975), less than 0.05 μg m^{-1}.

EFFECTS ON EMERGENCE OF RESISTANT MUTANTS

At times, antibacterials are given in combination, especially in the treatment of tuberculosis, in order to decrease the rate of emergence of resistant mutants. The basis for using combinations for this purpose is that, provided the resistant mutation for each drug is genetically distinct, resistance to both drugs arises from double mutation and the chances of this occurring is the product of the mutation rates of the individual drugs. Such data have not been documented for TMP and SMX, but the recorded observations of Darrell, Garrod and Waterworth (1968) show that the presence of a sulphonamide undoubtedly lessens the development of resistance to TMP. They found that although organisms from light inocula on ditch plates containing TMP showed little change in sensitivity to TMP even after 25 transfers, those from heavy inocula in broth containing increasing concentrations of the drug showed, even after only five transfers, decreases ranging from 32-fold to greater than 124-fold. However, when the sulphonamide was present at 10 times the concentration of TMP there were only small decreases in sensitivity even with large inocula, provided the organisms were sulphonamide-sensitive.

Bushby (1971) examined 19 strains of varying degrees of sensitivity to SMX and found that when they were exposed to both drugs the rate of emergence of TMP-resistant mutants depended upon the degree of sulphonamide resistance, the repressive effect being less with the more resistant strains. The clinical significance of these resistant mutants is doubtful. The majority of the variants grew as abnormally small colonies and many of them showed antigenic changes, associated with autoagglutination, which strongly suggests that the acquisition of TMP-resistance by this means will usually be associated with loss of virulence.

Probably more important than the development of resistance by mutation is the acquisition of resistance by R-factors. Organisms becoming resistant to TMP by this method are resistant to 1000 μg or more TMP per ml (Grüneberg *et al.*, 1975). This resistance is due to an alteration in the dihydrofolate reductase that reduces its affinity for TMP (Sköld and Widh, 1974; Amyes and Smith, 1974) and, according to Grüneberg (1975) these plasmid-carrying strains do not show enhanced susceptibility to the combination, thus contrasting with other TMP-resistant strains. Transference of TMP-resistance by this method was first recorded by Lebek (1972) but there is no convincing evidence that resistance to TMP–SMX through it has become widespread, at least in Britain, where the combination has been available since 1968 (Jobanputra and Datta, 1974). However, because resistance is transferred independently of the presence of the drugs, combining TMP and SMX cannot influence the development of resistance by this means, although the use of the drug will select the resistant strains when present.

Mention should be made of an alternative mechanism by which organisms can become resistant to TMP–SMX. This is by an alteration in metabolism by which the organism avoids, under certain conditions, the consequences of interference with the biosynthesis of tetrahydrofolate. TMP has been used as a tool by biochemists since 1965 for selecting thymidine-dependent mutants (Stacey and Simson, 1965). These mutants are deficient in thymidylate synthetase which, in association with the specific folate coenzyme, converts deoxyuridylate to thymidylate, and they overcome this requirement by using exogenous thymidine or thymine; these organisms are therefore resistant to TMP provided, as is usual, the other antagonists are present. Such thymidine/thymine-dependent mutants have been isolated from patients undergoing therapy with TMP–SMX (Barker, Healing and Hutchison, 1972; Okubadejo and Maskell, 1974; Tanner and Bullin, 1974; Tapsall, Wilson and Harper, 1974) and from animals (Devriese and Hommez, 1974). In practice, they are recognized by their ability to grow in the primary isolation medium, which contains adequate amounts of thymidine, but not on the TMP–SMX-susceptibility-testing medium which has very low thymidine content. Barker and his colleagues suggested that the occurrence of these mutants may be more common than is generally supposed because they are not often recognized. However, the high efficacy of TMP–SMX with its low relapse rate indicates that they are rarely of clinical significance, perhaps because under usual conditions the thymidine content in tissues, etc. is too low to support their growth or, alternatively, because they are pathogenically 'cripples' and are readily eliminated by the host. These suggestions are supported by the findings of Okubadejo and Maskell (1974) and by Smith and Tucker (1976). Okubadejo and Maskell, despite a very careful watch since 1972, isolated only one thymine-dependent strain from 75 000 samples of urine; this organism was a strain of *E. coli* and was from a patient with gross pyuria and renal calculi. However, more recently these investigators (Maskell, Okubadejo and Payne, 1976) reported that since 1971, they have isolated eight such strains from patients on prolonged treatment with TMP–SMX. Except for one, which was from sputum of a patient with chest infection, each strain was from urine of patients with renal calculi and, by physical means, the presence of a thymine-like substance was demonstrated in the urine of five of these patients but not in control samples from patients infected with normal bacteria or from healthy adults. Smith and Tucker (1976) demonstrated that thymine-dependent strains of salmonella had reduced virulence for chickens and mice. Therefore, it would seem that both explanations for the rarity of these mutants being causal may operate.

INCIDENCE OF RESISTANCE TO TMP AND SMX

Because errors that occur in TMP–SMX susceptibility testing are almost always due to the presence in the medium of thymidine, which leads to sensitive strains being reported as resistant, the reported incidence of resistant strains to the combination tends to be an overestimation. However, in spite of this tendency, published evidence indicates that there has not been an important increase in the incidence of infections by resistant strains except perhaps in hospital-acquired infections (Hunter, 1972; Nakhla, 1972; Lewis and Lacey, 1973; Ball and Wallace, 1974; Freunsgaard and Korner, 1974; Grüneberg, 1976). The increased resistance in these hospital strains appears to be mainly confined to members of the genera *Enterobacter, Proteus* and *Klebsiella,* each of which had a higher incidence of TMP-resistant strains than had other genera before the introduction of the combination.

TMP AND SULPHONAMIDE-RESISTANT STRAINS

The rational use of the TMP–SMX combination depends on the sulphonamide reducing the amount of dihydrofolate synthesized by the infecting organism, thus lowering the amount of TMP needed to inhibit growth through blocking the conversion of the folate to its active form. Justification for using the combination therefore depends upon the causal organism being sensitive to SMX, but 'sensitive' under these circumstances must be distinguished from 'sensitive' when the sulphonamide is used alone.

When examined by conventional susceptibility methods, an organism is regarded as resistant when its macroscopic growth is not affected by the sulphonamide. 'Resistance' by this definition does not necessarily mean that the sulphonamide has not affected the folate biosynthesis of the organism. Although there are now records of direct estimations of the amount of dihydrofolate in cells of sulphonamide-resistant bacteria grown in the presence and absence of a sulphonamide, these organisms are known to contain altered dihydropteroate synthetases. Pato and Brown (1963) showed that these enzymes of *E. coli*, made resistant to sulphonamides by serial passage, combined less effectively with the sulphonamide than did those of the parent strain, and Wise and Abou-Donia (1975) showed that strains carrying sulphonamide-resistant genes or plasmids contained two similar enzymes. One of these enzymes was the enzyme present in sensitive strains, and it was inactive in the presence of the sulphonamide while the other was active in its presence.

The effects of the sulphonamide on the dihydropteroate synthetase activity of the strains examined by Wise and Abou-Donia varied quantitatively and so the TMP-sensitivity of many of the sulphonamide-resistant strains may be expected to be increased in the presence of a sulphonamide because the amount of substrate against which TMP competes will be reduced. The effect of sulphonamides on the inhibitory action of TMP on the growth of sulphonamide-resistant strains was described by Bushby (1969). He showed that with *Strep. faecalis*, an organism often regarded as being indifferent to the presence of SMX, the sulphonamides markedly enhanced the suppressive effects of TMP. Similar effects were also observed with two strains of sulphonamide-resistant *E. coli* (*Table 5.3*). The

Table 5.3 The effects of sulphamethoxazole (SMX) on the growth of sulphonamide-resistant organisms. These strains showed no sign of inhibition with 300 μg sulphonamide disc. Medium: Oxoid Sensitivity broth plus 2% lysed horse blood

Organism	*Concentration* (μg ml^{-1}) *TMP*	*SMX*	*Percentage of control growth after 7 h*
Escherichia coli	–	30	93
S2127	0.03	–	63
	0.03	30	12
Escherichia coli	–	30	100
S2117	0.03	–	45
	0.03	30	23
	0.03	100	17
Streptococcus faecalis	–	30	97
H371	0.003	–	58
	0.003	30	7
Streptococcus faecalis	–	30	100
CN478	0.01	–	88
	0.01	30	45

potentiation by SMX can also be demonstrated by diffusion methods, for although a sulphonamide sensitivity disc produces no zone of inhibition with *Strep. faecalis,* discs containing 23.75 μg SMX plus 1.25 μg TMP, produce larger zones of inhibited growth with this organism than do discs containing 1.25 μg of TMP, and the difference in size is abolished by the presence of *p*-aminobenzoic acid.

Pechère (1971) similarly confirmed with sulphonamide-resistant strains of *E. coli* that the increased activity is due to the sequential blockade by abolishing it with *p*-aminobenzoic acid.

Reports concerning the detection of synergy by conventional susceptibility testing methods with sulphonamide-resistant strains are conflicting, but failure to demonstrate potentiation by these methods with a particular strain does not necessarily exclude its occurring *in vivo*; this is because neutralizing substances may be present in the medium, or an inappropriate ratio of TMP and SMX may have been used. The results of tests specifically designed to detect the interaction indicate that such strains are more susceptible to the action of the combination than to TMP alone although, with the more highly resistant strains, it may be that the degree of the potentiation is not of clinical importance.

The enhanced susceptibility of these strains has been demonstrated *in vivo*; it was reported by Grunberg (1973) and by Böhni (1973) in mice infected with sulphonamide-resistant strains. Also, Sourander, Saarimaa and Arvilommi (1972) reported that of 55 patients with long-lasting urinary infections due to sulphonamide-resistant bacterial strains, 21 out of 24 treated daily with 1.6 g SMX plus 320 mg TMP were cured, which compared with 8 out of 19 treated daily with 320 mg TMP and 1 out of 12 treated daily with 1.6 g SMX.

The question of whether potentiation occurs with TMP-resistant strains is of less clinical importance for these strains are relatively rare, and of those that do exist the majority have apparently arisen from mutation and are not due to R-factors; for example, of 95 TMP-resistant strains of enterobacteria from clinical specimens and examined by Jobanputra and Datta (1974), only 10 were found to be due to plasmids.

Synergy Under Clinical Conditions

Trimethoprim is a potent antibacterial in its own right and it also possesses the most unique property of being present in tissues and in body fluids, such as those of the prostate and vagina, in concentrations higher than those in plasma. So the question arises as to its clinical effectiveness when used alone. Protective experiments in mice suggest that TMP is a poor chemotherapeutic agent as compared with the sulphonamides; *in vitro* TMP is, on a weight basis, some twenty times more active than is SMX, yet its ED50 for mice is usually higher than that of SMX. This apparent contradiction can, however, be explained by the very short half-life of TMP in the mouse: it is only about 1 h which is several times shorter than the half-life of SMX.

The advantage claimed for using TMP with a sulphonamide have frequently been stated and, provided TMP does not increase unwanted side-effects of sulphonamide therapy, it seems rational to take advantage of them. However, only by clinical studies with TMP alone can their true value be assessed. Perhaps the strongest case for using TMP alone is in urinary infections where, with the current standard doses, its concentrations in the urine are well above the MIC for most pathogens. There are a few published results of studies in which TMP was compared with the combination but the number of patients in each study was small and the doses were not standard; strict comparison can therefore not be made but it is apparent that the therapeutic results obtained with TMP alone did not differ greatly from those obtained with the combination. In other infections, there is a stronger case for using the combination because the concentrations of the drugs at the site of infection are usually close to or even below the MIC of the individual drugs. However, Schneider *et al.* (1965) reported that TMP alone in doses of 400 to 800 mg per day (the normal dose when given with SMX is 320 mg per day) was very effective in the treatment of proteus infections in 31 patients with neoplastic disease.

The strongest objection to using TMP alone is probably the risk of resistance to it developing rapidly but, during the course of time, the strength of the objection has weakened. The combination has been used in Britain for eight years; it has frequently been given to patients infected with enterobacteria carrying plasmids which confer high sulphonamide-resistance, and in these patients it can be argued that TMP has been virtually used alone without causing a marked increase in resistance. If this is the case, then there seems no more justification for using the combination with this objective than any other combination of antibacterials.

In my opinion, the synergy of TMP and sulphonamides was always the main advantage of using the combination rather than the individual components and, except perhaps for urinary infections, this would still appear to be true.

References

ACAR, J.F., GOLDSTEIN, F. and CHABBERT, Y.A. (1973). *J. inf. Dis.,* **128** suppl., S470

AMYES, S.G.B. and SMITH, J.T. (1974). *J. med. Microbiol.,* **7**, 143

ANDERSON, J.D., LACEY, R.W., LEWIS, E.L. and SELLIN, M.A. (1974). *J. clin. Path.,* **27**, 619

ANGEHRN, P. and THEN, R. (1973). *Arzneimittel-Forsch.,* **23**, 447

ANGIER, R.B., BOOTHE, J.H., HUTCHINGS, B.L., MOWAT, J.H., SEMB, J., STOKSTAD, E.L.R., SUBBAROW, Y. and WALLER, C.W. (1946). *Science,* **103**, 667

BAKER, B.R. and BENG-THONG HO. (1964). *J. Pharmacol. Sci.,* **53**, 1137

BALL, A.P. and WALLACE, E.T. (1974). *J. Int. Med. Res.,* **2** suppl., 18

BARKER, J., HEALING, D. and HUTCHISON, J.G.P. (1972). *J. clin. Path.,* **25**, 1086

BASFORD, F.R., CURD, F.H.S., HOGGARTH, E. and ROSE, F.L. (1947). *J. Chem. Soc.,* 1354

BISHOP, A. and McCONNACHIE, E.W. (1948). *Nature,* **162**, 541

BOHNI, E. (1969a). *Chemotherapy,* **14** suppl., 1

BOHNI, E. (1969b). *Postgrad. Med. J.,* **45** suppl., 18

BOHNI, E. (1969c). *Schweiz. Med. Wschr.,* **99**, 1505

BOHNI, E. (1973). *Progress in Chemotherapy, Proceedings of the 8th Int. Cong. of Chemotherapy,* **2**, 204

BROWN, G.M. (1962). *J. biol. Chem.,* **237**, 536

BURCHALL, J.J. and HITCHINGS, G.H. (1965). *Mol. Pharmacol.,* **1**, 126

BUSHBY, S.R.M. (1969). *Postgrad. Med. J.,* **45** suppl., 10

BUSHBY, S.R.M. (1971). *Advances in Antimicrob. and Antineop. Chemotherapy, Proceedings of 7th Int. Cong. of Chemotherapy,* **1/2**, 847

BUSHBY, S.R.M. (1973a). *J. inf. Dis.,* **128** suppl., S442

BUSHBY, S.R.M. (1973b). *Med. J. Aust. Special Suppl.,* **1**, 10

BUSHBY, S.R.M. (1973c). *Brit. Med. J.,* **3**, 50

BUSHBY, S.R.M. (1975). *Canadian Med. Assoc. J.,* **112**, 63S

BUSHBY, S.R.M. and BARNETT, M. (1967). *Proc. V Int. Cong. of Chemotherapy,* **A1-6/11**, 753

BUSHBY, S.R.M. and BARNETT, M. (1969). *Proc. 6th Int. Cong. of Chemotherapy,* **1**, 1008

BUSHBY, S.R.M. and BUSHBY, M.B. (1973). *Progress in Chemotherapy, Proceedings of the 8th Int. Cong. of Chemotherapy,* **1**, 281

BUSHBY, S.R.M. and HITCHINGS, G.H. (1968). *Brit. J. Pharmacol. Chemother.,* **33**, 72

CARRINGTON, H.C., CROWTHER, A.F., DAVEY, D.G., LEVI, A.A. and ROSE, F.L. (1951). *Nature,* **168**, 1080

CUMMINGS, D.J. and MONDALE, L. (1967). *J. Bacteriol.,* **93**, 1917

CURD, F.H.S., DAVEY, D.G. and ROSE, F.L. (1945). *Ann. trop. Med.,* **39**, 157

DANIEL, L.J. and NORRIS, L.C. (1947). *J. biol. Chem.,* **170**, 747

DARRELL, J.H., GARROD, L.P. and WATERWORTH, P.M. (1968). *J. clin. Path.,* **21**, 202

DEVRIESE, L.A. and HOMMEZ, J. (1974). *Zbl. Vet. Med. B.,* **21**, 211

ELION, G.B., SINGER, S. and HITCHINGS, G.H. (1954). *J. biol. Chem.,* **208**, 477

EYLES, D.E. and COLEMAN, N. (1953). *Antibiotics and Chemotherapy,* **3**, 483

EYLES, D.E. and COLEMAN, N. (1955). *Antibiotics and Chemotherapy,* **5**, 529

FALCO, E.A., GOODWIN, L.G., HITCHINGS, G.H., ROLLO, I.M. and RUSSELL, P.B. (1951). *Brit. J. Pharmacol.,* **6**, 185

FERONE, R., BUSHBY, S.R.M., BURCHALL, J.J., MOORE, W.D. and SMITH. D. (1975). *Antimicrob. Agents and Chemother.,* **7**, 91

FRUENSGAARD, K. and KORNER, B. (1974). *Chemotherapy,* **20**, 97

GARROD, L.P. and WATERWORTH, P.M. (1968). *Brit. J. vener. Dis.,* **44**, 75

GRACE, M.E., BUSHBY, S.R.M. and SIGEL, C.W. (1975). *Antimicrob. Agents and Chemother.,* **8**, 45

GREENBERG, J. (1949). *J. Pharmacol. and exp. Therap.,* **97**, 238

GREENBERG, J., BOYD, B.L. and JOSEPHSON, E.S. (1948). *J. Pharmacol and exp. Therapy,* **94**, 60

GREENBERG, J. and RICHESON, E.M. (1950). *J. Pharmacol and exp. Therapy,* **99**, 444

GRUNBERG, E. (1973). *J. inf. Dis.,* **128** suppl., S478

GRUNBERG, E. and DELORENZO, W.F. (1967). *Proc. 6th Interscience Conference of Antimicrob. Agents and Chemother., Philadelphia, Pa.* (Amer. Soc. for Microbiology, Oct. 1966), 430

GRUNBERG, E., PRINCE, H.N. and DELORENZO, W.F. (1970). *J. clin. Pharmacol.,* **10**, 231

GRUNEBERG, R.N. (1976). *J. clin. Path.,* **29**, 292

GRUNEBERG, R.N., LEAKEY, A., BENDALL, M.J. and SMELLIE, J.M. (1975). *Kidney International,* **8**, S122

HARPER, G.J. and CAWSTON, W.C. (1945). *J. Path. and Bacteriol.,* **57**, 59

HARVEY, R.J. (1973). *J. Bacteriol.,* **114**, 309

HAWKING, F. and PERRY, W.L.M. (1948). *Brit. J. Pharmacol.,* **3**, 320

HITCHINGS, G.H. (1952). *Trans. R. Soc. Trop. Hyg.,* **46**, 467

HITCHINGS, G.H. (1955). *Amer. J. clin. Nutrit.,* **3**, 321

HITCHINGS, G.H. (1971). *Ann. N.Y. Acad. Sci.,* **186**, 444

HITCHINGS, G.H. and BUSHBY, S.R.M. (1961). *V Int. Cong. of Biochem.,* Section 7, 165

HITCHINGS, G.H., ELION, G.B., FALCO, E.A., RUSSELL, P.B., SHERWOOD, M.B. and VANDERWERFF, H. (1949). *J. biol. Chem.,* **183**, 1

HITCHINGS, G.H., ELION, G.B., FALCO, E.A., RUSSELL, P.B., VANDERWERFF, H. (1950). *Ann. N.Y. Acad. Sci.,* **52**, 1318

HITCHINGS, G.H., ELION, G.B., VANDERWERFF, H. and FALCO, E.A. (1948). *J. biol. Chem.,* **174**, 765

HITCHINGS, G.H., FALCO, E.A., VANDERWERFF, H., RUSSELL, P.B. and ELION, G.B. (1952). *J. biol. Chem.,* **199**, 43

HULL, R., LOVELL, B.J., OPENSHAW, H.T., PAYMAN, L.C. and TODD, A.R. (1946). *J. Chem. Soc.,* 357

HUNTER, I.J. (1972). *Med. J. Aust.,* **1**, 442

JOBANPUTRA, R.S. and DATTA, N. (1974). *J. med. Microbiol.,* **7**, 169

KOCH, A.E. and BURCHALL, J.J. (1971). *Appl. Microbiol.,* **22**, 812

LAMPEN, J.O. and JONES, M.J. (1946). *J. biol. Chem.*, **166**, 435
LEBEK, G. (1972). *Hippokrates,* **43**, 45
LEWIS, E.L. and LACEY, R.W. (1973). *J. clin. Path.*, **26**, 175
LUX, R.E. (1954). *Antibiot. and Chemother.*, **4**, 971
MASKELL, G., OKUBADEJO, O.A. and PAYNE, R.H. (1976). *Lancet,* **i**, 834
MITCHELL, H.K., SNELL, E.E. and WILLIAMS, R.J. (1941). *J. Amer. Chem. Soc.*, **63**, 2284
MOWAT, J.H., BOOTHE, J.H., HUTCHINGS, B.L., STOKSTAD, E.L.R., WALLER, C.W., ANGIER, R.B., SEMB, J., COSULICH, D.B. and SUBBAROW, Y. (1948). *J. Amer. Chem. Soc.*, **70**, 14
NAKHLA, L.S. (1972). *J. clin. Path.*, **25**, 708
NICHOL, C.A. and WELCH, A.D. (1950a). *Proc. Soc. exp. Biol. and Med.*, **74**, 52
NICHOL, C.A. and WELCH, A.D. (1950b). *Proc. Soc. exp. Biol. and Med.*, **74**, 402
OKUBADEJO, O.A. and MASKELL, R.M. (1974). *Brit. Med. J.*, **2**, 227
OSBORN, M.J., FREEMAN, M. and HUENNEKENS, F.M. (1956). *Proc. Soc. exp. Biol. and Med.*, **97**, 429
OSBORN, M.J. and HUENNEKENS, F.M. (1958). *J. biol. Chem.*, **233**, 969
PATO, M.L. and BROWN, G.M. (1963). *Arch. Biochem. and Biophys.*, **103**, 443
PECHERE, J.C. (1971). *Path. Biol.*, **19**, 621
POTTER, V.R. (1951). *Proc. Soc. exp. Biol. and Med.*, **76**, 41
ROTH, B., FALCO, E.A., HITCHINGS, G.H. and BUSHBY, S.R.M. (1962). *J. Med. pharmacol. Chem.*, **5**, 1103
SAUBERLICH, H.E. (1949). *J. biol. Chem.*, **181**, 467
SCHNEIDER, M., SCHWARZENBERG, L., CATTAN, A., SCHLUMBERGER, J.R., AMIEL, J.L. and MATHE, G. (1965). *La Presse Medicale,* **73**, 893
SEYDEL, J.K., WEMPE, E., MILLER, G.H. and MILLER, L. (1972). *Chemotherapy,* **17**, 217
SKOLD, O. and WIDH, A. (1974). *J. biol. Chem.*, **249**, 4324
SMITH, H.W. and TUCKER, J.F. (1976). *J. Hyg.*, **76**, 97
SNELL, E.E. and MITCHELL, H.K. (1941). *Proc. Nat. Acad. Sci.*, **27**, 1
SNELL, E.E. and PETERSON, W.H. (1940). *J. Bact.*, **39**, 273
SOURANDER, L., SAARIMAA, H. and ARVILOMMI, H. (1972). *Acta Med. Scand.*, **191**, 1
STACEY, K.A. and SIMSON, E. (1965). *J. Bact.*, **90**, 554
STOKSTAD, E.L.R. (1941). *J. biol. Chem.*, **139**, 475
TANNER, E.I. and BULLIN, C.H. (1974). *J. clin. Path.*, **27**, 565
TAPSALL, J.W., WILSON, E. and HARPER, J. (1974). *Pathology,* **6**, 161
THEN, R. (1973). *Zbl. Bakt. Hyg., I. Abt. Orig. A.*, **225**, 34
THEN, R. and ANGEHRN, P. (1973). *J. Gen. Microbiol.*, **76**, 255
THEN, R. and ANGEHRN, P. (1974). *Biochem. Pharmacol.*, **23**, 2977
THEN, R. and ANGEHRN, P. (1975). *Biochem. Pharmacol.*, **24**, 1003
WISE, E.M. and ABOU-DONIA, M.M. (1975). *Proc. Nat. Acad. Sci.*, **72**, 2621
WOOD, R.C., FERONE, R. and HITCHINGS, G.H. (1961). *Biochem. Pharmacol.*, **6**, 113
WOOD, R.C. and HITCHINGS, G.H. (1959a). *J. biol. Chem.*, **234**, 2377
WOOD, R.C. and HITCHINGS, G.H. (1959b). *J. biol. Chem.*, **234**, 2381

6

TRIMETHOPRIM PLUS SULPHAMETHOXAZOLE: SYNERGIC OR ANTAGONISTIC COMBINATION?

D. GREENWOOD
Department of Microbiology, University of Nottingham, City Hospital, Nottingha

The synergic interaction between trimethoprim and sulphonamides is now well established, but important questions regarding the nature and significance of synergy remain to be clarified. In an attempt to throw some further light on the interaction of these compounds we have looked at the kinetics of response of *Escherichia coli* (strain ECSA 1, a clinical isolate) to trimethoprim (TMP) and sulphamethoxazole (SMX) in two turbidimetric systems. In the first of these, a twelve-channel bacterial growth monitoring device (Mackintosh *et al.*, 1973) was used to follow the response of *E. coli* to TMP and SMX under growth conditions similar to those of conventional minimum inhibitory concentration (MIC) titration tests. In the second system dense populations of *E. coli* were exposed to the drugs in an *in vitro* model designed to simulate the hydrokinetic features of the urinary bladder (O'Grady *et al.*, 1973; Greenwood, 1976a).

Static Turbidimetric System

When *E. coli* is exposed to sulphonamides, growth continues normally for several generations before any antibacterial effect is obtained (Kohn and Harris, 1941; Seydel *et al.*, 1972). This effect was also demonstrated by continuous turbidimetric monitoring of cultures in Wellcotest broth containing various concentrations of SMX (*Figure 6.1*). Monitoring growth in this way also revealed a marked antibacterial effect at SMX concentrations below the conventionally determined 'MIC' with recovery during the overnight period from drug concentrations able to inhibit growth for long periods. Sub-inoculation of the regrowing culture into fresh drug-containing broth showed that the bacterial population was now resistant to the SMX concentration to which it had originally been exposed, but that it remained susceptible to higher drug concentrations; such 'resistance' was found to be unstable on passage in antibiotic-free broth.

A very similar situation, with adaptation to phenotypic resistance occurring at sub-MIC levels, was seen with TMP, but in this case inhibitory concentrations had a relatively rapid effect on growth (*Figure 6.2*).

Continuous turbidimetric monitoring also provides a simple means of examining the action of antibacterial agents in terms of the smallest concentration able

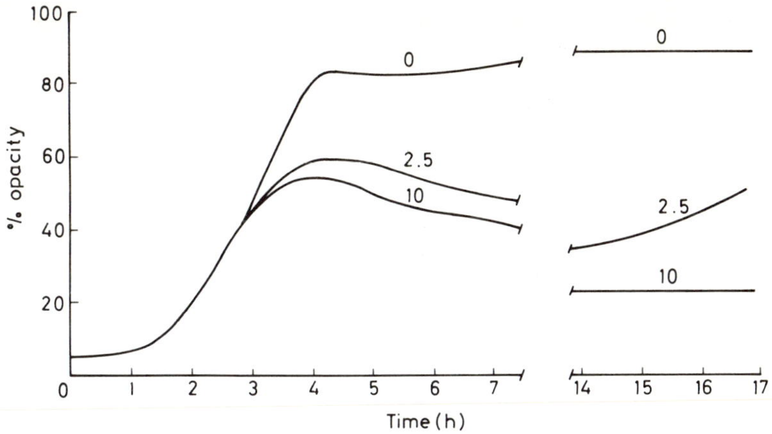

Figure 6.1 Continuous opacity records of E. coli. *Broth containing SMX at the concentrations ($\mu g\ ml^{-1}$) shown was inoculated with* ca *5×10^5 bacteria ml^{-1} at time 0*

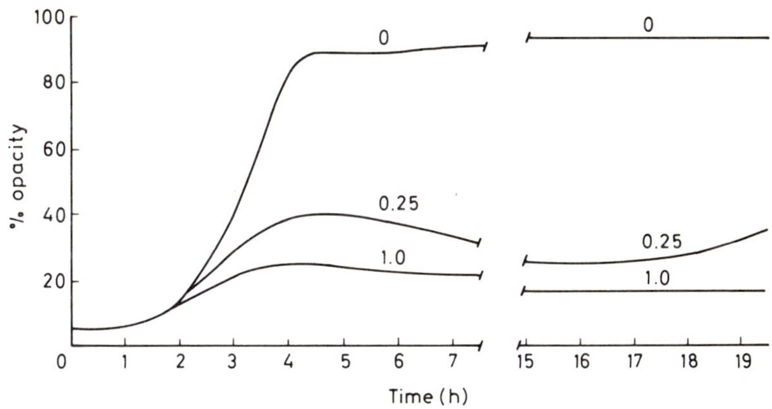

Figure 6.2 Continuous opacity records of E. coli. *Broth containing TMP at the concentrations ($\mu g\ ml^{-1}$) shown was inoculated with* ca *5×10^5 bacteria ml^{-1} at time 0*

to produce a deviation from the normal growth curve, the minimum antibacterial concentration (MAC) (Lorian, 1975). When TMP and SMX were examined in this way, synergy was clearly demonstrated in that sub-MAC concentrations of the two drugs could combine to produce an antibacterial effect that neither agent could produce alone, but the degree of synergy was not so striking as would be estimated by conventional chessboard titration: the lowest concentration of both agents just able to inhibit growth was MAC/2 TMP + MAC/8 SMX

Table 6.1 Synergy between TMP and SMX expressed as a fraction of the minimum antibacterial concentration

*Fraction of MAC** TMP*	*SMX*	*Degree of inhibition***
MAC	0	±
0	MAC	±
MAC/2	MAC	+++
MAC/2	MAC/2	++
MAC/2	MAC/4	++
MAC/2	MAC/8	+
MAC/2	MAC/16	0
MAC/4	MAC	++
MAC/4	MAC/2	+
MAC/4	MAC/4	0
MAC/8	MAC	+
MAC/8	MAC/2	0

*The minimum antibacterial concentration (MAC), defined as the lowest concentration of each drug to cause a deviation from the normal growth curve in the turbidimetric system, was 0.06 μg TMP ml^{-1} and 0.6 μg SMX ml^{-1} (MIC/16 in each case).

**Plusses represent estimates of degrees of inhibition judged by rapidity and maintenance of suppression of growth; +++ = suppression of growth for $>$12 h; 0 = no deviation from the normal growth curve.

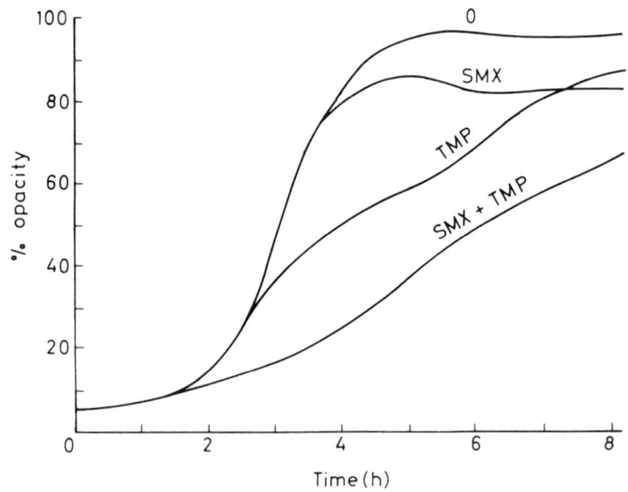

Figure 6.3 Continuous opacity records of E. coli. *Broth containing: no antibiotics; SMX (0.6 μg ml^{-1}; MAC); TMP (0.06 μg ml^{-1}; MAC); SMX (MAC) + TMP (MAC/8); was inoculated with ca 5×10^5 bacteria ml^{-1} at time 0*

or MAC/4 TMP + MAC/2 SMX (*Table 6.1*), compared to the MIC-related values (lowest concentrations able to suppress growth completely overnight) of MIC/16 TMP + MIC/8 SMX or MIC/8 TMP + MIC/32 SMX. Interestingly, inhibition of growth by combinations of TMP and SMX was always manifested by the delayed growth characteristic of trimethoprim action, not the sulphonamide-associated effect in which growth followed the normal curve for several hours before an antibacterial effect was seen. This held true even when the concentration of the trimethoprim component was extremely low (*Figure 6.3*) and offers empirical evidence for the theoretical prediction that SMX potentiates the action of TMP rather than vice versa.

Conventional MIC tests determine only the status of visible growth at the time of inspection. The demonstration that adaptation to resistance occurs at sub-MIC concentrations of both TMP and SMX (i.e. that the MIC end-point is partly governed by the ability of the bacteria to adapt to otherwise inhibitory levels of drug) suggests that mutual suppression of such phenotypic variation may be an important component of the overall synergic interaction as recorded in conventional chessboard titrations. Specific potentiation of TMP action, directly referable to the biochemical effect of SMX earlier in the same metabolic pathway, may be distinctly less than has generally been supposed. A more realistic estimate of the degree of such potentiation may be offered by the MAC-related values shown in *Table 6.1.*

Bladder Model

In bacterial cystitis – a condition for which co-trimoxazole is commonly used – the bladder urine frequently contains a bacterial population exceeding 10^8 bacteria ml^{-1}; the bacterial 'culture' is continually diluted by the secretion of fresh urine (which may contain antibiotic) and is periodically discharged on micturition. The response of bacteria to antibiotics in such complex dynamic circumstances is difficult to predict and an *in vitro* model was developed in order to investigate this problem (O'Grady *et al.,* 1973). The experimental design and the interpretation of results generated by the model have been described in detail elsewhere (O'Grady *et al.,* 1973; Greenwood, 1976a; Greenwood and O'Grady, 1974; 1975; 1976a, b). In the present experiments, 20 ml of a fully-grown broth culture of *E. coli* was diluted with fresh broth at a rate of 1 ml min^{-1} (the normal diurnal ureteric urine flow rate) and at hourly intervals a 'micturition' episode emptied the system leaving a 20 ml residual volume.

Of particular interest in the present study were the questions of whether the density of the bacterial population would influence the activity of TMP and SMX in the fluctuating conditions of the bladder as it does in conventional *in vitro* tests, and whether synergy could still be demonstrated when the drug levels achieved exceeded the conventionally determined MIC. In order to answer the first question TMP and SMX, alone and in combination, were introduced into the system as a single pulse, or in a second type of experiment, were included in the broth used to infuse the system. In these conditions a single pulse of SMX to achieve an initial concentration of 500 $\mu g\ ml^{-1}$ (50 MIC) had no effect on the normal growth/dilution response whereas TMP at an initial concentration of 50 $\mu g\ ml^{-1}$ (50 MIC) was able to exert a transient effect (Greenwood and O'Grady,

1976b). When continuously infused with the diluent broth, SMX, which is notoriously affected by inoculum size in conventional *in vitro* tests, was found to be able to suppress growth of the dense bacterial population ($>10^8$ organisms ml^{-1}) after several hours' exposure, even at concentrations below the conventionally determined MIC (*Figure 6.4*). This suggests that the inoculum effect seen

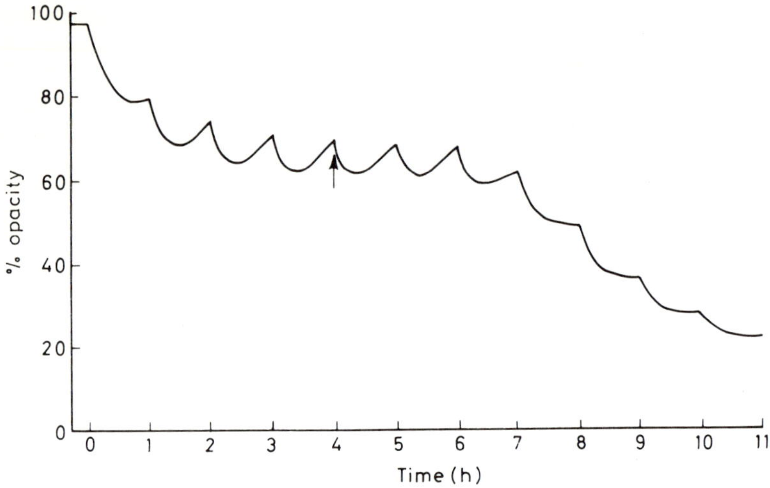

Figure 6.4 Continuous opacity record of E. coli *in the bladder model. After 4 cycles of dilution and hourly 'micturition', dilution was continued with broth containing 5 μg SMX ml*$^{-1}$

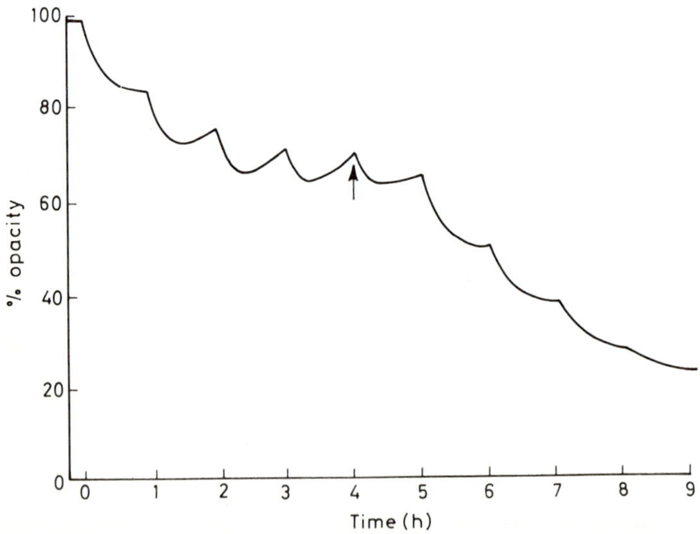

Figure 6.5 Continuous opacity record of E. coli *in the bladder model. After 4 cycles of dilution and hourly 'micturition', dilution was continued with broth containing 0.25 μg TMP ml*$^{-1}$

with SMX is entirely due to the presence of a folate pool which must be diluted out by bacterial growth and division before the sulphonamide activity can take effect. In conventional tests, dense populations presumably achieve visible proportions before inhibition occurs and in extreme cases enter the stationary growth phase before the drug is able to act (Greenwood, 1976b). When TMP was infused with the diluent broth an immediate effect was observed as the concentration of TMP in the culture reached an inhibitory level and a progressive decline in opacity subsequently occurred (*Figure 6.5*). In experiments in which SMX and TMP were added together, either as a pulse or as a continuous infusion, the form of the opacity trace was always identical to that obtained with TMP alone. This indicates that the additional presence of SMX fails to enhance the hydrokinetic clearance of infection, but does not exclude the possibility that the sulphonamide contributes to the overall antibacterial effect in some other way, for example by potentiating the bactericidal activity of TMP or by prolonging the bacteristatic effect. A further experiment was therefore devised in which the drugs, alone and in combination, were infused into the culture for 8 h after which dilution was continued with fresh broth. The time taken, following the switch to drug-free broth, for recovery of the culture to occur (judged by a rise in turbidity) was then measured. Any antibacterial activity of the combination, over and above that achieved by the components alone, should in this way be reflected by an increase in the time taken for recovery to occur. Typical results are shown in *Table 6.2.* At concentrations above the conventionally-determined

Table 6.2 Comparison of the ability of cultures of *E. coli* to recover following exposure to SMX and/or TMP for 8 h, in the bladder model

Antibacterial agent	*Concentration* (μg ml^{-1}) *in infusion*	*Time* (h) *to regrowth after switch to drug-free broth*
SMX	5	1.5
TMP	0.25	1.5
SMX + TMP	5 + 0.25	3
SMX	100	3
TMP	5	6
SMX + TMP	100 + 5	6

SMX = sulphamethoxazole; TMP = trimethoprim..

MIC the additional presence of SMX failed to delay recovery seen following exposure to TMP alone, but at sub-MIC concentrations a small additional suppression of growth was achieved.

As demonstrated in both the static turbidimetric system and the bladder model, the action of TMP is very rapid, presumably because its effect of trapping folate in the dihydrofolate form quickly halts crucial metabolic processes of the cell (Hitchings, 1973). Sulphonamides, in contrast, have a delayed effect because even when the folic acid supply is cut off at source, preformed tetrahydrofolate can still fulfil the needs of the cell until growth and division have diluted the concentration to below a functional level. When TMP is present in sufficient concentration, its relatively rapid effect in inhibiting growth means that the folate pool itself does not become depleted and even if a sulphonamide is also present it does not have the opportunity to exert its effect. In this sense TMP may be said to antagonize the action of sulphonamides.

Synergy between SMX and TMP appears to be very much an MIC-associated phenomenon. Undeniably, potentiation of TMP action by SMX occurs, but altering the criterion of measurement to the MAC rather than to the MIC reduces the scale of the potentiating effect. Furthermore, at concentrations exceeding the MIC no synergic interaction could be demonstrated in the model system used here, and on theoretical grounds one would predict that SMX would be antagonized by the presence of inhibitory concentrations of TMP. In infections of the urinary tract, where relatively high concentrations of TMP can easily be achieved and maintained, it is difficult to see what advantage the additional presence of SMX may confer, unless it be to prevent the possible emergence of spontaneously occurring TMP-resistant mutants. However, in other therapeutic situations, where drug levels at the site of infection are more difficult to achieve and maintain, the potentiating effect may be of positive value.

Acknowledgment

Figures 6.1, 6.2, 6.4 and *6.5* and *Table 6.2* are taken from Greenwood and O'Grady (1976b) and are reproduced by kind permission of the Editor of *The Journal of Clinical Pathology.*

References

GREENWOOD, D. (1976a). In *Chemotherapy,* vol. 2, p. 241. Ed. Williams, J.D. and Geddes, A.M., Plenum Publishing Corporation, New York and London

GREENWOOD, D. (1976b). *J. antimicrob. Chemother.,* **2**, 87

GREENWOOD, D. and O'GRADY, F. (1974). *Brit. J. exp. Pathol.,* **55**, 245

GREENWOOD, D. and O'GRADY, F. (1975). *Brit. J. exp. Pathol.,* **56**, 167

GREENWOOD, D. and O'GRADY, F. (1976a). *Brit. J. exp. Pathol.,* **57**, 303

GREENWOOD, D. and O'GRADY, F. (1976b). *J. clin. Pathol.,* **29**, 162

HITCHINGS, G.H. (1973). In *Trimethoprim/Sulphamethoxazole in Bacterial Infections,* p. 7. Ed. Bernstein, L.S. and Salter, A.J., Churchill Livingstone, Edinburgh

KOHN, H.I. and HARRIS, J.S. (1941). *J. Pharmacol. exp. Ther.,* **73**, 343

LORIAN, V. (1975). *Bull. N.Y. Acad. Med.,* **51**, 1046

MACKINTOSH, I.P., O'GRADY, F., GREENWOOD, D., WATSON, B.W., CRICHTON, T.C., PIPER, R. and FERRER, A. (1973). *Biomed. Eng.,* **8**, 514

O'GRADY, F., MACKINTOSH, I.P., GREENWOOD, D. and WATSON, B.W. (1973). *Brit. J. exp. Pathol.,* **54**, 283

SEYDEL, J.K., WEMPE, E., MILLER, G.H. and MILLER, L. (1972). *Chemotherapy,* **17**, 217

7

SYNERGIC ACTIVITIES OF PENICILLIN COMBINATIONS

R. SUTHERLAND
Beecham Pharmaceuticals, Betchworth

The use of combinations of antibiotics is commonplace in clinical practice despite the disapprobation of many authorities. Combined therapy is usually based on a desire to extend the antibacterial spectrum but in a number of cases it is also hoped that the individual agents may interact to produce synergistic effects. Penicillins are often combined with other antibiotics and this report describes examples where antibacterial synergy may arise from penicillin combinations.

Synergy between Pencillins and Aminoglycosides against Enterococci

Perhaps the best known example of synergism between antibiotics is that demonstrated by penicillins and aminoglycosides against enterococci. Enhancement of the bactericidal activity of benzylpenicillin against *Streptococcus faecalis* by streptomycin was studied by Jawetz and his collaborators in their early studies on antibiotic interactions (Jawetz, Gunnison and Coleman, 1950) and the value of combined penicillin/aminoglycoside therapy in the treatment of enterococcal endocarditis is well established.

Enterococci are moderately sensitive to benzylpenicillin, amoxycillin and ampicillin and the growth of the organisms is inhibited by relatively low concentrations of the penicillins (*Table 7.1*). Aminoglycoside antibiotics are notably

Table 7.1 Distribution of minimum inhibitory concentrations (MICs) of penicillins and aminoglycosides against 55 strains of enterococci (after Russell and Sutherland, 1975)

	Number of strains with an MIC (μg ml^{-1}) *of*											
Antibiotic	*0.25*	*0.5*	*1.25*	*2.5*	*5.0*	*12.5*	*25*	*50*	*125*	*250*	*500*	*>500*
Amoxycillin	5	49	1	0	0	0	0	0	0	0	0	0
Ampicillin	0	25	29	1	0	0	0	0	0	0	0	0
Benzylpenicillin	0	2	49	4	0	0	0	0	0	0	0	0
Gentamicin	0	0	1	19	26	7	2	0	0	0	0	0
Kanamycin	0	0	0	0	5	19	22	5	2	0	0	2*
Streptomycin	0	0	0	0	0	7	9	21	2	0	1	15*

*MIC >5000 μg ml^{-1}

less active than the penicillins against these organisms, but newer compounds such as gentamicin and tobramycin show a marked improvement in activity compared with streptomycin (*Table 7.1*). The penicillins are bactericidal in action against *S. faecalis*, but less so than against most other bacteria, and a significant number of survivors persist in cultures exposed to penicillins. However, when the penicillin is combined with an aminoglycoside, at a concentration of the latter which is itself ineffective, a marked synergistic action occurs with many strains of enterococci resulting in a striking increase in the bactericidal activity of the penicillin (Sonne and Jawetz, 1968; Watanakunakorn, 1971; Russell and Sutherland, 1975).

Thus, results in *Table 7.2* show the Minimum Bactericidal Concentrations (MBCs) of amoxycillin against enterococci alone and in combination with sublethal concentrations of streptomycin, kanamycin and gentamicin. The bactericidal activities of the combinations were much greater than those of amoxycillin

Table 7.2 Minimum bactericidal concentrations (MBCs) of amoxycillin and aminoglycosides alone, and in combination, for 12 strains of enterococci (after Russell and Sutherland, 1975)

Penicillin	*Aminoglycoside and its concentration* (μg ml^{-1})	*Number of strains with an MBC* (μg ml^{-1})* *of* 0.25	0.5	1.0	2.5	5.0	10	25	50	100	>100
Amoxycillin	None	0	0	0	0	0	0	0	0	0	12
	Streptomycin (20)	1	0	2	2	0	0	0	0	0	7†
	Kanamycin (20)	0	5	4	1	0	0	0	0	0	2‡
	Gentamicin (10)	6	3	3	0	0	0	0	0	0	0

*For an inoculum size *ca* 10^6 cells ml^{-1} of medium.
†Streptomycin MIC >5000 μg ml^{-1}.
‡Kanamycin MIC >5000 μg ml^{-1}.

alone provided that the test organism was sensitive to the aminoglycoside. In these tests, streptomycin-resistant strains were resistant to amoxycillin + streptomycin but were killed by combinations containing kanamycin or gentamicin and, similarly, kanamycin-resistant strains were not killed by amoxycillin + kanamycin but were sensitive to the combination with gentamicin. It should be noted that although amoxycillin appeared to show poor bactericidal activity against enterococci in these tests to measure MBCs, this was because the test was particularly stringent, requiring the viable count to fall from the initial inoculum of 10^6 cells ml^{-1} to less than 10^2 cells ml^{-1}, i.e. 99.99% kill. When the inoculum was reduced to 10^4 cells ml^{-1}, amoxycillin readily reduced the bacterial count to less than 10^2 cells ml^{-1} (99.0% kill), and the MBCs were of the same order as the Minimum Inhibitory Concentrations (MICs).

The bactericidal activity of amoxycillin against *S. faecalis* and its enhancement in combinations with aminoglycosides is illustrated in greater detail in *Figure 7.1*, which shows the effects of combinations of amoxycillin + streptomycin and amoxycillin + kanamycin against a streptomycin-resistant strain, *S. faecalis* 816 (MIC >5000 μg streptomycin ml^{-1}). Amoxycillin was bactericidal at a concentration of 1.0 μg ml^{-1} over the first 6 h and reduced the viable count by 99.9% but this was followed by a resumption of growth to visible levels. Streptomycin (20 μg ml^{-1}) had no effect on the growth of the organisms while kanamycin (20 μg ml^{-1}) was bactericidal for 6 h but at 24 h growth equalled that of the control antibiotic-free culture. The combination of streptomycin and

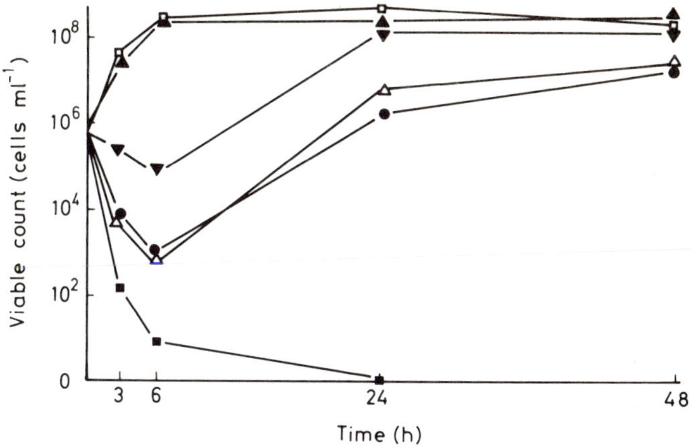

Figure 7.1 Bactericidal activity of amoxycillin, alone and in combination with streptomycin and kanamycin, against Streptococcus faecalis *816.* □ = *Control;* ▲ = *streptomycin 20 μg ml^{-1}; = kanamycin, 20 μg ml^{-1};* △ = *amoxycillin + streptomycin, 1.0 + 20 μg ml^{-1};* ● = *amoxycillin, 1.0 μg ml^{-1};* ■ = *amoxycillin + kanamycin, 1.0 + 20 μg ml^{-1}*

amoxycillin was no more effective than amoxycillin alone, which is not unexpected in view of the high level of resistance of the organism to streptomycin, whereas amoxycillin + kanamycin caused a 99.99% kill by 6 h and had sterilized the culture after 24 h incubation.

It has been suggested that the mechanism of synergism between penicillin and streptomycin against enterococci is that the penicillin induces the formation of enterococcal L-forms that are more sensitive to the aminoglycoside than the parent strains (Hewitt, Seligman and Deigh, 1966). An alternative mechanism is proposed from the results of studies with radio-labelled streptomycin which have shown that enterococci are relatively impermeable to the compound, but that uptake of the aminoglycoside is greatly enhanced by the presence of penicillin (Moellering and Weinberg, 1971). Uptake of streptomycin was also enhanced in cells with a high level of resistance to streptomycin and it appears that the failure of penicillin + streptomycin to produce synergy against these strains is due to the resistance of the ribosomes to the aminoglycoside (Zimmerman, Moellering and Weinberg, 1971).

Combined therapy with benzylpenicillin and streptomycin has long been regarded as the treatment of choice for severe enterococcal infection on the basis of the bactericidal synergy that can be demonstrated *in vitro*, and the use of this antibiotic combination is the most widely accepted example of clinical synergism (Jawetz, 1968). However, a significant proportion of strains of enterococci are resistant to the combined effects of penicillin + streptomycin (Standiford, de

Maine and Kirby, 1970; Moellering, Wennersten and Weinberg, 1971) and there is increasing interest in the activity of combinations of penicillins with newer aminoglycosides such as gentamicin, tobramycin and amikacin (Watanakunakorn, 1971; Moellering, Wennersten and Weinstein, 1973; Iannini, Ehret and Eickhoff, 1976). Nevertheless, the treatment of choice for enterococcal infection remains an appropriate penicillin/aminoglycoside combination.

Penicillin/Aminoglycoside Combinations against *Pseudomonas aeruginosa*

Serious infections due to Gram-negative bacilli now constitute a major problem in hospital practice and infections due to *Pseudomonas aeruginosa* are particularly difficult to treat because of the resistance of this opportunistic pathogen to most antibiotics. Carbenicillin was the first penicillin to show clinically useful anti-pseudomonas activity and gentamicin has been the aminoglycoside of choice for the treatment of pseudomonas infections for a number of years. Early studies showed that combinations of carbenicillin and gentamicin provided synergistic antibacterial effects against *Ps. aeruginosa in vitro* (Brumfitt, Percival and Leigh, 1967; Rolinson and Sutherland, 1968) and synergism has been demonstrated against experimental infections in laboratory animals (Andriole, 1971). Combinations of the compounds have been used with significant success in the treatment of serious infections (Klastersky, Cappel and Debusscher, 1971; Schimpff *et al.*, 1971; Yuce and Van Rooyen, 1971), although there are few controlled studies to show that combined therapy is distinctly better than the use of either drug alone.

More recently, a number of penicillins active against *Ps. aeruginosa* and other Gram-negative bacteria have been introduced, for example sulbenicillin and ticarcillin, and there has been a proliferation of new, active aminoglycosides, namely, amikacin, sisomicin and tobramycin. Synergy, similar to that originally reported with carbenicillin and gentamicin has also been described in laboratory studies *in vitro* and *in vivo* with various combinations of these newer penicillins and aminoglycosides (Klastersky, Nyamubeya and Vandenborre, 1974; Klastersky, Hensgens and Debusscher, 1975; Wald *et al.*, 1975; Kelly and Matsen, 1976).

Table 7.3 Comparative activities of penicillin/aminoglycoside combinations against 3 strains of *Ps. aeruginosa*

	Minimum Inhibitory Concentration (μg ml^{-1})		
Antibiotic	*R2*	*986*	*HT1*
Ticarcillin	31	31	62
Carbenicillin	62	125	250
Tobramycin	0.12	0.25	0.12
Gentamicin	0.5	1.0	1.0
Ticarcillin/tobramycin	8 + 0.03	8 + 0.06	16 + 0.03
Ticarcillin/gentamicin	8 + 0.12	16 + 0.12	16 + 0.06
Carbenicillin/tobramycin	8 + 0.12	31 + 0.06	62 + 0.03
Carbenicillin/gentamicin	31 + 0.12	62 + 0.25	31 + 0.50

Results in *Table 7.3* show the effects demonstrated by a number of penicillin/aminoglycoside combinations against three strains of *Ps. aeruginosa*. The antibacterial activities were determined by a modified chess-board system using the microtiter technique as shown in *Figure 7.2*. The action of the test combination

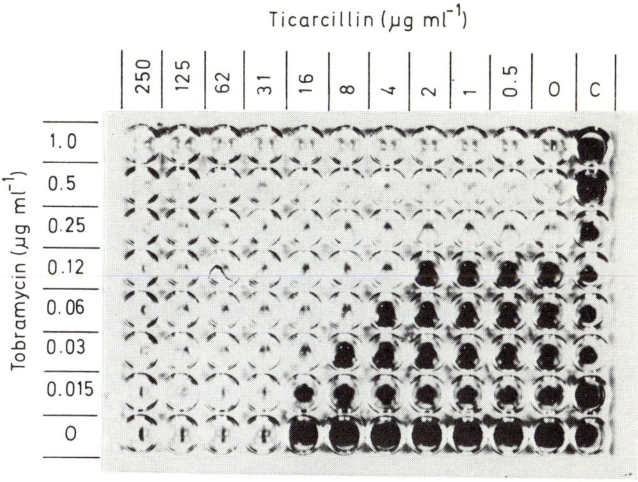

Figure 7.2 Microtiter chess-board technique to demonstrate synergism between ticarcillin and tobramycin against Pseudomonas aeruginosa

of antibiotics was considered synergistic when the MIC of each compound was at least four times as effective in combination as the MIC of that drug alone. It can be seen that in most cases synergy was demonstrated and that combinations of ticarcillin and tobramycin produced the greatest activity against the test strains, which might be expected since these compounds were the most active of the penicillins and aminoglycosides tested. The synergistic bactericidal action of a combination of ticarcillin and tobramycin against *Ps. aeruginosa* is illustrated in *Figure 7.3*, which shows that neither compound produced significant bacteri-

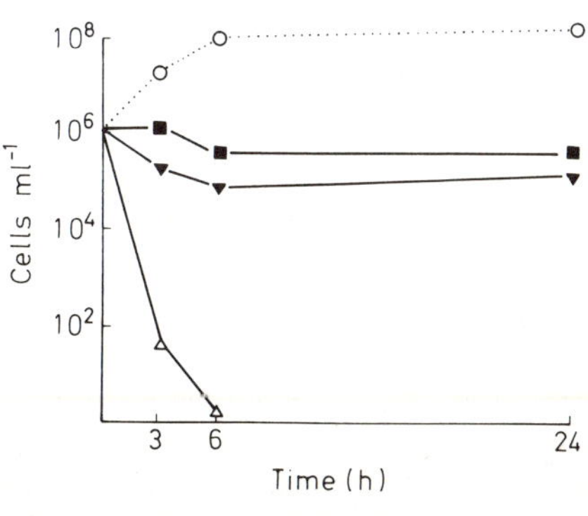

Figure 7.3 Bactericidal synergy between ticarcillin and tobramycin against Pseudomonas aeruginosa. ○–○ = *Control;* ■–■ = *ticarcillin (100);* ▼–▼ = *tobramycin (1.0);* △–△ = *ticarcillin (100) + tobramycin (1.0)*

cidal effects on its own but that a combination of the two antibiotics reduced the viable count to zero within 6 h.

Although the combination of carbenicillin and gentamicin is used successfully in the treatment of clinical infection, inactivation of gentamicin by carbenicillin which is readily demonstrable *in vitro* has also been reported to occur during therapy (McLaughlin and Reeves, 1971) and fears have been expressed that the value of this combination might be limited because of the interaction between the two drugs. However, it is now generally accepted that the combination of drugs should not be withheld from patients with normal renal function (Riff and Jackson, 1972).

The mechanism of the synergy between penicillins and aminoglycosides is not known, but may involve an enhancement of the uptake of the aminoglycoside into the bacterial cell in the presence of the penicillin, which acts by inhibiting cell-wall synthesis, as has been suggested for the effects produced by penicillin–aminoglycosides against enterococci. Whatever the mechanism, the evidence does suggest that combined therapy may well produce enhanced clinical effects in the treatment of infections due to *Ps. aeruginosa.*

Mecillinam Combinations

Penicillins lacking an acyl group in the 6-position of the nucleus are normally devoid of significant antibacterial activity but mecillinam is an example of a non-acyl penicillin with unusual antibacterial properties *in vitro* (Lund and Tybring, 1972; Neu, 1976). For example, the antibacterial spectrum of mecillinam differs from that of conventional penicillins in that the compound shows a high level of activity against certain Gram-negative bacilli but is quite inactive against Gram-positive bacteria. In addition, mecillinam has been shown to have a different mode of action which is readily evident from the morphological responses provoked by mecillinam against sensitive bacteria. Bacterial cells are converted to large spherical forms which are relatively stable in normal media compared with the spheroplasts induced by penicillins (Greenwood and O'Grady, 1973; Melchior *et al.,* 1973).

It has been suggested that, because mecillinam and penicillins have different binding sites, combinations of the compounds would exert synergistic effects (Park and Burman, 1973; Matsuhashi *et al.,* 1974; Spratt, 1975). In practice, synergy has been reported when mecillinam was combined with ampicillin but the extent of synergism appeared to be variable and was greatly influenced by inoculum size and the osmolality of the medium (Tybring and Melchior, 1975). According to these workers synergy arises because the spherical bacterial forms induced by mecillinam are particularly sensitive to ampicillin.

The morphological effects produced by mecillinam were studied in some detail by Greenwood and O'Grady (1973), who reported interesting results when mecillinam was combined with the cephalosporin antibiotic, cephalexin. In a turbidimetric system, neither mecillinam nor cephalexin produced any obvious effect on the growth of *Escherichia coli,* but when the two agents were combined, rapid lysis ensued (*Figure 7.4*) similar to the effects produced by penicillins in this system. Microscopic examination of the various cultures showed the round cell-forms produced by mecillinam and the filament formation

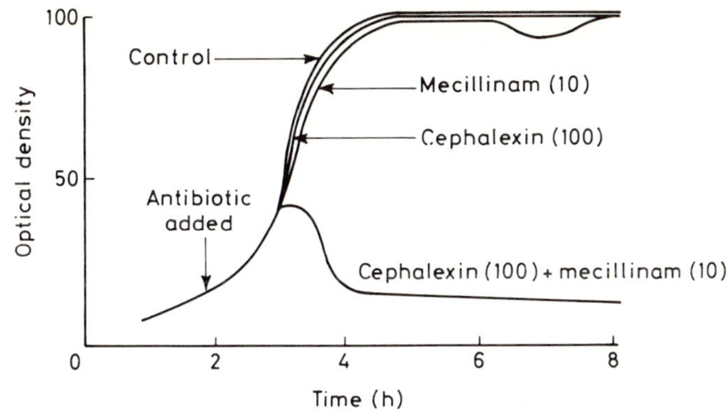

Figure 7.4 Bacteriolytic activities of cephalexin and mecillinam against E. coli, *alone and in combination*

associated with cephalexin, but in the presence of the combination of compounds, spheroplasts similar to those induced by penicillins were observed (*Figure 7.5*).

These results show that two β-lactam antibiotics, each of which produces different morphological effects in sensitive bacteria, presumably by functioning against different sites in the bacterial cell, can interact to produce the classical lytic effects associated with penicillins. The clinical significance of the interaction of mecillinam with other β-lactam antibiotics is uncertain as yet but the phenomenon observed in the laboratory is of considerable interest.

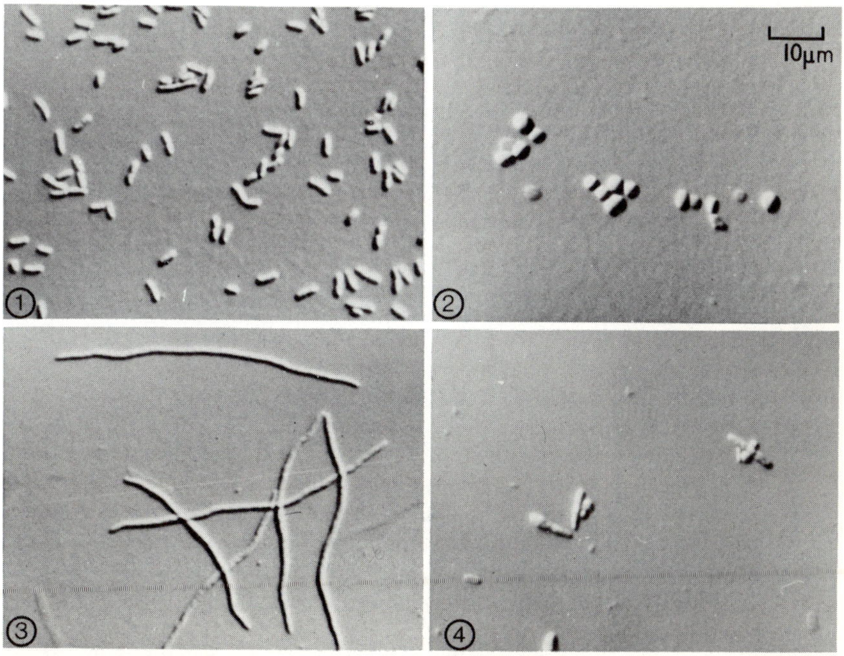

Figure 7.5 Photomicrographs showing the morphological effects produced by cephalexin and mecillinam against E. coli. *(1) Control; (2) mecillinam, 10 μg ml^{-1}; (3) cephalexin 100 μg ml^{-1}; (4) mecillinam 10 μg ml^{-1} + cephalexin 100 μg ml^{-1}*

Synergy arising by Inhibition of β-Lactamase

An entirely different example of synergy involving penicillins, for which the mechanism appears to be clearly established, is that depending upon competitive inhibition of β-lactamase whereby synergism may be demonstrated between pairs of β-lactam antibiotics. The resistance of Gram-negative bacilli to broad-spectrum penicillins or cephalosporins is often associated with β-lactamase activity and the ability of these bacteria to destroy the β-lactam antibiotics (Smith, Hamilton-Miller and Knox, 1969; Richmond and Curtis, 1974). Certain combinations of broad-spectrum penicillins, e.g. ampicillin or amoxycillin, and β-lactamase-stable penicillins, e.g. methicillin or cloxacillin, exhibit synergistic antibacterial effects which are due to inhibition of the β-lactamase by the stable penicillin (Hamilton-Miller and Smith, 1964; Sutherland and Batchelor, 1964). The β-lactamase-stable compounds have little antibacterial activity against Gram-negative bacilli but have a relatively high affinity for their β-lactamases and are able to protect the labile broad-spectrum penicillin by inhibition of the enzyme.

Table 7.4 Synergistic activity of a combination of ampicillin against ampicillin-resistant bacteria, *in vitro* and *in vivo*

	MIC (μg ml^{-1})			*CD*$_{50}$* (mg kg^{-1}) *(oral)*		
Organism	*Ampicillin*	*Cloxacillin*	*Ampicillin + cloxacillin*	*Ampicillin*	*Cloxacillin*	*Ampicillin + cloxacillin*
Escherichia coli 487	250	500	25 + 25	>5000	>1000	320 + 320
Shigella sonnei 3606	250	500	12.5 + 12.5	>5000	>1000	90 + 90
Proteus morganii 718	125	1000	12.5 + 12.5	>5000	>1000	80 + 80

*Mice infected by the intraperitoneal route were dosed immediately after infection with a single dose of the compound or combination.

The results in *Table 7.4* illustrate examples of synergy between β-lactam antibiotics and show the antibacterial activities *in vitro* and *in vivo* of a combination of equal parts of ampicillin and cloxacillin against three cultures of β-lactamase-producing bacteria. Both penicillins were relatively inactive against the organisms (MIC 125–1000 μg ml^{-1}) but the combination of penicillins was notably more active (MIC 25–50 μg ml^{-1}). The synergistic antibacterial activity of ampicillin + cloxacillin was also exhibited against experimental infections caused by these β-lactamase-producing bacteria. Ampicillin and cloxacillin were ineffective in preventing death of infected mice whereas the combination of the two penicillins demonstrated marked protective effects.

Inhibition of β-lactamase activity is illustrated in *Figure 7.6* which shows the bactericidal activities of ampicillin and ampicillin + cloxacillin against a β-lactamase-producing strain of *E. coli.* Ampicillin (10 μg ml^{-1}) produced a slight inhibition of growth for the first 3 h of the test but by 6 h the concentration of ampicillin had fallen to 2 μg ml^{-1} and the viable count was similar to that of the control culture. At a higher concentration (100 μg ml^{-1}), ampicillin was active during the early part of the experiment but at 24 h the concentration had fallen to 4 μg ml^{-1} and the viable count had increased to greater than 10^6 cells ml^{-1}. In the presence of cloxacillin, however, which was itself relatively ineffective, the bactericidal effects of ampicillin were greatly increased and a combination of 10 μg ampicillin ml^{-1} + 10 μg cloxacillin ml^{-1} was significantly more active than 100 μg ampicillin ml^{-1} during the first 6 h of the test. A higher concentration of cloxacillin (100 μg ml^{-1}) almost completely prevented destruction of ampicillin (10 μg ml^{-1}) and caused a total bactericidal effect at 24 h. The combination containing 100 μg ml^{-1} of each penicillin sterilized the culture and there was no obvious destruction of ampicillin at the end of 24 h.

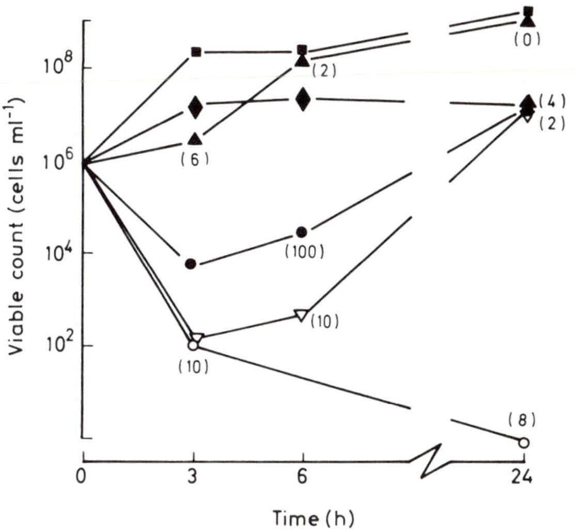

Figure 7.6 Bactericidal activities of ampicillin and ampicillin/cloxacillin combinations against E. coli *425.* ■ = *Control;* ♦ = *cloxacillin, 100 μg ml^{-1};* ▲ = *ampicillin, 10 μg ml^{-1};* ● = *ampicillin, 100 μg ml^{-1};* ▽ = *ampicillin, 10 μg ml^{-1} + cloxacillin, 10 μg ml^{-1};* ○ = *ampicillin, 10 μg ml^{-1} + cloxacillin, 100 μg ml^{-1}*

Although there has been considerable interest in applying the principle of β-lactamase inhibition as a means of treating resistant bacteria, clinical application of combinations of pencillins for this purpose has been limited (Sabath *et al.*, 1967; Riff, Olexy and Jackson, 1970; Klastersky, Debusscher and Ruhl, 1972). This is largely because no one compound has been found to be an effective and potent inhibitor of the more important of the wide range of β-lactamases produced by Gram-negative bacilli. Nevertheless, penicillins which are much more effective inhibitors of β-lactamases than the compounds clinically available have been described (Cole, Elson and Fullbrook, 1972) and one compound studied in detail, BRL 1437, an analogue of nafcillin, demonstrated impressive synergy in combination with other β-lactam antibiotics (Greenwood and O'Grady, 1975). Moreover, reports appearing in the literature describing potent mould-metabolite β-lactamase inhibitors (Ohno *et al.*, 1973; Umezawa *et al.*, 1973; Brown *et al.*, 1976) suggest the possibility of clinically useful substances being introduced to potentiate the efficacy of existing penicillins and cephalosporins against infections due to β-lactamase-producing bacteria.

Conclusion

Although the casual use of combinations of antibiotics is to be deprecated, there are numerous clinical settings which justify combined therapy with penicillins. The bactericidal synergy demonstrated *in vitro* between penicillins and aminoglycosides against enterococci is considered to have clinical significance and is generally accepted to provide an example of clinical synergism. The use of combinations of carbenicillin and aminoglycosides for the treatment of infections due to Gram-negative bacilli, particularly *Ps. aeruginosa,* is also widely accepted, largely on the grounds of the synergy that can be demonstrated *in vitro*, although clinical evidence is less readily available. The application of β-lactamase inhibitors to clinical therapy is limited as yet but there is evidence that proper use of this principle to produce synergy with β-lactam antibiotics has significant clinical potential.

Acknowledgments

I wish to thank my colleagues, D.F. Lawson and D.A. Wilson, for providing the photomicrographs illustrated in *Figure 7.5.*

References

ANDRIOLE, V.T. (1971). *J. infect. Dis.*, **124**. Suppl., S46

BROWN, A.G., BUTTERWORTH, D., COLE, M., HANSCOMB, G., HOOD, J.D., READING, C. and ROLINSON, G.N. (1976). *J. Antibiot.*, **25**, 668

BRUMFITT, W., PERCIVAL, A. and LEIGH, D.A. (1967). *Lancet,* **1**, 1289

COLE, M., ELSON, S. and FULLBROOK, P.D. (1972). *Biochem. J.*, **127**, 295

GREENWOOD, D. and O'GRADY, F. (1973). *J. infect. Dis.*, **128**, 791

GREENWOOD, D. and O'GRADY, F. (1975). *Chemotherapy,* **21**, 330

HAMILTON-MILLER, J.M.T. and SMITH, J.T. (1964). *Nature, Lond.*, **201**, 999

HEWITT, W.L., SELIGMAN, S.J. and DEIGH, R.A. (1966). *J. lab. clin. Med.*, **67**, 792

IANNINI, P.B., EHRET, J. and EICKHOFF, T.C. (1976). *Antimicrob. Agents Chemother.*, **9**, 448

JAWETZ, E. (1968). *Ann Rev. Pharmacol.*, **8**, 151

JAWETZ, E., GUNNISON, J.B. and COLEMAN, V.R. (1950). *Science, N.Y.*, **111**, 254

KELLY, M.T. and MATSEN, J.M. (1976). *Antimicrob. Agents Chemother.*, **9**, 440

KLASTERSKY, J., CAPPEL, R. and DEBUSSCHER, L. (1971). *Curr. ther. Res.*, **13**, 17

KLASTERSKY, J., DEBUSSCHER, L. and RUHL, D. (1972). *Chemother.*, **17**, 382

KLASTERSKY, J., HENSGENS, C. and DEBUSSCHER, L. (1975). *Antimicrob. Agents Chemother.*, **7**, 640

KLASTERSKY, J., NYAMUBEYA, B. and VANDENBORRE, L. (1974). *J. med. Microbiol.*, **7**, 465

LUND, F. and TYBRING, L. (1972). *Nature, New Biol.,* **236**, 135

McLAUGHLIN, J.E. and REEVES, D.S. (1971). *Lancet,* **1**, 261

MATSUHASHI, S., KAMIRYO, T., BLUMBERG, P.M., LINNETT, P., WILLOUGHBY, E. and STROMINGER, J.L. (1974). *J. Bact.,* **117**, 578

MELCHIOR, N.H., BLOOM, J., TYBRING, L. and BIRCH-ANDERSON, A. (1973). *Acta. Pathol. Microb. Scand.,* Sect. B., **81**, 393

MOELLERING, R.C. JR., and WEINBERG, A.N. (1971). *J. clin. Invest.,* **50**, 2580

MOELLERING, R.C. JR., WENNERSTEN, C. and WEINBERG, A.N. (1971). *J. infect. Dis.,* **124**, Suppl., S207

MOELLERING, R.C. JR., WENNERSTEN, C. and WEINSTEIN, A.J. (1973). *Antimicrob. Agents Chemother.,* **3**, 526

NEU, H.C. (1976). *Antimicrob. Agents Chemother.,* **9**, 793

OHNO, H., MATSUMAE, A., IWAI, Y., NAKAE, M., OMURA, S. and HATA, T. (1973). *Antimicrob. Agents Chemother.,* **4**, 226

PARK, J.T. and BURMAN, L. (1973). *Biochem. Biophys. Res. Commun.,* **51**, 863

RICHMOND, M.H. and CURTIS, N.A.C. (1974). *Ann. N.Y. Acad. Sci.,* **235**, 553

RIFF, L.J. and JACKSON, G.G. (1972). *Arch. intern. Med.,* **130**, 887

RIFF, L.J., OLEXY, V. and JACKSON, G.G. (1970). *Antimicrob. Agents Chemother.,* **1969**, 405

ROLINSON, G.N. and SUTHERLAND, R. (1968). *Antimicrob. Agents Chemother.,* **1967**, 609

RUSSELL, E.J. and SUTHERLAND, R. (1975). *J. med. Microbiol.,* **8**, 1

SABATH, L.D., McCALL, C.E., STEIGBIGEL, N.H. and FINLAND, M. (1967). *Antimicrob. Agents. Chemother.,* **1966**, 149

SCHIMPFF, S., SATTERLEA, W., YOUNG, V.M. and SERPICK, A. (1971). *N. Engl. J. Med.,* **284**, 1061

SMITH, J.T., HAMILTON-MILLER, J.M.T. and KNOX, R. (1969). *J. Pharm. Pharmacol.,* **21**, 337

SONNE, M. and JAWETZ, E. (1968). *Appl. Microbiol.,* **16**, 645

SPRATT, B.G. (1975). *Proc. Nat. Acad. Sci. U.S.A.,* **72**, 2999

STANDIFORD, H.D., DE MAINE, J.B. and KIRBY, W.M.M. (1970). *Archs. intern. Med.,* **126**, 255

SUTHERLAND, R. and BATCHELOR, F.R. (1964). *Nature, Lond.,* **201**, 868

TYBRING, L. and MELCHIOR, N.H. (1975). *Antimicrob. Agents Chemother.,* **8**, 271

UMEZAWA, H., MITSUHASHI, S., HAMADA, M., LYOBE, S., TAKAHASHI, S., UTAHARA, R., OSATO, Y., YAMAZAKI, S., OGAWARA, H. and MAEDA, K. (1973). *J. Antibiot.,* **26**, 51

WALD, E.R., STANDIFORD, H.C., TATEM, B.A., CALIA, F.M. and HORNICK, R.B. (1975). *Antimicrob. Agents Chemother.,* **7**, 336

WATANAKUNAKORN, C. (1971). *J. infect. Dis.,* **124**, 581

YUCE, K. and VAN ROOYEN, C.E. (1971). *Canad. med. Ass.,* **105**, 919

ZIMMERMAN, R.A., MOELLERING, R.C. JR. and WEINBERG, A.N. (1971). *J. Bact.,* **105**, 873

III

ANTIBIOTICS, ANTIBIOSIS AND FOOD

8

NISIN AND ITS APPLICATIONS

EWA LIPIŃSKA
Institute of Dairy Industry, Warsaw, Poland

Introduction

The aim of this paper is to present the progress in the problem of nisin and its applications since the 1962 Easter School on 'Antibiotics in Agriculture'.

Nisin is an antibiotic produced by certain *Str. lactis* strains, usually occurring in milk. This is a collective name representing several closely related substances: i.e. A, B, C, D and E nisins, which – though exhibiting a similar amino acid composition – differ in the antibiotic activity. All amino acids, except for the unusual lanthionine and β-methyllanthionine, show the normal L-configuration.

Nisin is used as an aid in heat preservation of foods. Other possibilities of its application include, for example, rennet cheese production and animal feeding; they will be discussed later. When added to food, nisin allows moderation of heat treatment from the normally applied F_0 range of 4–40 to F_0 = 3, this representing the minimum thermal process required for destruction of *Cl. botulinum* spores without any risk of food poisoning. Nisin prevents the outgrowth of most thermophilic bacteria from spores remaining in food after the minimum thermal process. Nisin can also be applied for prolongation of the shelf-life of semi-preserves. Its use improves the nutritional value, organoleptic properties and keeping quality as well as increasing the plant capacity.

To begin with, I should like to stress that being a microbiologist in cheese-making, I am aware of the food canning problems only from the standpoint of nisin.

Properties of Nisin

STRUCTURE AND PHYSICO-CHEMICAL PROPERTIES

During the last decade the structure of nisin and its biosynthesis by bacteria have been studied by modern methods of molecular biology. Recent investigations resulted in a deeper insight into the composition and structure of nisin (Gross and Morell, 1967, 1969, 1970, 1971). They revealed the presence of two α, β-unsaturated amino acids, dehydroalanine and β-methyldehydroalanine, and showed that dehydroalanyllysine is the –COOH terminal sequence of nisin while isoleucine is the N–final amino acid. A novel bicyclic structure of identical ring size, formed by sulphide bridges of lanthionine and β-methyllanthionine, was assigned to nisin. Thirteen-membered ring structures with one sulphur atom are new in peptide chemistry. The two remaining rings of nisin are larger in size, being composed of 16 to 22 members. They suggested that nisin acted by competition with metabolically important compounds, such as sulphhydryl-containing enzymes, glutathione or coenzyme A (*Figure 8.1*);

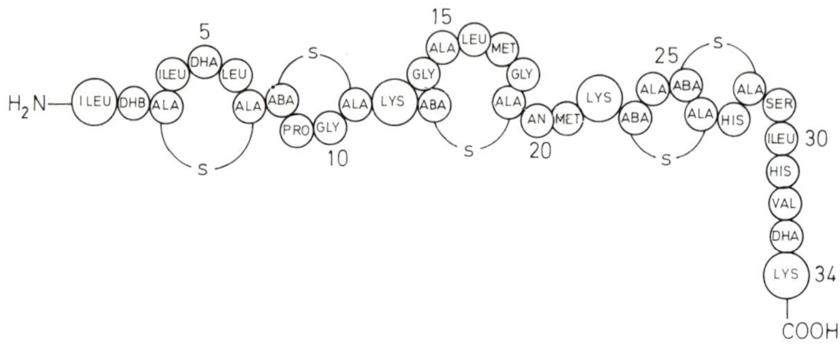

Figure 8.1 The structure of nisin: ABA = aminobutyric acid; DHA = dehydroalanine; DHB = dehydrobutyrine (β-methyldehydroalanine) (Gross and Morell, 1971)

Steps of the biosynthesis of the two unusual amino acids were also elucidated; serine and cysteine were shown to be precursors of lanthionine, and threonine and cysteine precursors of β-methyllanthionine (Ingram, 1969).

Determinations of the molecular weight of nisin gave different results, depending on the methods used. However, the resulting values were always multiples of about 3500. Nisin with molecular weight of 3510 was obtained by dinitrophenylation and counter-current separation (Gross and Morell, 1967). By separation on polyacrylamide gel, values of 14000 and 7000 were obtained (Ingram, Tombs and Hurst, 1967); this in some measure confirmed the earlier values based on the determination of the diffusion coefficient and amino acid composition. By ultracentrifugation and molecular filtration, the molecular weight of primary nisin was shown to be 7000. Under definite conditions nisin either may split into two subunits of a molecular weight 3500 each, or may form a dimer of molecular weight of 14000. All three forms exhibit biological activity (Jarvis, Jeffsoat and Cheeseman, 1968).

Some properties of nisin closely depend on pH. Its solubility ranges from 12% at pH 2.5 to 4% at pH 5.0 (Hall, 1966). As regards its resistance to heating, sterilization at pH 2 does not affect the activity, at pH 5.0 and 6.8 the percentage of inactivation is about 40% and 90%, respectively. However, in the presence of proteins the destruction of nisin by drastic heating is less dramatic (Tramer, 1966). These properties are essential for the nisin activity in food products undergoing thermal treatment at different pH values. Since nisin is only a weak bactericide, being rather a bacterio- and sporostatic substance, treated food must contain an adequate amount of nisin to allow for any losses of this antibiotic, which may occur during heat processing and subsequent storage.

Table 8.1 Nisin residues in foods after different thermal treatments, at various pH values (Fowler, 1968)

(a) Nisin residues from 100 units g^{-1} added before processing

Product	*pH*	*Heating process*	*Nisin residues* (units g^{-1})
Green peas	6.4	30 min/116°C	22.0
Mushrooms	6.0	18 min/121.1°C	32.7
Tomatoes	4.5	40 min/100°C	72.4
Processed cheese	5.8	12 min/to 90°C	82.0

(b) Nisin residues in skimmed milk (pH 6.5) *heated at various temperatures*

	Nisin residues (%) after heating		
Temperature (°C)	3 *min*	11 *min*	40 *min*
110	84	57	19
116	67	38	7
121.1	60	34	4

(c) Nisin residues in canned green peas (pH 6.4) *stored at* 8–21°C

Storage period (months)	*Nisin residues (%)*	*Storage period (months)*	*Nisin residues (%)*
3	93	18	43
6	90	21	44
9	84	24	48
12	81	27	44
15	62	30	42

Table 8.1 shows some interrelations between the factors decisive of the activity of nisin (Fowler, 1968).

MODE OF ACTION

Effect on spores

The outgrowth of bacteria from spores proceeds in three stages: (*a*) germination swelling, (*b*) pre-emergency swelling, and (*c*) emergency and elongation; nisin is regarded as a factor preventing pre-emergency swelling (Gould, 1964; Attwell, Cross and Gould, 1972). *Figure 8.2* illustrates the stages of growth arrest by nisin and some other preservatives. The manner of spore-coat opening seems to be correlated with the resistance to nisin. Species (e.g. *B. subtilis*) which open their spore-coats by mechanical pressure (type M) are sensitive to 2–10 i.u. nisin ml^{-1}, while large-spore species (e.g. *B. cereus*) opening their spore-coats by lysis (type L) are much more resistant (even to as much as 100 i.u. nisin ml^{-1}).

Though nisin is often referred to as an agent reducing the heat resistance of bacterial spores, experimental data show that spores damaged by heat are characterized by increased nisin sensitivity (*Figure 8.3*) (Heinemann, Voris and Stumbo, 1965). All agents either injuring bacterial cells and spores (or adversely affecting the vital processes of the vegetative cells) can be considered potential synergists of nisin. This concerns, for example, γ-rays (Porretta, Campanini and

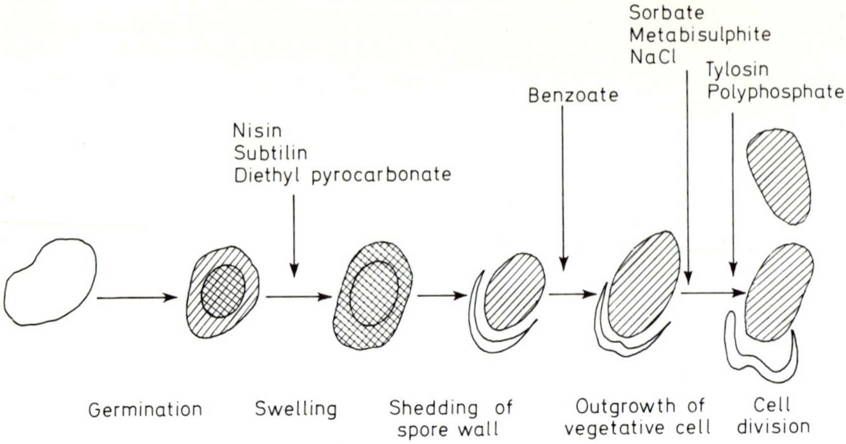

Figure 8.2 Growth of a spore into vegetative cells and stages of growth arrested by nisin and other preservatives (Gould, 1964)

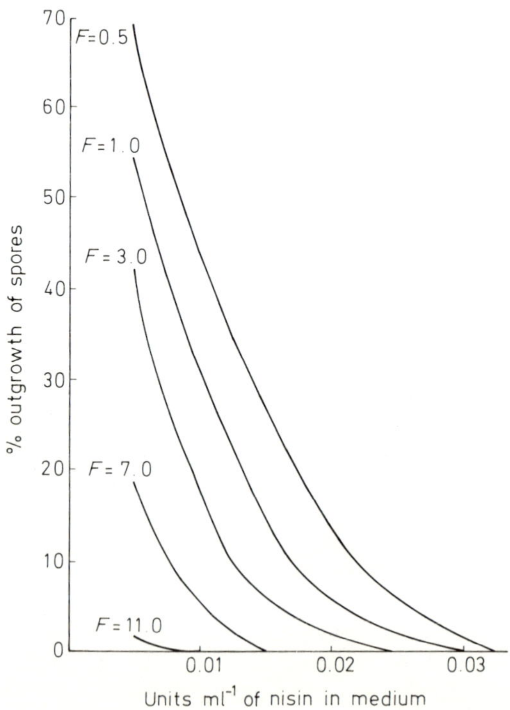

Figure 8.3 Variation of the nisin sensitivity of spores with degree of heat damage (Heinemann, Voris and Stumbo, 1965; quoted by Hall, 1966)

Casolari, 1970), sodium chloride (Pulay and Krasz, 1968), polyphosphates used as melting salts in processed cheese (Ruf, 1969) and, probably, curing salts.

In contrast, nisin is apparently inactivated by compounds enhancing spore germination, such as Mg^{++} and Ca^{++} ions (Gupta, Sidhu and Yadav, 1971), monosaccharides (glucose is most active), and polysaccharides (Gupta, Sidhu and Yadav, 1972), α-alanine, phenylalanine and pyruvate (Mikolajcik, Reeves and Harper, 1965; Gupta, 1974). Probably the same holds true for citrates which may act as agents enhancing spore germination in nisin-treated processed cheese. Milk fat is another non-typical inhibitor of the nisin activity (Jones, 1974).

Spores of different types of bacteria and even of strains of one species differ in their sensitivity to nisin. The effect of nisin depends also on the spore load in the medium.

In this connection it is necessary to stress the importance of the carry-over of nisin in investigations on the sensitivity of spores to this antibiotic. Nisin fails to be firmly bound to the spore (Tramer, 1966); however, there are contrary views on this subject (Ramseier, 1960).

Effect on vegetative cells

Fundamental studies on the effect of nisin on vegetative cells are scarce. In growing bacterial cultures of *Cl. butyricum,* with nisin added, bacteriolysis takes place; this process is most intense during the logarithmic phase of growth (Ramseier, 1960). Lysed bacterial cells release substances absorbing at 260 nm (*Figure 8.4*). Cell lysis is caused by irreversible destruction of the cytoplasmic membrane which regulates the osmotic pressure in the cell. The high rate of the bactericidal action of nisin on vegetative cells can be explained by changes in the

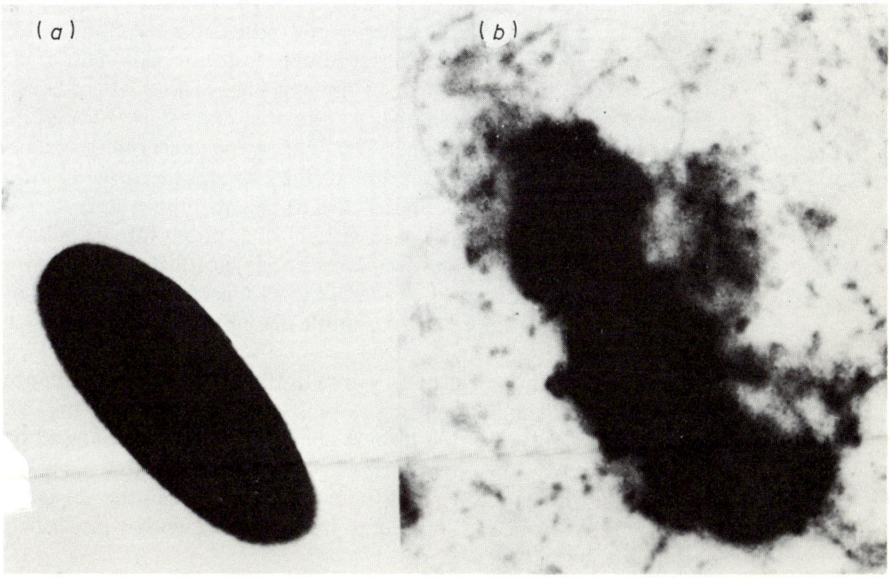

Figure 8.4 Action of nisin on vegetative 6 h-old Cl. butyricum *cells; (a) culture medium without nisin, (b) culture medium with nisin added, magn.* × *8100 (Ramseier, 1960)*

surface tension on the cytoplasmic membrane, which cause disturbances in cell permeability leading to bacteriolysis. However, as shown in studies of inhibitors of the peptidoglycan synthesis, nisin can also inhibit the synthesis of the rigid structures of the *B. stearothermophilus* cell wall (Linnett and Strominger, 1973).

ANTIBIOSIS AND SYNERGISM

Many approaches to this problem are possible; the oldest one concerns nisin as a secondary metabolite of some *Str. lactis* strains, usually weak lactic acid-producers, presumably formed by bacteria as an aid for their survival.

Nisin was discovered as a consequence of the accidents sometimes provoked by nisin-producing streptococci in ripening cheese manufacture. This happens even now when these strains, multiplying too intensely in milk, inhibit the growth of cheese starters, owing to the antibiotic produced.

To these natural antibiosis phenomena, some new man-made ones are added. Nisin-producing streptococci used as a starter in milk during ripening rennet cheese production, constitute a new factor in the multiplicity of antibiosis and synergistic phenomena occurring naturally. Some of them are favourable and others are antagonistic to nisin; only a few of them, presenting a practical interest, are an object of investigations. This concerns (*a*) the control of spore-forming bacteria in cheese by nisin, (*b*) the influence of nisin on the cheese starter, and (*c*) the nisin destruction ability of some bacteria surviving pasteurization or derived from milk recontamination or else from the starter.

Nisin is a weak, but very specific, bacterial antagonist; moreover, it is inactivated by nisinase. It is astonishing to observe its potent effect in a nearly natural environment, especially when cheese is produced under poor hygienic conditions. The effect observed is enhanced by synergistic phenomena and naturally occurring factors. In other words, nisin shifts the equilibrium of the biological system in a direction unfavourable to the development of clostridia. Thus, it prevents butyric blowing of ripening hard and semi-hard cheeses.

When nisin is used as an adjunct in a thermal process, it gives rise in the food product to antagonistic and synergetic phenomena concerning a much lower number of bacterial species, or rather of their spores, surviving the heat process. However, these phenomena concern also some environmental factors (pH, temperature, etc.) and perhaps also certain other properties of foods, with texture playing an important role. For example, heating may simultaneously act as antagonist (inactivation of nisin) and as synergist (impairment of spores), the final effect being the result of a subtle equilibrium between these two activities.

The mode of action of nisin as a growth-stimulating factor remains unclear. It does not influence the intestinal flora. It may be thought, as suggested by Gross and Morell (1967), that nisin in competition with a biological substance (e.g. coenzyme A) causes the observed growth stimulation.

The antibiositic and synergistic phenomena involving nisin are taken up through this paper. In addition, some studies dealing with nisin-destroying enzymes will be surveyed.

Nisinase, as inducible specific enzyme occurring in different spores and bacteria (including lactic acid bacteria, micrococci and others) is the most important nisin antagonist. Nisinase of *B. cereus* has been extensively studied (Jarvis and Farr, 1971). There is an extremely high correlation between the nisin-resistance of spores and the intensity of nisinase production; M-type spores being more nisin-sensitive are weak nisinase producers, while the L-type spores, which are more nisin-resistant, produce nisinase more actively. Nisinase acts by way of reducing the double bond of dehydroalanyllysine located in the terminal –COOH sequence of nisin. This shows that nisinase is a dehydropeptide reductase.

Nisinase produced by *B. cereus* (and *B. polymyxa*) is active also against subtilin which is known to contain a similar amino acid residue, but does not influence polymyxin, gramicidin, bacitracin, penicillin, erythromycin, neomycin, streptomycin and tylosin (Jarvis, 1967).

The previous views on nisin inactivation by pancreatin and trypsin have to be changed in the light of the most recent investigations on the effect of proteolytic, digestive and other enzymes on this antibiotic (Jarvis and Mahoney, 1969; Tiemann and Belitz, 1969). It was found that only α-chymotrypsin inactivates nisin. Carboxypeptidase A, trypsin, elastase, pepsin and erepsin and similarly proteases of *Aspergillus oryzae* and *Aspergillus parasiticus*, fail to destroy nisin. It is assumed that the activity exhibited by pancreatin and trypsin is due to traces of α-chymotrypsin. Thus far it has been claimed that nisin is inactivated by ptyalin of the saliva (Hawley, 1958). The absence of nisin in the human oral cavity 10 minutes after ingestion of milk containing 200 i.u. nisin ml^{-1} may also support this opinion (Claypool *et al.*, 1966; Covell, Allen and Jarvis, 1971).

BIOSYNTHESIS

According to the literature, the problem of nisin biosynthesis can be approached from the standpoint of mechanisms operating either in a single cell or in a bacterial population.

The biosynthesis of polypeptide antibiotics has not so far been fully elucidated. They may be synthesized enzymatically, via a non-ribosomal mechanism, since the invariant genetic code does not permit ribosomal synthesis of antibiotics containing unusual amino acids (Bodansky and Perlman, 1964). However, data regarding the nisin biosynthesis inhibition by protein synthesis inhibitors, such as chloramphenicol, puromycin and chlortetracycline, support the validity of a ribosomal mechanism of nisin synthesis (Ingram, 1970). Moreover, investigations on the effect of proflavine, ethidium bromide, as well as of heating, on nisin-producing *Str. lactis* strains furnish evidence that the genes responsible for nisin production may be located in plasmids (Kozak *et al.*, 1975). These data point to a very complex mechanism of nisin biosynthesis, which could involve ribosomal reactions controlled by the invariant gentic code and reactions depending on plasmid-located genes.

Nisin produced by streptococci is partially released to the culture medium; the ratio of cell-bound and released nisin depends on the pH value, this fact being utilized in industrial nisin-producing fermentation (Hurst and Dring, 1968; White and Hurst, 1968; Hurst and Kruse, 1970). Its biosynthesis by bacteria is most intensive during the logarithmic phase of growth (Hurst, 1966; Oberman and Pabis, 1975). Lactic streptococci which are not nisin producers synthesize a 'nisinoid' basic peptide which is electrophoretically similar to nisin, except for the antibiotic activity (Hurst, 1967). Cell extracts from nisin-producing strains incubated with the 'nisinoid' peptide preparations generate an antibiotic believed to be nisin (Hurst and Patterson, 1971). These results point to the possibility of a half-synthetic way of nisin synthesis.

There is widespread interest, also in geographic terms, in the nisin biosynthesis by lactic streptococci *in situ,* during cheesemaking, as well as in the production of nisin preparations. The search for efficient natural nisin producers is in progress (Pyanitsina, 1968; Kalra and Dudani, 1973). In order to obtain mutants with increased nisin production yield, u.v., γ- and x-rays were applied (Oberman, 1968; Hylmar, Teply and Tesarkova, 1970a; Jakubczyk, Lipińska and Szadkowska, 1973; Kalra, Kuila and Ranganathan, 1973). Mutants with a 10-fold increase in nisin output were selected, this new feature being sufficiently persistent for industrial purposes. Nisin biosynthesis under industrial conditions is closely related to the very high sensitivity of nisin-producing streptococci to bacteriophages. The bacteriophage-caused disturbances occur more often during cheese making in open vats (Lipińska, Domanska and Soltys, 1971a). Some nisin-producing *Str. lactis* strains are lysogenic and release phages after u.v.-irradiation (Kozak, Rajchert-Trzpil and Dobrzanski, 1973). Attempts at the development of phage-resistance in nisin-producing streptococci were made (Lipińska *et al.,* 1976b).

For optimal nutrient broths for the biosynthesis of nisin, almost all known substances involved in the streptococcal metabolism (sugars, fatty acids, amino acids, peptone, yeast extracts, vitamins and mineral components) were investigated. Other investigations were aimed at the detection of growth factors stimulating nisin biosynthesis in cheap whey culture media. The suitability of pancreatin-hydrolysed wastes from insulin production and pepsin-hydrolysed milk cultures of lactic acid bacteria was investigated (Shkundova, 1967; Baranova and Egorov, 1967; 1969; 1970; Matosic, Tamburasev and Jukič, 1971; Egorov, Baranova and Silvestrova, 1972; Matelova and Brečka, 1972; El-Gendy and El-Badavi, 1972; Egorov *et al.,* 1973; Baranova, Egorov and Silverstrova, 1973; Baranova *et al.,* 1974; Szadkowska *et al.,* 1974).

Some papers deal with the production and characterization of nisin preparations. A cell-extracted nisin preparation was found to be very active (Bailey and Hurst, 1971). Laboratory microdevices for nisin concentration by the flotation method, as well as large-scale production of nisin-enriched (up to 20 000 i.u. g^{-1}) milk powder were described (Lipińska *et al*., 1973b; Peterkova and Hylmar, 1974). Tests for evaluation of the storage stability of British, Polish and Russian nisin preparations revealed that Nisaplin of British make was most stable (Tokmakova, 1972; Gudkov *et al*., 1973).

HEALTH AND LEGAL ASPECTS

The data published direct attention to several aspects such as toxicological data, hazards due to pathogenic and nisin-resistant bacteria, as well as the legal aspects of nisin-treated food.

Toxicological data

Extensive toxicological work on nisin was reported in Japan (Hara *et al.*, 1962) and USSR (Ignatyev, 1965; Dinerman and Ignatyev, 1966; Shillinger, Bogoroditskaya and Osipova, 1969; Shtenberg and Ignatyev, 1971). Observations on this subject were also made as a part of some studies on nisin application in food processing (Pesquera, 1966; Gross and Morell, 1967; Gontzea *et al.*, 1973). Commercial British and Russian nisin preparations were examined either alone or in comparison with other food preservatives. Toxicological tests comprised many generations of rats and mice administered normal levels and overdoses of nisin. They concerned a wide range of biological properties: carcinogenicity, survival, reproduction, blood chemistry, kidney function, brain capacity, effects of stress factors, pathology in the organs of animals, etc. Results of these experiments consistently confirm the non-toxicity of nisin and slight, if any, effect on some of the properties examined. Exceptions in this respect comprise the shorter survival of mice administered overdoses of nisin (Ignatyev, 1965) as well as erythrocyte lysis and lysosome release by nisin (Gross and Morell, 1971).

Hazards caused by pathogenic and nisin-resistant bacteria

Sterilization of nisin-containing low-acid foods (pH 4.5 or more) at $F_0 = 3$ (effective against *Cl. botulinum* spores) should rule out completely the hazard of botulinum poisoning. From the theoretical point of view, nisin-treated foods should not entail any risk of bacterial food poisoning, on account of the high hygienic standards recommended when nisin is used. There are only few data on this subject. In Cheddar cheese nisin did not affect the development of *Salmonella* spp. (Hargrove, McDonough and Mattingby, 1969). In a total of 11 *Staph. aureus* strains tested, nisin inhibited only 2 strains (Sahani, 1962). In sweetened condensed milk *Staph. aureus* was not inhibited by 500 i.u. nisin g^{-1}, probably owing to insufficient mixing (Jarchowska *et al.*, 1974), whereas in bakery dough nisin was effective at levels of 200–750 i.u. g^{-1} (Ticha, 1970). In processed cheese *Cl. perfringens* strains were inhibited by 200 i.u. nisin g^{-1} (Tsugo, 1962). These observations emphasize the need for more work on pathogenic bacteria in nisin-treated foods. This applies particularly to new developments in food distribution and storage, e.g. to hot-vending trade.

Nisin-resistant mesophilic micrococci and lactobacilli were isolated from nisin-treated bacon (Gibbs and Hurst, 1964) but strains of these species, as nisinase producers, are often found to be naturally resistant to nisin. Furthermore, it was reported that a selected nisin-resistant, food-spoiling *B. coagulans* strain lost nisin-resistance after a few transfers in nisin-free medium (Ovcharova and Maslennikova, 1969).

Nisin-resistant lactic acid bacteria selected for industrial purposes exhibited no cross-resistance with medical antibiotics, such as penicillin, streptomycin, erythromycin, chloramphenicol, tetramycin and aureomycin. As compared with the parent strains, they were much more sensitive to medical antibiotics (Lipińska and Strzalkowska, 1964), and more sensitive to adverse factors, such as drastic heating, as well as high salt and bile concentrations (Lipińska, 1975).

Nutritional value of nisin-treated foods

The information on the nutritional value of nisin-treated foods is very scarce. Studies on nisin-treated unsweetened evaporated milk and Edam cheese, as compared with control products, indicated, among others, higher contents of vitamins A, B_1, B_2 and C, whey proteins and free amino acids (Gregory, Henry and Kon, 1964; Karlikanowa, Gudkov and Trofimova, 1970a; Gontzea *et al.,* 1973; Radacva, Anatskaya and Efimova, 1975).

Acceptance of nisin as food additive

The use of nisin as food additive is now permitted in more than 20 countries. There are differences in the admissible levels as well as in the products to which it can be added; nevertheless, wide international acceptance is noted. This is expressed by the conclusion of the Joint F.A.O./W.H.O. Experts' Committee on Food Additives (1969a): 'Use of nisin should be considered as acceptable, the unconditional average daily intake (ADI) being 0–33 000 units per kg of body weight'.

ANALYTICAL METHODS

During the last decade, three important events concerning the analytical problems of nisin took place: (*a*) the definition of a unit of nisin in terms of a standard preparation, (*b*) establishment of an International Reference Preparation of Nisin, under F.A.O./W.H.O. protection, (*c*) the inclusion of methods for estimation and differentiation of nisin in the 'Specification for Identity and Purity of some Antibiotics', edited by F.A.O./W.H.O. (*see* Specification, 1969). In this monograph, the Tramer and Fowler (1964) plate diffusion method, with *M. flavus* as test organism, is suggested for quantitative determination of nisin. For semi-quantitative estimation, the reverse-phase disc assay technique using *B. stearothermophilus* spores is recommended. Moreover, for the differentiation of nisin and other common antibiotics in food a nisin-producing *Str. lactis* culture is used. This method of differentiation was later supplemented by a reference method based on an incubation assay with nisinase extracted from *B. cereus* (British Standards Institution, 1974). Another method for nisin differentiation, seems to be simpler; it consists of acidity estimation in milk cultures of nisin-sensitive and nisin-resistant *Str. lactis* strains, with the tested product added – it is used for sorting purposes. The bio-autographic method using *S. lutea* as a test organism for differentiation of nisin, penicillin, streptomycin and erythromycin on the grounds of differences in shape, size and location of the inhibition zones is applied as reference method (Lipińska, Jakubczyk and Szadkowska, 1971b).

Two papers on this subject concern the Tramer and Fowler method (Hernandez, 1972; Jakubczyk, Lipińska and Kosikowska, 1973), as well as the Epstein and Friedman method (Gudkov *et al*., 1973); others the newly developed methods (Egorov and Shkundova, 1964; Stumbo *et al*., 1964; Kalra, Dudani and Laxminaryana, 1973).

Practical Applications

CANNED AND SEMI-PRESERVED FOOD

Figure 8.5 presents the general possibilities offered by nisin as an adjunct in thermally processed food (Vas, 1964). As will be seen, nisin is effective against

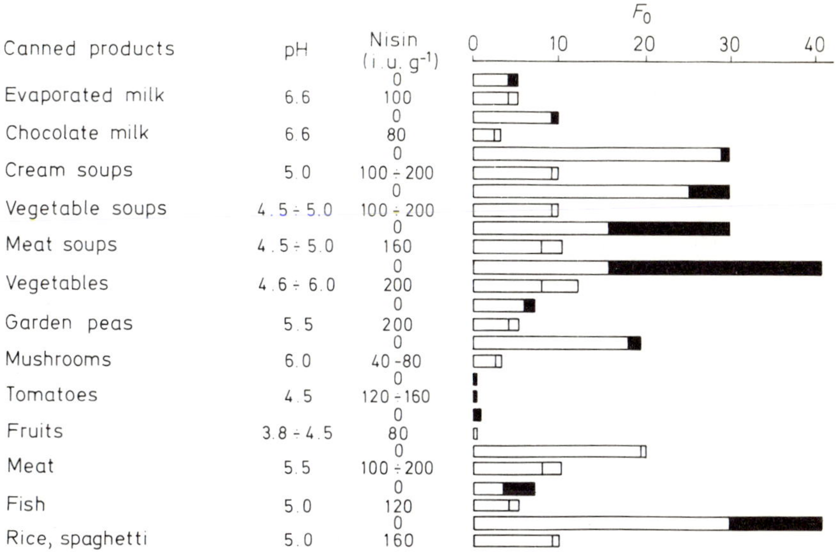

Figure 8.5 Possibilities of moderation of heat processing in the presence of nisin (Vas, 1964). ▬ = range of heat treatment without nisin; ▭ = range of heat treatment with nisin added

thermophilic flat-souring and other bacteria even if the process is drastically reduced. However, in individual cases spoilage due to mesophilic sporeformers was not controlled in underprocessed or semi-preserved food.

Sterilized and flavoured milks

Experimental work and industrial usage show that nisin at levels of 100–200 i.u. g^{-1} allows processing of evaporated milk at moderate temperatures, with improved nutritional value and prolonged shelf-life (Gregory, Henry and Kon, 1964; Efimowa, 1974; Radaeva, Anatskaya and Efimova, 1975). Trials performed in the U.S.S.R. comprised over a million milk containers manufactured in three dairies. In pilot-scale trials sterilized milk and chocolate-flavoured milk contaminated either naturally or with sporeformers (*B. subtilis* and *B. stearothermophilus*) and containing 10–100 i.u. nisin ml^{-1}, were processed at $F_0 = 3$, instead of usually applied $F_0 = 9$; both nisin-treated milks did not spoil with 6-month storage at 37°C, and 3-weeks storage at 55°C. The moderate heat treatment was favourable to the flavour and taste of the products (Heinemann, Stumbo and

Scurlock, 1964; Pesquera, 1966; Wajid and Kalia, 1974). Moreover, there are possibilities of nisin application in recombined and reconstituted evaporated milk (Fowler and McCann, 1971).

Processed cheese and spreads

The published data stress the well known utility of nisin in controlling clostridia. Studies of the role of some substances (glycine, leucine, calcium propionate and nisin) in the prevention of butyric blowing in processed cheese, revealed the undoubted superiority of nisin (Pulay and Krasz, 1966). The latter authors pointed to the synergistic effect of nisin and salt on sporeformers in processed cheese (Pulay and Krasz, 1968). Extensive investigations on the effect of nisin on the keeping quality of processed cheese prepared with the use of different contents of sodium chloride, melting salts (*see* earlier) and fat as well as at various pH values and melting temperature, constitute a virtual vade-mecum in processing of nisin-treated cheese. The authors recommend addition of nisin at levels of 150–200 i.u. g^{-1} to products intended either for storage and sale at more than 10°C, or for long-term storage; the same nisin levels are to be used when the cheese mix contains more than 100 spores g^{-1}, as well as when its fat content is high and salt content low (Gudkov *et al.*, 1969). Further findings obtained in Japan (Tsugo, 1962), U.S.S.R. (Rudavskaya, Orlova and Kutoval, 1971), India (Kalra, Laxminarayana and Dudani, 1973), and Czechoslovakia (Hylmar, 1975) confirm the utility of nisin in cheese processing under different conditions. In only one case no significant effect of 100–400 i.u. nisin g^{-1} on the keeping quality of cheese processed on a laboratory scale was observed (Wegner, 1969). The use of nisin also proved beneficial in prolongation of the shelf-life of low-fat spreads (Goel, Calbert and Marth, 1969).

Tomatoes, green peas, other vegetables and fruits

An interesting nisin application consists in the protection of the texture and appearance of products, with regard to canned peppers (Duran, Hernandez and Flores, 1964), a Hungarian speciality 'Lecso' comprising peppers in concentrated tomato juice (Vas, 1963), as well as peeled tomatoes in tomato juice or in salt brine. Nisin at levels of 100–200 i.u. g^{-1} allows reduced heat treatment without impairing the keeping quality (Mateyev and Strandjev, 1963; Hall, 1966; Shkundova and Kulieva, 1967). A new development, the additive effect of γ-rays and nisin, was observed in tomato juice artificially infected with *Cl. pasteurianum* (Porretta, Campanini and Cassara, 1968; Casolari and Cassara, 1970; Porretta, Campanini and Casolari, 1970). Nisin together with sorbic acid prolonged shelf-life of heated tomato pulp, during long-term transport in a hot climate (Ovcharova and Maslennikova, 1969).

The previous reports on the utility of nisin at levels of 100–200 i.u. g^{-1} in permitting mild heat treatment of garden peas, were confirmed in commercial pack trials (10000 cans). An improvement in the appearance, taste and a good keeping quality was observed (Shkundova and Kulieva, 1966), as in pilot-scale trials using raw material naturally and artificially spoiled by *B. stearo-*

thermophilus (Nekhotenova and Kulieva, 1966; Vas, Kiss and Kiss, 1967; Casolari, Campanini and Pezzani, 1967; Kiss *et al.*, 1970; Seeger, 1970).

Pears and pineapples, particularly sensitive to contamination with *Cl. pasteurianum* and *Cl. butyricum*, were protected against spoilage by using 80–100 i.u. nisin g^{-1}. The same amount of antibiotic permitted the moderation of the sterilization conditions for cherries, apples and peaches, with benefit to the fruit texture and other organoleptic properties (Heinemann, Voris and Stumbo, 1965).

Only one report of the Findus company stated that the milder heat treatment allowed by nisin was not advantageous to the organoleptic quality of green peas on account of off-flavours, although the flat-sour fermentation was controlled, Furthermore, nisin at the price prevailing at that time seemed unprofitable (Findus, 1964). There are some single reports on the efficacy of nisin applied in milder heated carrots with green peas, carrot purée as baby food, beets, salsify, semi-raw potatoes, asparagus and spinach (Vas, 1964; Maslenikova and Lokshina, 1968; Seeger, 1970).

Puddings, hot-vended meals, soups and sauces

The increasing scope of food technology processes as well as the hot-vending sales systems gives rise to many previously unknown problems, in the solving of which efforts have been undertaken to use nisin. In the industrial production of canned puddings with rice, sago, semolina, tapioca and macaroni, an addition of nisin (50–100 i.u. g^{-1}) permits less drastic heating, improving the organoleptic properties and shelf-life (Fowler and McCann, 1971). With food packed in foil, destined for sale in hot-vending machines, pilot scale production of chicken chow mein, macaroni, and cream-style corn infected with flat-sour sporeformers and nisin added (100–200 i.u. g^{-1}) was effective. These trials proved the possibility of nisin application in this field (Wheaton and Hays, 1964; Heinemann, Voris and Stumbo, 1965).

It is the same in the prolongation of shelf-life of mildly sterilized vegetable and meat or fish or mushroom soups by using nisin. Concentrated soups such as vegetable and groat, borsh, sauerkraut, are nisin-treated (150–200 i.u g^{-1}) on an industrial scale (Shornikova *et al.*, 1972). But one case with rapid inactivation of nisin during storage, at 55°C, of lentil soup prepared from heavily contaminated raw material was reported (Gibbs and Hurst, 1964).

Finally, various low-acid sauces infected with *B. coagulans* and *B. stearothermophilus*, mildly heated in the presence of 100 i.u. nisin g^{-1}, exhibited a shelf-life equal to that of a severely heated product with better appearance and flavour in pilot-scale trials (Nekhotenova and Kulieva, 1966).

Meat, fish and meat pies, sausages and sandwich pastes

High-protein products of this type are subjected to thermal treatment ensuring commercial sterility, for example in the case of sandwich pastes or ox-tongues. Pasteurization is applied when the texture and appearance of products such as ham and caviar may be changed as a result of stronger heating.

Experiments on the prolongation of shelf-life of pre-packed pasteurized bacon at nisin levels of 200–500 i.u. g^{-1} proved unsuccessful on account of the development of mesophilic micrococci and lactobacilli, which are, moreover, reported to have acquired nisin-resistance (Gibbs and Hurst, 1964). Attempts at the stabilization of nisin in brine by ultrasonics are an example of the difficulties encountered in the search for better ways of its application in ham (Koniečny, Minks and Cervenka, 1970). The keeping quality of hamburgers with nisin addition (200 i.u. g^{-1}) to sausage-meat was prolonged owing to the protection against greening caused by lactobacilli (Stankiewicz-Berger, 1969). Nisin allows moderation, by about 45%, of the heating process of ox-tongues and sandwich pastes made of poultry or other meats, fish and crabs; and, at levels of 80 i.u. g^{-1}, is extremely valuable in canned mushrooms (Vas, 1964; Tramer, 1966).

A specific case is presented by caviar which requires very mild heat processing conditions. When 0.5% of nisin and 5% of salt were added, pasteurization at 60°C for 120 min ensured 12 months shelf-life upon storage at −2°C to 4°C, while packs without nisin became spoiled (Ushakova, 1972). Nisin was also applied to protect bakers' yeast fermentation against lactobacilli infection (Kozlova and Kobrina, 1971).

RENNET CHEESE PRODUCTION

In 1951, a group of British and French scientists succeeded in controlling butyric blowing of Emmental cheese. Nisin-producing lactic streptococci were used as a starter. At that time butyric blowing in hard and semi-hard rennet cheeses became widespread in all countries in which these cheese varieties were manufactured. It was due to the increasing use of silage fodder, not always of high quality. From such silages, *Clostridium* spp. – the agent causing delayed gas-production in cheese – pass into milk and then into cheese. Mild heat treatment (pasteurization) of milk does not destroy them. A considerable amount of research work was devoted to the methods of avoiding butyric blowing in hard and semi-hard rennet cheeses; nevertheless, all the means offered at this time to the cheesemakers were of limited efficiency and often harmful to the quality of cheese.

Much progress in both silage production and cheese technology in the countries with developed agriculture and dairying, are the main reasons for clostridial spoilage of such cheeses being no longer any real economic problem. The Harvestone equipment, when properly used, results in entirely safe silage. The bactofugation technique removes the clostridia sporeformers from milk. Unfortunately, this equipment is very expensive and in the poorer countries nisin-producing starters may be valuable.

There are two distinct periods in the research work concerning the use of nisin-producing streptococci as starters (NP-starter). In the first, lasting until about 1960, the NP-starter alone or together with the usual starter (U-starter) was applied in cheesemaking. Moreover, the properties of nisin-producing streptococci were extensively investigated.

Detailed evaluation of the above-mentioned investigations as well as of cheesemaking trials, mainly Edam cheese, carried out in many countries (Austria, Czechoslovakia, France, Holland, Hungary, Denmark, Poland, Spain, Sweden) is presented elsewhere (Ritter, 1957; Lipińska, 1966; Lipińska *et al.*, 1972; Hurst, 1972) and reference will be only to the general conclusions.

The major part of the cultural features of nisin-producing *Str. lactis* strains does not differentiate them from other lactic streptococci, except for a somewhat slower rate of lactic acid production.

Nisin is effectively bacteriostatic and/or bactericidal towards clostridia isolated from blown cheese, and – unfortunately – also to the bacteria present in the usual starters, all Gram-positive. Some bacterial species present in raw milk and even certain starter bacteria produce the nisin-destroying nisinase.

The results of cheese-making trials were as follows:

(1) Nisin produced *in situ* by NP-starter effectively controlled clostridial blowing of cheese. When cheese was produced from pasteurized milk, nisin persisted till the end of the maturation period. In raw-milk cheese the nisin content rapidly decreased.

(2) Cheese with NP starters often presents quality defects typical of a slow rise in acidity during the manufacture and ripening period, namely high pH values, irregular eyes, even coliform gassiness. The same defects, though expressed much more strongly, are observed in the hard rennet cheese such as Emmental.

(3) The NP starter is highly sensitive to bacteriophage attack.

These results reduced the interest in use of nisin-producing streptococci as starters. They were applied only in Holland for preparation of cheeses destined for melting.

In the early sixties the industrial application of bactofugation was at its beginning. It still seemed worthwhile to look for a new approach to the use of nisin-producing starters in cheese-making. The above trials showed that the inhibitory action of NP starters on the usual (U) starters was the main reason of the poor quality of cheeses. One could be justified in expecting that a starter composed of nisin-resistant and nisin-producing bacteria would ensure a substantial rise in acidity, in the presence of nisin, which would inhibit the sporeformers in cheese. Among the bacterial species used as starters, there are no strains naturally resistant to the levels of nisin found in cheese prepared with NP starters. Moreover, they were supposed not to produce nisinase.

The second period of research on nisin-producing starters began when training of some starter strains was undertaken, in order to adapt them to grow and to ferment lactose at a nearly normal rate in the presence of nisin (Ritter, 1957; Lipińska and Strzalkowska, 1959). The major parts of the successful experiments were carried out by subculturing in media with increasing quantities of nisin (Lipińska and Strzalkowska, 1959; Hylmar, Teplý and Tesarkova, 1970b; Oberman and Libudzisz, 1973).

The behaviour of different species of bacteria and even of different strains of the same species varied widely, from the impossibility of obtaining nisin resistance without a total loss of acidifying ability (e.g. *L. helveticus* spp.) or without a sharp rise in nisinase production (e.g. *Str. thermophilus* spp.), to the greater ease of training of mesophilic starter bacteria.

The nisin-resistant strains selected (two *Str. lactis,* one *Str. cremoris,* one *Str. diacetilactis,* one *L. casei* and two *Propionibacterium*) were first examined as starters in pilot-scale trials.

The selected strains were considered nisin-resistant if they presented the following features essential for their future use: (*a*) acidification ability in the presence of about 300 i.u. nisin ml^{-1} of medium (similar to that of the parent strain), (*b*) nisin-resistance lasting for more than one month, (*c*) no nisinase production. Nisin-resistant strains were found to exhibit the following properties: at nisin concentrations largely exceeding the levels to which the strains were trained, their metabolic activity could be impaired (Hylmar, Teplý and Tesarkova, 1970b). Their cell size was larger than that of the parent cells (Karlikanova, Gudkov and Trofimova, 1970; Karlikanova and Gudkov, 1970).

Nisin-resistant streptococci did not differ from the parent strains in the major part of the cultured features considered in the physiological classification, except for the lower resistance to adverse factors such as elevated temperature and higher bile concentration. They had a longer lag-phase and a lower cell mass than the nisin-sensitive parent strains when grown in the same culture medium. At the same time, their metabolic activity was more intense when expressed as lactic acid, diacetyl or acetoin production, CO_2 accumulation and proteolytic activity (*Figure 8.6* and *Table 8.2*). They were also more sensitive to medical antibiotics

Table 8.2 Metabolic activity of nisin-sensitive and nisin-resistant *Str. lactis* strains in milk (Lipińska, 1975)

		Str. lactis	
Property	*Units*	*Nisin-sensitive strain*	*Nisin-resistant strain*
Bacterial count*	10^9 ml^{-1}	1.7	0.6
Acidity*	°SH	40	39.5
Diacetyl*	mg l^{-1}	0.56	1.70
Acetoine*	mg l^{-1}	5.0	5.8
CO_2†	mg l^{-1}	87.0	120.0
Proteolytic activity*	μm tyrosine ml^{-1}	3.13	11.73

*Incubation: 20 h at 23°C.
†Incubation: 7 days at 30°C.

than the parent strains (*see* earlier). Similar properties were found in nisin-resistant *Propionibacterium shermanii* strains, with respect to their propionic acid, acetic acid and CO_2 production and to the respiratory rate determined by the Warburg technique (*Figure 8.7*) (Lipińska *et al.*, 1973b). CO_2 production by nisin-resistant and parent strains of *P. shermanii* grown in cell-free substrates fermented by various contaminating and starter bacterial species was also investigated (Jakubczyk, Kosikowska and Lipińska, 1974; Kosikowska, Jakubczyk and Lipińska, 1974).

There were some differences in the amino acid composition of extracts from nisin-sensitive and nisin-resistant *Str. lactis* cells. The higher content of threonine, valine and aspartic acid (precursor of threonine) in the nisin-resistant strains was the most striking fact; these amino acids are essential for the biosynthesis of the cytoplasmic proteins of bacteria (Lipińska and Tomaszewska, 1965).

The above results seem to show that the acquirement of nisin-resistance is accompanied by deep changes in the bacterial cell. This is a general phenomenon. A lower bacterial cell count was observed also in a tetramycin-resistant *Str. lactis* strain (Sahani, 1959). According to Dean and Hinshelwood (1966), the higher metabolic activity of a strain with acquired resistance to a substance disturbing

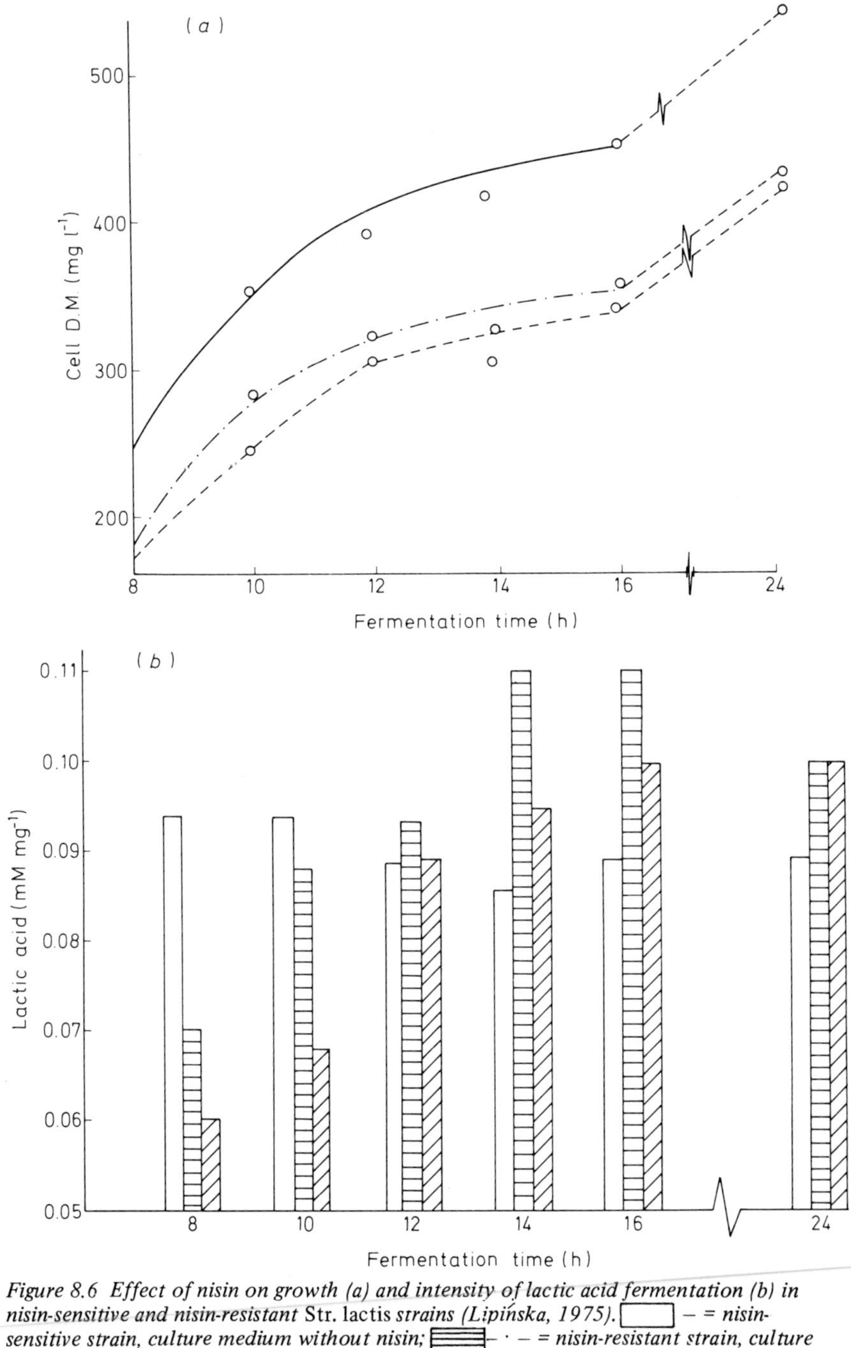

Figure 8.6 Effect of nisin on growth (a) and intensity of lactic acid fermentation (b) in nisin-sensitive and nisin-resistant Str. lactis *strains (Lipińska, 1975).* [open bar] *— = nisin-sensitive strain, culture medium without nisin;* [horizontally hatched bar] *— · — = nisin-resistant strain, culture medium without nisin;* [diagonally hatched bar] *- - - - = nisin-resistant strain, culture medium with 300 i.u. nisin ml*$^{-1}$*. (In the graphs no consideration is given to the nisin-sensitive* Str. lactis *strain in nisin-containing medium, because of complete inhibition of bacterial growth by the antibiotic)*

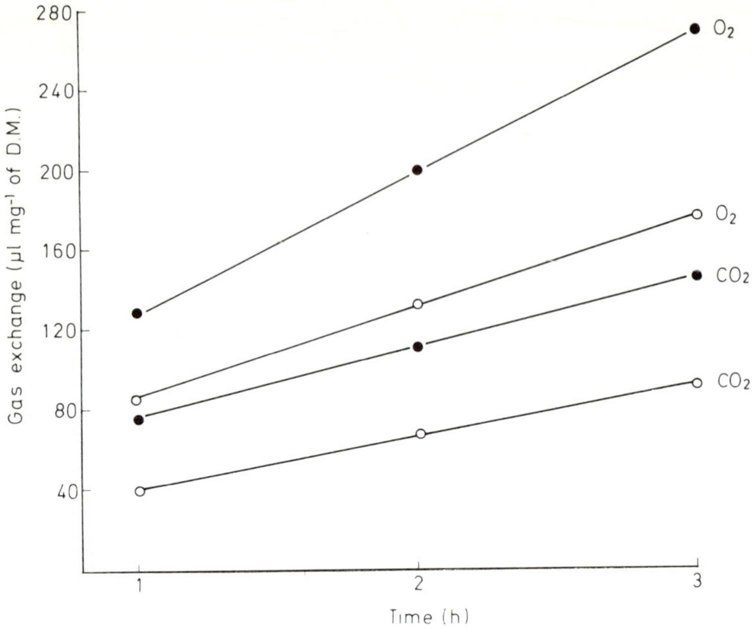

Figure 8.7 Effect of nisin on gas exchange in nisin-sensitive and nisin-resistant Propionibacterium shermanii *strains.* ○–○ = *nisin-sensitive strain;* ●–● = *nisin-resistant strain, culture medium with 200 i.u. nisin ml*$^{-1}$ *(Lipińska* et al., *1973a)*

its activity could be an expression of the stabilized form of a modified enzymic system formed during the training, to the end of survival in the presence of increasing quantities of the disturbing substance (nisin, in our case).

The higher sensitivity of nisin-resistant streptococci to adverse factors (bile, elevated temperature, medical antibiotics), as compared with the parent strains, together with what is actually known on the cytoplasmic membrane as being the site of the action of nisin on vegetative bacteria (Ramseier, 1960), suggests that the observed higher metabolic activity is a feature of some importance; namely, this enhanced metabolic activity could allow the cell to overcome the disturbances occurring when the cell membrane is changed, thus presumably being more permeable to toxic substances.

If the changes in the bacteria, resulting from nisin-resistance, act in opposite directions (e.g. lower bacterial count and higher acidification capacity), they finally lead to metabolic activity approximating to that of the parent strain. Nevertheless, there are some changes in the cell's features which do not facilitate the use of these strains as starters among others, they include: prolonged lag-phase increasing their sensitivity to bacteriophages; lower heat-resistance causing in an extreme case of a *L. acidophilus* strain resistant to 200 i.u. nisin ml^{-1} the inability to grow in milk with an addition of 20 i.u. nisin ml^{-1} at 55°C (i.e. the scalding temperature of hard rennet cheese) (Lipińska *et al.,* 1976a).

Edam cheese pilot-scale production with the use of NP and NR starters was initiated in Poland (Lipińska, 1961) and then carried out in the U.S.S.R. (Karlikanova, Gudkov and Trofimova, 1970; Karlikanova and Gudkov, 1970). Pasteurized milk was naturally and artificially infected with clostridia spores. Nisin produced *in situ* by the NP starter in the presence of the NR starter controlled butyric blowing in cheese. The resulting products were of the first quality in taste, aroma, and texture, except that the eyes were smaller and not as regular as in U starter cheeses prepared from milk free of sporeformers. Nisin level of NP + NR starter cheeses was very high (400–1000 i.u. g^{-1}).

The acidification capacity (rate of lactose fermentation) of NP + NR starters was lower, as compared with U starters, but sufficiently high to ensure quite normal ripening of cheese (*Figure 8.8*). In NP + NR cheeses the total bacterial

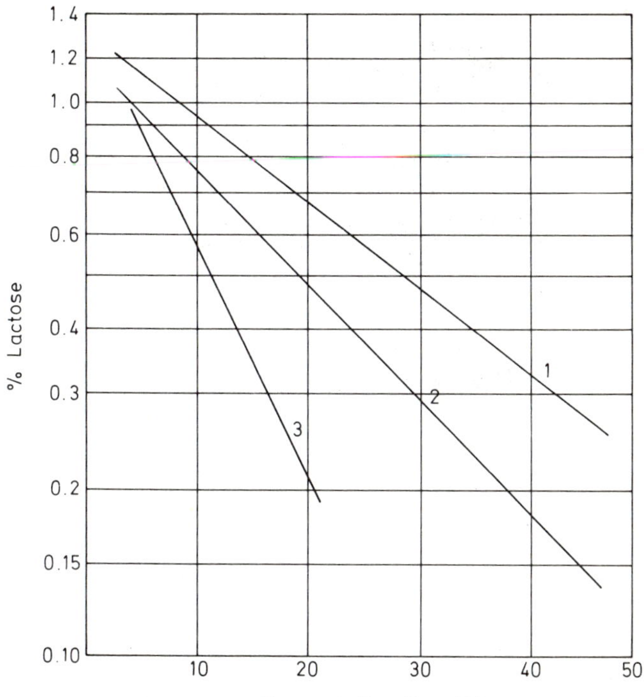

Figure 8.8 Intensity of lactose fermentation in cheese with different starters added. 1 = Nisin-producing NP + normal U starters; 2 = NP (nisin-producing) + NR (nisin-resistant) starters; 3 = U-starter only (Lipinska, 1961)

count was lower, citric acid persisted longer and the free amino acid content was higher, in comparison with U-starter cheeses. NP + NR starters controlled butyric blowing also in cheese with low salt content (1.5–2.5%).

Some pilot-scale trials (120 l batches) using a commercial nisin preparation (10^6 i.u. g^{-1}) and a nisin-resistant NR starter were carried out. Tilsit cheeses in which there are no eyes formation problems, were of first class quality when produced from pasteurized milk heavily contaminated with clostridia spores, with an addition of 10–15 i.u. nisin ml^{-1} and 0.6–0.8% of NP starters. Parallel U starter cheeses produced without nisin were all blown. It is stressed that any nisin added to milk at levels exceeding 30–35 i.u. ml^{-1} passes into the whey during cheese making (Lipińska *et al.*, 1966).

Edam cheeses prepared using the same levels of the nisin preparation and NP starter were of poor quality (Gontzea *et al.*, 1973). By increasing the NR starter content up to 2.0–2.5% and maintaining the same nisin level, the defects caused by the slow acidity rise were eliminated, while the nisin added controlled butyric blowing of cheese (Lipińska *et al.*, 1976a) (*Figure 8.9*).

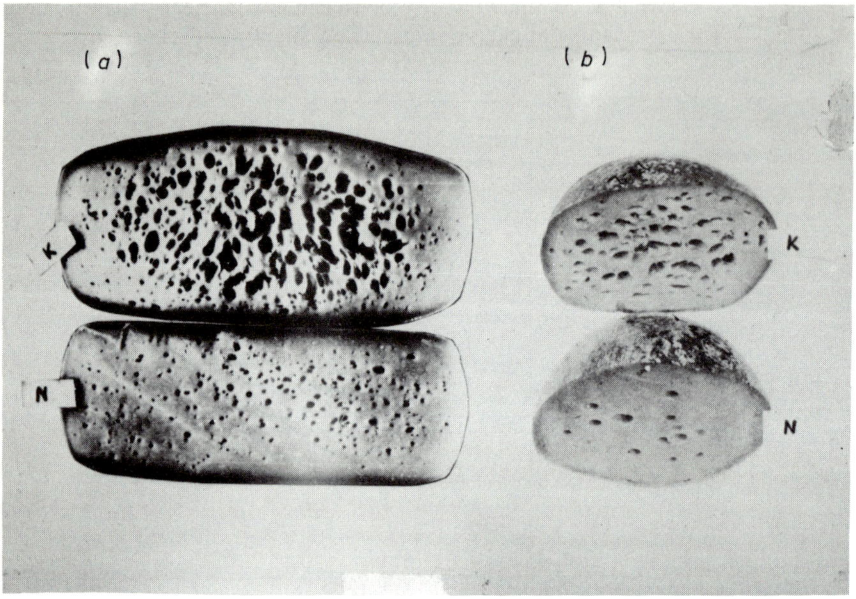

Figure 8.9 Effect of nisin on clostridial blowing in rennet ripening cheese. (a) Tilsit cheese with nisin preparation added (10–15 i.u. ml^{-1} milk); (b) Edam cheese obtained with NP + NR starters. N = nisin-treated; K = without nisin (Lipińska, 1961; Lipinska et al., *1966)*

In view of the impossibility of selecting nisin-resistant strains of *L. helveticus* spp. and *Str. thermophilus* spp. for use as starters in hard rennet cheese, trials selected strains of related species, already used as starters for the Emmental cheese production (Demeter, *et al.*, 1959). Pilot-scale trials using a starter composed of *L. acidophilus* and *Str. lactis* var. *taette* strains, resistant to 200 i.u. nisin ml^{-1}, showed the inability of the former strain to survive the synergistic effect of low levels of nisin (20 i.u. ml^{-1}) and heating at 55°C (i.e. the scalding temperature of hard rennet cheese). As recently reported in Italy, a nisin-resistant *L. helveticus* strain was selected and successfully applied in pilot-scale production of Provolone cheese (Senesi, Emaldi and Casenio, 1975).

In Poland, Gouda cheese was comparatively produced with NP + NR starters and U starter in 5000 l batches, during 100 days, from pasteurized milk naturally infected with sporeformers. Potassium nitrate was added (Lipińska, Domanska and Soltys, 1971). In the U.S.S.R., industrial trials were carried out under the same conditions for 50 days in two cheese-making dairies (Gudkov and Dolidze, 1974). Application of the NP + NR starters doubled the quantity of first-class cheeses and reduced the amount of third-class quality and rejected cheeses by about a half.

All cheeses, except one, contained nisin till the end of maturation. There was a correlation between the cheese quality and nisin content. Even in the presence of high coliform contamination the NP + NR starters controlled butyric blowing of cheese. There were several bacteriophage accidents, the NR starter being more sensitive than the NP starter (*Figure 8.10*).

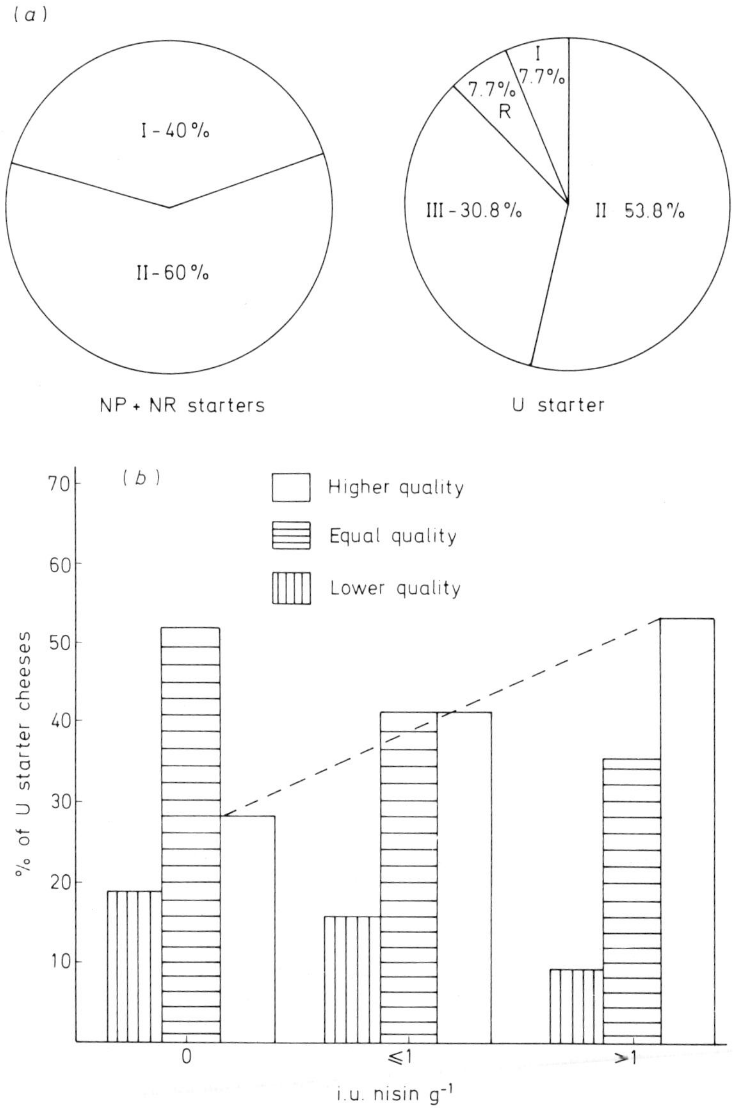

Figure 8.10 The effect of nisin on cheese quality. (a) Effect of NP + NR starters on quality of heavily contaminated cheeses (700 000 coliforms g^{-1} and 10–100 sporeformers g^{-1}); (b) effect of nisin content on cheese quality; I, II, III, R (rejected) = quality classes of cheese (Lipińska et al., *1971)*

In industrial trials performed in the U.S.S.R., 90% of cheeses prepared with the NP + NR starter were of high quality, while 59% of cheeses with the U starter were blown. The use of NP + NR starters permitted in Poland a saving of 4200 zl per ton and in the U.S.S.R. of 91 Rb per ton.

GROWTH-PROMOTING ABILITY

The first attempts at an application of nisin for growth-promoting were unsuccessful (Coates *et al.*, 1951; Barber, Braude and Hirsch, 1952). Moreover, no attention was given to the high gains in body weight of laboratory animals fed nisin in toxicological trials (Shtenberg and Ignatyev, 1971; Gontzea *et al.*, 1973). Four feeding experiments, using over 100 calves and two using about 100 piglets were carried out in Poland and Czechoslovakia. In the major part of these trials nisin-enriched milk-powder was fed. The results consistently testified to the growth-promoting properties of nisin (Lipińska and Strzalkowska, 1964; Namiotkiewicz *et al.*, 1966; Korniewicz, 1970; Jasiorowski *et al.*, 1971; Prokop *et al.*, 1973; Lipińska *et al.*, 1974). Nisin-fed calves and piglets exhibited a significant (over 10% higher) gain in body weight, lower susceptibility to diseases and better utilization of food, as compared with controls. No nisin was found in the muscles, blood and urine of calves. In nisin-fed calves 3 h before slaughter, 30% of the antibiotic was detected chiefly in the abomasum, whereas only 1% was present in the intestine. There were no differences in coliform and enterococci titres, nor in lactobacilli and anaerobic total counts in faeces between nisin-fed and control calves (Jasiorowski *et al.*, 1971).

Conclusions

Undoubtedly, the results surveyed in this paper, together with the previous studies on nisin, permit a deeper insight into the problems of this antibiotic. Nisin is an interesting, biologically active compound, and many of the published papers deal with its structure, properties and mechanism of biosynthesis. The results suggest, among others, the possibility of nisin production by semi-synthesis, if the economic advantage of such a procedure could be demonstrated.

The question arises to what extent the research work carried out since 1962 complies with the suggestions formulated regarding this topic at the previous Easter School. Among the three antibiotics: nisin, subtilin and tylosin, widely discussed by Hawley (1962), only nisin has gained fairly broad acceptance. Subtilin, a very interesting biological inhibitor, has not yet recovered from the set-back which it suffered in the early fifties. The status of tylosin, defined at the session of F.A.O./W.H.O. Experts (1969a), is expressed as follows: 'Although tylosin cross-resistance is not complete with all macrolides, the incidence of cross-resistance to medically important macrolides is sufficiently significant to preclude the use of tylosine as a direct food additive, unless it can be used to solve an extremely important problem'. It is stressed that during the last 15 years no important data on new antibiotics applicable in food processing have been published. This seems to express the strong objections against the use of medical antibiotics for other than health purposes. This feeling extends to include all antibiotics, and is justified by the discovery of the extrachromosomal infectious resistance in bacteria.

The publications surveyed fulfilled the previously formulated need for studies on the analytical problems of nisin, its stability at various heat treatments and at different pH values as well as the problems of synergism and antibiosis. These publications confirm some suggestions made at the previous Easter School, namely: the importance of carry-over of nisin in investigations on the resistance of bacteria and spores, the relationship between nisin and the true heat resistance of spores, the stage of spore outgrowth at which the action of nisin takes place, as well as the synergistic effect of heat and nisin on spores.

The data on the practical application of nisin point to the progress achieved. The most valuable concerns testing of commercial packs of nisin-treated food. Attention was focused on certain canned products. It should, however, be emphasized that the majority of trials were performed on a pilot-scale, mainly with artificial infections. The shortcomings of such trials are well known. In these trials much attention was given to the organoleptic properties and keeping quality of nisin-treated foods. Less attention was directed to the very important problem of the higher nutritional value of nisin-treated foods, compared with nisin-free ones. There are also few economic analyses on the application of nisin, taking into consideration all its previously mentioned advantages. More information should be obtained on pathogenic bacteria in nisin-treated foods. Knowledge of nisin applications in canning calls for a continuation of research work.

In view of the relatively great number of aspects to be studied, the question arises as to whether it is worthwhile undertaking such expensive and labour-consuming effort. The following facts would seem to support such a necessity: (*a*) ultra-high temperature (UHT) treatment proves to be unsatisfactory for many products, (*b*) economic integration on a world scale creates new needs with respect to the transport and storage of food in hot climate zones and newly exploited areas as well as for military purposes. Moreover, from the standpoint of improvement of the quality of food and prevention of waste, it seems worthwhile continuing investigations on nisin. This conclusion is valid if, indeed, the present opinion on the harmlessness of nisin is not refuted and if nisin is not used for medical purposes (e.g. in the treatment of malaria, *see* Gross and Morell, 1967).

The fact that the attempts so far made in an application of nisin-producing and nisin-resistant starters for control of sporeformers in semi-hard and hard rennet cheese were not always successful should not stop further experiments in this field. Application of these starters should now be much easier, owing to the progress in the methods of preparation and protection of starters.

Nisin-producing and nisin-resistant starters would, even now, be cheaper and thus more attractive than the expensive modern equipment for the production of milk free of sporeformers and for their removal, if present, from milk destined for cheese-making.

Finally, there is the problem of the application of nisin-enriched milk-powder, now the least expensive nisin preparation, as a growth stimulant in young animals. It has to be established whether the observed lack of cross-resistance to medical antibiotics and the lower viability of nisin-resistant bacteria justify this application.

In addition to these problems many more questions should be answered by future investigations on nisin.

References

ATTWELL, R.W., CROSS, T. and GOULD, G.W. (1972). *J. Gen. Microbiol.*, **73** (3), 471

BAILEY, F.J. and HURST, A. (1971). *Can. J. Microbiol.*, **17** (1), 61

BARANOVA, I.P. and EGOROV, N.S. (1967). *Antibiotiki*, **12** (1), 66

BARANOVA, I.P. and EGOROV, N.S. (1969). *Priklad. Bioch. i Mikrobiol.*, **5** (2), 175

BARANOVA, I.P. and EGOROV, N.S. (1970). *Antibiotiki*, **15** (8), 686

BARANOVA, I.P., EGOROV, N.S. and SILVESTROVA, O.I. (1973). *Prikl. Bioch. Mikrobiol.*, **9** (1), 55

BARANOVA, I.P., EGOROV, N.S., KOZLOVA, YU. I. and MAKSIMOV, W.N. (1974). *Biol. Nauki*, **17** (10), 94

BARBER, R.S., BRAUDE, R. and HIRSCH, A. (1952). *Nature (Lond.)*, **159**, 200

BODANSKY, M. and PERLMAN, D. (1964). *Nature (Lond.)*, **204**, 840

BRITISH STANDARDS INSTITUTION: 'Methods for the estimation and differentiation of nisin in processed cheese' (1974). British Standard, **BS 4020**, 1974

CASOLARI, A., CAMPANINI, M. and PEZZANI, G. (1967). *Ind. Cons.*, **42**, 97

CLAYPOOL, L., HEINEMANN, B., VORIS, L. and STUMBO, C.R. (1966). *J. Dairy Sci.*, **49**, 314

COATES, M.E., HARRISON, G.F., KON, S.K., MANN, M.E. and ROSE, C.D. (1951). *Biochem. J.*, **48**, XII

COVELL, N.D., ALLEN, A.R. and JARVIS, B. (1971). *J. appl. Bact.*, **34** (4), 787

DEAN, A.C.R. and HINSHELWOOD, C. (1966). *Growth, Function and Regulation in Bacterial Cell.* The Clarendon Press, Oxford

DEMETER, K.J., KUNDRAT, W., LOCATELLI, C. and PORTA, A. (1959). *XV Int. Dairy Cong.*, **2**, 854. Richard Clay, London

DINERMAN, A.A. and IGNATYEV, A.D. (1966). *Gig. i Sanit.*, **9**, 38

DURAN, L., HERNANDEZ, E. and FLORES, J. (1964). *Rev. Agr. Tec. Alimentos*, **4**, 87

EFIMOVA, W.A. (1974). *Nauchn. Trudy Omsk. Sielsko. Inst.*, **121**, 59

EGOROV, N.S., BARANOVA, I.P., MAKSIMOV, W.N. and SILVESTROVA, O.Y. (1973). *Izv. Akad. Nauk SSSR, Ser. Biol.*, **1**, 99

EGOROV, N.S., BARANOVA, I.P. and SILVESTROVA, O.Y. (1972). *Mikrobiologia*, **41** (5), 805

EGOROV, N.S. and SHKUNDOVA, Y.V. (1964). *Antibiotiki*, **9**, 88

EL-GENDY, S.M. and EL-BADAWI, S.M. (1972). *Assiut Journ. of Agricult. Sci.*, **3** (3)

FINDUS REPORT (1964). 'The use of Nisin with tinned peas', *Techn. Inform.*, Aplin and Barrett

FOWLER, G.G. (1968). *Conf. Inst. Food Sci. Technol.*, Sutton Bonington

FOWLER, G.G. and McCANN, B. (1971). *Austr. J. Dairy Techn.*, **26** (2), 44

GIBBS, B.M. and HURST, A. (1964). In *Microbial Inhibitors in Food,* IV Int. Symp. Food Microbiol. Almquist & Wiksell, Stockholm

GOEL, M.C., CALBERT, H.E. and MARTH, E.H. (1969). *J. Milk Food Technol.*, **32**, 312

GONTZEA, J., TOMA, C., BARDUTA, Z., MOLDOVAN, E., CALINESCU, S. and MAVROMATI, E. (1973). *Lait,* **LIII** (521), 40
GOULD, G.W. (1964). In *Microbial Inhibitors in Food.* IV Int. Symp. on Food Microbiol. Almquist & Wiksell, Stockholm
GREGORY, MARGARET E., HENRY, KATHLEEN M. and KON, K. (1964). *J. Dairy Res.,* **31** (1), 113
GROSS, E. and MORELL, J.L. (1967). *J. Amer. Chem. Soc.,* **89**, 2791
GROSS, E. and MORELL, J.L. (1970). *J. Amer. Chem. Soc.,* **92**, 2919
GROSS, E. and MORELL, J.L. (1971). *J. Amer. Chem. Soc.,* **93**, 4634
GROSS, E., MORELL, J.L. and CRAIG, N.L. (1969). *Proc. Nat. Acad. Sci.,* **62**, 952
GUDKOV, A.W. and DOLIDZE, G.G. (1974). *Molochn. Promyshl.,* **40** (7), 13
GUDKOV, A.W., KUDRYASHEVA, M.M., KOSTRITSKAYA, N.P. and RAMAZANOVA, D.P. (1969). *Molochn. Promyshl.,* **35** (3), 21
GUDKOV, A.W., LUBIMOVA, L.A., TROFIMOVA, T., SILEVA, M.W. and LITVINOVA, M.N. (1973). *Antibiotiki,* **18** (4), 346
GUPTA, K.G. (1974). *IV Int. Congress Sci. Technol. Food, Madrid,* **4b**, 50
GUPTA, K.G., SIDHU, R. and YADAV, N.K. (1971). *J. Food Sci.,* **36** (6), 896
GUPTA, K.G., SIDHU, R. and YADAV, N.K. (1972). *J. Food Sci.,* **37** (6), 971
HALL, R.H. (1966). *Process Biochem.* (12)
HARA, S., KEIDO, Y., KOJI, M., TAKAKO, T., TATSUNORI, K., MASACHIRO, S., ZIRO, I. and TAKESHI, S. (1962). *Dept. Pharm. Rep. Tokyo Medical College*
HARGROVE, R.E., McDONOUGH, F.E. and MATTINGBY, W.A. (1969). *J. Milk Food Technol.,* **32**, 480
HAWLEY, H.B. (1958). *Milchwiss.,* **13**, 253
HAWLEY, H.B. (1963). In *Antibiotics in Agriculture.* Ed. Woodbine, M. Butterworths, London
HEINEMANN, B., STUMBO, C.R. and SCURLOCK, A. (1964). *J. Dairy Sci.,* **47** (1), 8
HEINEMANN, B., VORIS, L. and STUMBO, C.R. (1965). *Food Technol.,* **19** (2), 92
HERNANDEZ, BRIZ S. (1972). *Anal. Bromatol.,* **24** (2), 217
HURST, A. (1966). *Can. J. Gen. Microbiol.,* **44**, 209
HURST, A. (1967). *Nature,* **214**, 1232
HURST, A. (1972). *J. Milk Food Technol.,* **35** (7), 418
HURST. A. and DRING, G.J. (1968). *J. Gen. Microbiol.,* **50**, 383
HURST, A. and KRUSE, H. (1970). *J. Gen. Microbiol.,* **16**, 1250
HURST, A. and PATERSON, G.M. (1971). *Bact. Proc.,* 127
HYLMAR, B. (1975). *Prum. Potr.,* **26** (4), 214
HYLMAR, B., TEPLY, M. and TESARKOVA, H. (1970a). *Prum. Potr.,* **21** (6), 186
HYLMAR, B., TEPLY, M. and TESARKOVA, H. (1970b). *Prum. Potr.,* **21** (12), 390
IGNATYEV, A.D. (1965). *Voprosy pitanya,* **5**, 61
INGRAM, L. (1969). *Bioch. Biophys. Acta,* **184**, 216
INGRAM, L. (1970). *Bioch. Biophys. Acta,* **224**, 263
INGRAM, L., TOMBS, M.P. and HURST, A. (1967). *Analyt. Biochem.,* **20**, 24
JAKUBCZYK, E., KOSIKOWSKA, M. and LIPINSKA, E. (1974). *XIX Int. Dairy Congr.,* **1E**, 395

JAKUBCZYK, E., LIPINSKA, E. and KOSIKOWSKA, M. (1973). *Rocz. Inst. Przem. Mlecz.*, **XV** (1/45), 27

JAKUBCZYK, E., LIPINSKA, E. and SZADKOWSKA, M. (1973). *Rocz. Inst. Przem. Mlecz.*, **XV** (2/46), 97

JARCHOVSKA, H., KOLAR, J., KATZER, B. and KRIKRYL, F. (1974). *Prum. Potr.*, **25** (6), 190

JARVIS, B. (1967). *J. Gen. Microbiol.*, **47**, 33

JARVIS, B. (1970). *Proc. Biochem. Soc.*, **119**, 56P

JARVIS, B. and FARR, J. (1971). *Bioch. Bioph. Acta*, **227**, 232

JARVIS, B., JEFFSOAT, JOAN and CHEESEMAN, G.C. (1968). *Bioch. Biophys. Acta*, **168** (1), 153

JARVIS, B. and MAHONEY, R.R. (1969). *J. Dairy Sci.*, **52**, 1448

JASIOROWSKI, H., ZIELINSKI, W., LIPINSKA, E., PIETRASZEK, A. and MALUSZYNSKA, G.M. (1971). *Biul. Inst. Gen. Hod. Zwierz. PAN*, **24** (51)

JONES, L.W. (1974). *Can. J. Microbiol.*, **20** (9), 1257

KALRA, M.S. and DUDANI, A.T. (1973). *Indian J. Dairy Sci.*, **26** (3), 208

KALRA, M.S., DUDANI, A.T. and LAXMINARYANA, H. (1973). *Indian J. Dairy Sci.*, **26** (2), 137

KALRA, M.S., KUILA, R.K. and RANGANATHAN, B. (1973). *Experientia*, **29** (5), 624

KALRA, M.S., LAXMINARYANA, H. and DUDANI, A.T. (1973). *J. Food Sci. Technol.*, **10** (3), 92

KARLIKANOVA, S.N. and GUDKOV, A.W. (1970). *XVIII Int. Dairy Congr.*, **A 4.6**, 385. Ramsay, Melbourne

KARLIKANOVA, S.N., GUDKOV, A.W. and TROFIMOVA, A.W. (1970). *Molochn. Promyshl.*, **31** (6), 6

KISS, I., KISS-KURTZ, N., FARKAS, J., FABRI, F. and VAS, K. (1970). *Food Sci. Technol. Abstr.*, **2** (8), 87784

KONIECNY, V., MINKS, J. and CERVENKA, J. (1970). *Acta Vet. (Czechoslovak)*, **39** (4), 485

KORNIEWICZ, A. (1970). *Med. Wet.*, **20** (9), 561

KOSIKOWSKA, M., JAKUBCZYK, E. and LIPINSKA, E. (1974). *XIX Int. Dairy Congr.*, **1E**, 397

KOZAK, W., RAJCHERT-TRZPIL, M. and DOBRZANSKI, W.T. (1973). *Bull. Acad. Polon. Sci., Sci. Biol.*, **12** (12), 811

KOZAK, W., RAJCHERT-TRZPIL, M., ZAJDEL, J. and DOBRZANSKI, W.T. (1975). *Appl. Microbiol.*, **25** (2), 305

KOZLOVA, M.A. and KOBRINA, YU.P. (1971). *Pishtsh. Tekhnol.*, **2**, 82

LINNETT, P.E. and STROMINGER, J.L. (1973). *Antimicrob. Agents Chemother.*, **4** (3), 231

LIPINSKA, E. (1961). *Prace Inst. Przem. Mlecz.*, **VIII** (1), 9

LIPINSKA, E. (1966). *Antybiotyki w mleczarstwie.* Zaklad Wydawnictw CRS, Warszawa

LIPINSKA, E. (1975). *Roczn. Inst. Przem. Mlecz.*, **XVII** (2/52), 15

LIPINSKA, E., DOMANSKA, M. and SOLTYS, W. (1971). *Przeglad Mleczarski*, **20** (4), 18

LIPINSKA, E., GUDKOV, A.W. and KARLIKANOVA, S.N. (1972). *Zastosowanie nizyny w serowarstwie.* Wyd. N.T. Warsaw

LIPINSKA, E., JAKUBCZYK, E. and SZADKOWSKA, M. (1971). *Roczn. Inst. Przem. Mlecz.*, **XIII** (3), 15

LIPINSKA, E., JAKUBCZYK, E., KOSIKOWSKA, M. and LIPNIEWSKA, D. (1973a). *Proc. Symp. Wydz. II Nauk Biolog. PAN. Poznan,* 131

LIPINSKA, E., KOSIKOWSKA, M., JAKUBCZYK, E. and LIPNIEWSKA, D. (1976b). *Roczn. Inst. Przem. Mlecz.*, in press

LIPINSKA, E., ROSLON, E., TOMASZEWSKA, J. and SWIATEK, A. (1966). *XVII Int. Dairy Congr. (Munich),* **D**, 633

LIPINSKA, E., SOLTYS, W., BIJOK, E., JAKUBCZYK, E., KOSIKOWSKA, M. and KURPIEWSKA, W. (1976a). *Roczn. Inst. Przem. Mlecz.*, in press

LIPINSKA, E. and STRZALKOWSKA, M. (1959). *XV Int. Dairy Congr.*, **2**, 572. Richard Clay, London

LIPINSKA, E. and STRZALKOWSKA, M. (1960). *Prace Inst. Przem. Mlecz.*, **VII** (1), 9

LIPINSKA, E. and STRZALKOWSKA, M. (1964). *Prace Inst. Przem. Mlecz.*, **X** (1), 59

LIPINSKA, E., SZADKOWSKA, M., JAKUBCZYK, E. and LIPNIEWSKA, D. (1973b). *Roczn. Inst. Przem. Mlecz.*, **XV**, 25

LIPINSKA, E. and TOMASZEWSKA, J. (1965). *Zesz. Probl. Post. Nauk Roln.*, **53**, 156

LIPINSKA, E., WAWRZYNCZAK, S., KOSIKOWSKA, M., JAKUBCZYK, E., KAMINSKI, S. and FILIPKOWSKI, S. (1974). *XIX Int. Dairy Congr.*, **1E**, 122

MASLENNIKOVA, N.M. and LOKSHINA, R.V. (1968). *Konservn. i Ovoshtshesush. Prom.*, **1**, 12

MATELOVA, V. and BRECKA, A. (1972). *Prum. Potr.*, **23**, 28

MATEYEV, A. and STRANDJEV, A. (1963). *Konservn. i Ovoshtshesush. Prom.*, **2**, 17

MATOSIC, S., TAMBURASEV, G. and JUKIC, N. (1971). *Mikrobiologija (Yugoslavia),* **8** (2), 267

MIKOLAJCIK, E.M., REEVES, C.B. and HARPER, W.J. (1965). *J. Dairy Sci.*, **48** (11), 1522

NAMIOTKIEWICZ, J., LIPINSKA, E., BOGATKO, J. and NAMIOTKIEWICZ, H. (1966). *Roczn. Nauk Roln.*, **88-B-2**, 147

NEKHOTENOVA, T.I. and KULIEVA, I.P. (1966). *Konservn. i Ovoshtshesush. Prom.*, **8**, 24

OBERMAN, H. (1968). *Zesz. Nauk. Polit. Lodzkiej, Chemia Spozywcza,* **116**, 16

OBERMAN, H. and LIBUDZISZ, Z. (1973). *Acta Microbiol. Polon. Ser. B., Microbiol. Appl.*, **5** (4), 151

OBERMAN, H. and PABIS, E. (1975). *Acta Aliment. Polon.*, **I(XXV)** (3–4), 221

OVCHAROVA, T.P. and MASLENNIKOVA, N.M. (1969). *Antibiotiki v piszczevoj promyshlennosti.* Piszczewaja Promyshlennost, Moscow

PESQUERA, T.I. (1966). *Rev. Esp. Lech.*, no. 59

PETERKOVA, L. and HYLMAR, B. (1974). *Prum. Potr.*, **25**, 377

PORRETTA, A., CAMPANINI, M. and CASOLARI, A. (1970). *Industria Conserv.*, **45** (4), 298

PORRETTA, A., CASOLARI, A. and CASSARA, A. (1968). *Ind. conserv,* **1**, 13

PROKOP, V., KRATKY, F., HLADIKOVA, Z. and DOLCZALEK, J. (1973). *Zivocisna Wyroba,* **18** (12), 893

PULAY, G. and KRASZ, A. (1966). *Elem. Iper.*, **20** (8), 259

PULAY, G. and KRASZ, A. (1968). *Tejpari. Kut. Kozl.*, **11** (1), 3

PYANITSINA, I.N. (1968). *Trudy Vsyes. N. Issl. Instit. Molochn. Prom.*, **26**, 30

RADAEVA, J.R., ANATSKAYA, A.A. and EFIMOVA, W.A. (1975). *Molochn. Prom.,* **41** (2), 20

RAMSEIER, H.R. (1960). *Archiv für Mikrobiologie,* **37**, 57

RITTER, P. (1957). *Zeitschr. Allg. Path.,* **20** (5), 458

RUDAVSKAYA, A.B., ORLOVA, N.YA. and KUTOVAL, KH.A. (1971). *Tovarovyeden.,* **5**, 55

RUF, F. (1969). *Monogr.,* **63**, 1125

SAHANI, K.M. (1959). *J. Dairy Sci.,* **42**, 1659

SAHANI, K.M. (1962). *J. Dairy Sci.,* **45**, 827

SEEGER, J. (1970). 'Effect of nisin on the bacteria associated with canned vegetables', *INACOL Bruxelles. Techn. Inform.,* Aplin & Barrett

SENESI, E., EMALDI, G.C. and CASENIO, J. (1975). *Latte,* **2**, 84

SHILLINGER, YU.I., BOGORODITSKAYA, V.P. and OSIPOVA, N.J. (1969). *Vopr. Pitan.,* **28**, 44

SHKUNDOVA, Y.V. (1967). *Antibiotiki,* **12** (7), 586

SHKUNDOVA, Y.V. (1968). *Prikl. Biokhimia i Mikrobiol.,* **4** (5), 599

SHKUNDOVA, Y.V. and KULIEVA, I.P. (1966, 1967). In *Ovcharova* (1969)

SHORNIKOVA, N.M., OVCHAROVA, T.P., MASLENNIKOVA, N.M. and RUBEN, T.M. (1972). *Kons. Ovoshch. Promyshl.,* **9**, 15

SHTENBERG, A.J. and IGNATYEV, A.D. (1971). *Food Cosm. Toxicol.,* **8**, 369

SPECIFICATIONS (1969a) for the identity and purity of food additives and their toxological evaluation. F.A.O./W.H.O., Rome

SPECIFICATIONS (1969b) for the identity and purity of some antibiotics. F.A.O./W.H.O., Rome

STANKIEWICZ-BERGER, H. (1969). *Acta Microbiol. Polonica, Ser. B.,* **1** (XVIII) (3/4), 121

STUMBO, C.R., VORIS, L., SKAGGS, B. and HEINEMANN, B. (1964). *J. of Food Sci.,* **26** (6), 859

SZADKOWSKA, M., LIPINSKA, E., JAKUBCZYK, E. and LIPNIEWSKA, D. (1974). *Rocz. Inst. Przem. Mlecz.,* **XVI** (1/48), 5

TICHA, A. (1970). *Mlynsko-Pekarensky Prumysl,* **16** (2), 37

TIEMANN, U. and BELITZ, H.D. (1969). *Z. Lebensmittel-Unters. Forsch.,* **141** (5), 260

TOKMAKOVA, V.N. (1972). *Trudy Vsgys. N. Issl. Inst. Kons. i Ovoshesush. Prom.,* **16**, 123

TRAMER, J. and FOWLER, G.G. (1964). *J. Sci. Fd. Agric.,* **15** (8), 522

TRAMER, J. (1966). *Chem. Ind.,* 446

TSUGO, T. (1962). *J. Food Hyg. Soc.,* 356

USHAKOVA, R.F. (1972). *Trudy. Vsyies. Nauchn. Issl. Inst. Morsk. Rybn. Khoz. i Okeanogr.,* **88**, 24

VAS, K. (1963). *Confructa, Fruchtsaft Industrie,* **8** (2), 73

VAS, K. (1964). *Lebensm. Rundsch.,* **60** (3), 63

VAS, K., KISS, I. and KISS, N. (1967). *Zeitsch. für Lebensm. Unters. Forsch.,* **133** (3), 141

WAJID, K. and KALRA, M.S. (1974). *XIX Int. Dairy Congr.,* **1E**, 545

WEGNER, K. (1969). *FBM Milch Standard,* **11** (2), 76

WHEATON, E. and HAYS, G.L. (1964). *Food Technol.,* **18** (4), 147

WHITE, R.J. and HURST, A. (1968). *J. Gen. Microb.,* **53**, 171

9

STRESS EFFECTS AND FOOD MICROBIOLOGY

L.D. WITTER
Z.J. ORDAL
Departments of Food Science and Microbiology, University of Illinois, U.S.A.

Food scientists have always been concerned with the effectiveness of processing operations in destroying unwanted microorganisms. Microbial survival and the factors influencing it, therefore, have always comprised a reasonably large proportion of the literature of food microbiology. In the earlier literature a bacterial cell was either alive or dead and the concept of recoverable injury was not included in contemplating the mechanisms of bacterial death. A reduction in the intensity of a process simply reduced the number of bacteria killed.

In the two decades prior to the 1960s, it was occasionally observed and reported that microorganisms exposed to a sublethal stress showed more restrictive conditions for growth. The growth supporting ranges of temperature, pH, water activity, oxidation–reduction potential or osmostic pressure for such stressed cells were detectably less. Such stressed cells were also more fastidious in nutrient requirements and more susceptible to selective agents or potentially toxic compounds. But these scattered observations did not lead to a clear concept of a recoverably injured cell.

It was during the 1960s that the nature of injury due to sublethal stresses became more clearly delineated by observing that injured cells recovered in the absence of growth. Injury and recovery can be monitored by a dual plating procedure. Plating the sublethally stressed culture on a non-selective medium enumerates the total viable microorganisms, plating simultaneously on a selective medium enumerates the microorganisms in the culture which are tolerant of the selective agent, and the difference between these two plate counts is the count of the microorganisms which are injured and unable to initiate growth in the presence of the particular selective agent. It was immediately recognized that with the ability to monitor recovery the testing of the effect of various inhibitors on the recovery was possible and would provide insight into what repairs were occurring and what the nature of the injury was in the first place.

Trends and Reviews

Ramifications of injury and recovery rapidly spread to all areas of food microbiology. Public health concern centered around the possibility that viable food pathogens might go undetected in foods when conventional selective media were used for their enumeration. This possibility of not properly enumerating injured microorganisms was also directed toward food spoilage organisms that might cause economic havoc, toward indicator organisms or total plate counts that might cause faulty conclusions in quality assurance programmes and toward cultures used in the food industry that might be unnecessarily discarded. Most of the earlier papers were content to define and redefine the various problem areas that might arise by virtue of injury and recovery, and only recently has greater attention been directed to solving the problem of including injured organisms in selective counting procedures.

Academic interests in injury and recovery were directed towards (*a*) defining the nature of the lesions that were produced by the various types of stress, (*b*) demonstrating and examining the repair of these lesions during recovery, and (*c*) looking for consistency in the patterns of injury produced by the various primary and secondary stresses in different organisms.

Most of the literature dealing with effect of stresses on microbial death, injury and repair can be located in a series of fine reviews. Each review varies slightly in emphasis and approach. Tomlins and Ordal (1976) covered thermal resistance, injury and recovery in their up-to-date review. They carefully dealt with the mechanisms of injury and recovery. Allwood and Russell (1970) also covered the mechanisms of thermal injury and provided a comprehensive look at the earlier literature. Busta (1976) summarized the practical implications of stress-induced injury and also provided the first review treatment of spores and injury. Ray and Speck (1973a) contributed a very thorough review of freezing and thawing injury; Gomez, Takano and Sinskey (1973) did the same for the stress of freeze-drying, while Morichi and Irie (1973) reported on repair of injury caused by these two types of stress. Corry (1973) made a progress report on heat resistance and water activity. Postgate (1967) covered the literature on the mild stresses encountered in bacterial aging, in adverse environments and during starvation; indeed, he describes the extreme difficulty of avoiding stressful situations. Consequently, with only a very few exceptions, we have avoided either citing or including in our reference list the many exciting papers written prior to 1973, since they are already amply documented.

General Considerations

Only two facts of general significance have emerged from the collective literature. First, bacteria subjected to sublethal stress produce repairable lesions. Secondly, bacteria subjected to sublethal stress become hypersensitive to secondary stresses.

When examined, injury has universally been accompanied by the leakage of cytoplasmic constituents into the suspending solution. This suggests that universal and collective lesion damages the cytoplasmic membrane. A second universally observed lesion is the degradation of ribosomes and ribosomal RNA. Although these two lesions have been consistently observed, one is reluctant to conclude that they are necessary for bacterial injury: that recoverable injury cannot exist without cytoplasmic membrane damage and ribosomes and ribosomal RNA degradation. Other lesions such as DNA breaks and enzyme inactivation have been less consistently observed and are unlikely candidates for the role as necessary causes of injury. But the evidence is convincing that DNA breaks and cellular injury correlate and that the repair of breaks in DNA mimics the repair of injured cells. Consequently, one comes to the not very informative conclusion that there are a number of possible different causes and modifiers of injury whose exact roles await further information.

Synergistic Interactions of Stresses

Since stressed bacteria are hypersensitive to secondary stresses, the various interactions of combinations of primary and secondary stresses should provide a rich opportunity to explore the theme of synergy in sublethal injury. Most of the investigations have used heat as the primary stress. Tsuchido *et al.* (1972) addressed the theme of synergism in their study of the interaction of antimicrobial chemicals and heat; Corry (1974) studied the interaction of possible protective chemicals and heat. She showed that the heat resistance of salmonellae was enhanced by increased concentrations of sucrose, glucose, fructose, sorbitol and glycerol. All of these solutes except glycerol showed a linear correlation between the logarithm of the D-value and the concentration of the solute. Such a linear relationship was not found between the water activity produced by these solutes and the D-value. Horner and Anagnostopoulos (1975) minimized the experimental variables by heating and recovering *in situ* on surface inoculated plates. The water activity of maximum survival was dependent upon whether sodium chloride, sucrose or glycerol was used to regulate the water activity. Also the effect of water activity on heat survival was dependent upon the test organism; *Salmonella senftenberg* was unaffected by reducing the water activity in the heating/recovery plates. Other investigators examining dual actions are Hurst, Collins-Thompson and Kruse (1973): heat and pH; Lee and Geopfert (1975): heat and solutes; Shibasaki and Tsuchido (1973): heat and chemicals; and Smolka, Nelson and Kelley (1974): heat and pH level and NaCl concentration, alone and in combination. Duitschaever and Jordan (1974) examined cells of *Streptococcus faecium* after recovery from heat injury to salt tolerance and found an increase in the unsaturated fatty acid composition of the cells. Further, these recovered cells showed an increased heat resistance and an increased tolerance to NaCl; they conjectured that this was a membrane phenomenon.

Synergism between primary stresses other than heat and secondary stresses has also been investigated. Minor and Marth (1972) examined the secondary roles of salt, heat and freezing on modifying the primary stress of acidification. Fay and Farias (1976) showed that preincubation at 0°C increased the bactericidal action of nonanoic and decanoic acid on *Escherichia coli*. They theorized that the lipopolysaccharide layer of the organism was the probable site of action. In a series of papers, Janssen and Busta (1973a, b, c) examined the influence of the milk constituents lactose, milk salts, casein, and whey proteins on the injury, repair and death of *Salmonella anatum.* They found that all of the constituents except whey proteins protected the cells from injury and promoted repair. Wu and Klein (1976), using starvation as the primary stress of *Escherichia coli,* evaluated the effect of mild heating. They showed that with prolonged starvation the cells became less sensitive to the secondary warming stress. This would appear to be, and perhaps is, a case where a primary stress reduces the sensitivity of the cells to a secondary stress, but it is not altogether clear that prolonging starvation is an increasingly stressful event. It might be productive to look further at starvation as a stress.

Starvation as a Stress

While the stress of starvation produces an injury type phenomenon that is amenable to recovery, a systematic study of injury and death by starvation has not produced systematic results. Whether a particular agent protects against or accelerates starvation death in a culture may be determined by the nature of the substrate that has limited growth of the culture. Postgate (1967) has reviewed some of these curious results. The substrate which limits growth of the culture may accelerate death of the culture when present in the starvation menstrum; this has been observed frequently enough to be given a name 'substrate-accelerated death'.

The stress of starvation has also provided an interesting example of negative synergy. A culture of *Enterobacter aerogenes,* that ceased growth because of exhaustion of glycerol, was sensitive to glycerol-accelerated death. This starved culture was also sensitive to the toxicity of 2,4-dinitrophenol. However, the presence of both 2,4-dinitrophenol and glycerol prevented both the glycerol-accelerated death and the toxicity of the 2,4-dinitrophenol.

Table 9.1 The use of starvation-stressed *E. coli* to study events of death and injury

Growth-limiting substrate	*Area of investigation*	*Reference*
Nitrogen-starved	Interrelationship of energy reserve and glycogen synthesis	Dietzler, Lais and Leckie (1974)
Guanine-starved	Synthesis and turnover of ribosomal RNA	Erlich, Gallant and Lazzarini (1975)
Carbon-starved	Fate of ribosomes and the degradation of RNA	Kaplan and Apirion (1974, 1975)
Glucose-starved	Ribosome degradation	Okamura, Muruyama and Yanggita (1973)
Amino acid-starved	Degradation of RNA by rifampin treatment	Rogerson and Ezekiel (1974)
Thymine-starved	Characterization of DNA	Nakayama and Hanawact (1975)
Carbon-starved	Sensitivity of secondary warming and nutrient addition	Wu and Klein (1976)

In order to give the flavour and scope of the possible exploitation of starvation-stress in the examination of death and injury phenomena, a brief sample of some of the current work on just the single organism, *Escherichia coli*, was assembled in *Table 9.1*.

Detection of Injured Microorganisms

Certainly the greatest concern of the practical food microbiologist is the inclusion of injured microorganisms in the procedures for enumeration. In the food industry, stressful situations abound for the bacterial cell. Injury can be produced by unfavourable oxidation–reduction potentials, chemicals in the food products, sanitizing agents and cleaning compounds. Bacteria may encounter any of the traditional preservative methods of heating, cooling, freezing, acidification, drying, sugaring, salting and even irradiating, all of which can produce a sublethal injury.

Once bacterial cells are injured, they are hypersensitive to secondary stresses which they may encounter in the enumeration procedure and not show up as viable. Such secondary stresses may be obvious, like selective agents and other challenges which border on being inhibitory to even non-stressed cells. Secondary stresses may also be more subtle, like the normally inocuous dilution water or warm agar.

The injury observed by Gray, Witter and Ordal (1973) produced by mild thermal stress of *Pseudomonas fluorescens* was subsequently found to be due to the secondary stress of the 0.1% peptone dilution water and could be relieved by using trypticase soy broth as a diluent. Years ago 0.1% peptone dilution water was recommended in the literature as a diluent for *P. fluorescens* and its suitability was separately confirmed for this particular strain, but when the organisms were injured, the 0.1% peptone dilution water was no longer satisfactory.

Ray and Speck (1973) reported on the heat stress of the warm agar used in pour plating. Klein and Wu (1974) showed that the transient warming stress of warm agar can be eliminated and the plate counts increased by using surface plating instead of pour plating for stressed cells.

Of course, the easiest way to enumerate injured organisms is simply to grow the culture in a rich, non-selective medium which poses no secondary stress. The Baird-Parker medium for selecting *Staphylococcus aureus* is the ideal exception: while it is highly selective and differential for *Staph. aureus*, it is also stress-free.

To detect most of the food pathogens or indicator organisms, however, it is necessary to use selective media. These media usually contain constituents which are inhibitory to the injured organisms but are not inhibitory to the unstressed or to the injury-recovered cells. Hence, before using such selective media for counting or growth, it is mandatory that any injured cells be allowed an opportunity to repair under non-selective and unstressful conditions. A number of schemes for the preincubation of injured cells on non-selective media to allow for recovery time have been suggested.

Preincubation in liquid non-selective media is adequate for the qualitative determination of a particular microorganism, but is less satisfactory in quantitation. If the preincubation is too long, it is difficult to distinguish between the repair of injured organisms and the growth of surviving and recovered organisms (Ray and Speck, 1973). Setting the time of preincubation short enough to assure no growth is not entirely satisfactory; times for recovery of a particular organism may vary as much as five hours. Monitoring the recovery by plating to determine the duration of the lag phase, which signals the end of the recovery period, makes for an unnecessarily burdensome procedure. These difficulties led to the use of solid media for preincubation (Hartman, Hartman and Lanz,

1975; Ray and Speck, 1973b; Speck, Ray and Read, 1975; Warseck, Ray and Speck, 1973).

One approach using solid media for preincubation is simply to surface plate the organism to be counted on a non-selective medium, incubate to allow for recovery and then overlay with the appropriate selective medium; Speck, Ray and Read (1975) used this approach to enumerate injured coliforms. The coliforms were surface plated on trypticase soy agar, incubated for 1–2 h at 25°C and overlayed with violet red bile agar. Hartman, Hartman and Lanz (1975) used a modification of this approach to enumerate injured coliforms. The coliforms were pour plated in a basal medium which had the composition of violet red bile agar except that the bile and dyes were removed. The pour plates were then overlayed with violet red bile agar containing double the usual concentration of bile salts, neutral red and crystal violet. Upon equilibration in the plate, the medium composition throughout is that of normal violet red bile agar. It is not necessary to incubate the plates between pouring and overlaying.

Another approach using solid media is the collection of the test organisms on a membrane filter, incubating the filter in contact with a non-selective recovery medium, then transferring the filter to the surface of an appropriate selective medium and incubating until colonies appear. The extreme flexibility of this method is immediately apparent, since the membrane filter with the organisms fixed in position can be easily transferred from one medium to another such that more than one non-selective medium might be used for recovery. Goff, Claydon and Iandolo (1972) tested repair using this membrane filter method on mix milk flora and Claydon (1975) adapted this method to pasteurized milk samples.

Appropriate supplementation of a selective medium may overcome the sensitivity of injured cells to the selective agents. This is apparently true of the Baird-Parker medium for staphylococci. In a like manner supplementation of various media with lysosyme appears to reverse the heat injury of *Clostridium perfringens* spores (Adams, 1974) and *Clostridium botulinum* spores (Alderton, Chen and Ito, 1974). When the germination system of *C. perfringens* spores is injured by heat the lysosyme serves as an artificial germination agent. Use of lysosyme allows an experimenter to bypass this injury lesion (Barach, Adams and Speck, 1974; Barach, Flowers and Adams, 1975).

The most probable number technique of counting is not usually suitable for enumerating injured organisms because a selective medium is usually needed in the tubes. If injured coliforms were to be determined by the most probable number technique, it would be necessary to use a non-selective medium in the tubes. After appropriate incubation for recovery, the tubes could be allowed to continue incubating and eventually each tube could be retested for coliforms, or alternatively, selective agents could be added and tubes eventually showing positive growth would be counted as positive.

Moran and Witter (1976) used the most probable number technique with a non-selective medium in the tubes to quantitatively enumerate injured and uninjured *E. coli.* The tubes were judged positive or negative after ten hours of incubation by measuring the presence of *E. coli*-produced glutamate decarboxylase with the Technicon Auto-Analyzer II system. This partially automated, rapid test is specific for *E. coli* and enumerates process-injured organisms.

References and Bibliography

ADAMS, D.M. (1974). *Appl. Microbiol.,* **27**, 797

ALDERTON, G., CHEN, J.K. and ITO, K.A. (1974). *Appl. Microbiol.,* **27**, 613

ALLWOOD, M.C. and HUGO, W.B. (1971). *J. appl. Bacteriol.,* **34**, 369

ALLWOOD, M.C. and RUSSELL, A.D. (1970). *Adv. appl. Microbiol.,* **12**, 89

ANDERSON, J.M. and BAIRD-PARKER, A.C. (1975). *J. appl. Bacteriol.,* **39**, 111

ANDREWS, W.H., DIGGS, C.D. and WILSON, C.R. (1975). *Appl. Microbiol.,* **29**, 130

BARACH, J.T., ADAMS, D.M. and SPECK, M.L. (1974). *Appl. Microbiol.,* **28**, 793

BARACH, J.T., FLOWERS, R.S. and ADAMS, D.M. (1975). *Appl. Microbiol.,* **30**, 873

BISSONNETTE, G.C., JEZESKI, J.J., McFETERS, G.A. and STUART, D.G. (1975). *Appl. Microbiol.,* **29**, 186

BOYLEN, C.W. (1973). *J. Bacteriol.,* **113**, 33

BUSTA, F.F. (1976). *J. Milk Technol.,* **39**, 138

CHEN, M. and ALEXANDER, M. (1973). *Soil Biol. Biochem.,* **5**, 213

CLAYDON, T.J. (1975). *J. Milk Food Technol.,* **38**, 87

CORRY, J.E.L. (1973). *Prog. Ind. Microbiol.,* **12**, 73

CORRY, J.E.L. (1974). *J. appl. Bacteriol.,* **37**, 31

DAVIES, R., SINSKEY, A.J. and BOTSTEIN, D. (1973). *J. Bacteriol.,* **114**, 357

DIETZLER, D.N., LAIS, C.L. and LECKIE, M.P. (1974). *Arch. Biochem. Biophys.,* **160**, 14

DUITSCHAEVER, C.L. and JORDAN, D.C. (1974). *J. Milk Food Technol.,* **37**, 382

ERLICH, H., GALLANT, J. and LAZZARINI, R.A. (1975). *J. biol. Chem.,* **250**, 3057

ERWIN, D.G. and HAIGHT, R.D. (1973). *J. Bacteriol.,* **116**, 337

FAY, J.P. and FARIAS, R.N. (1976). *Appl. environ. Microbiol.,* **31**, 153

FRANCIS, D.W., PEELER, J.T. and TWEDT, R.M. (1974). *Appl. Microbiol.,* **27**, 1127

FUNG, D.Y.C. and VANDEN BOSCH, L.L. (1975). *J. Milk Food Technol.,* **38**, 212

GOFF, J.H., CLAYDON, T.J. and IANDOLO, J.J. (1972). *Appl. Microbiol.,* **23**, 857

GOMEZ, R.F. and SINSKEY, A.J. (1973). *J. Bacteriol.,* **115**, 522

GOMEZ, R.F. and SINSKEY, A.J. (1975). *J. Bacteriol.,* **122**, 106

GOMEZ, R.F., SINSKEY, A.J., DAVIES, R. and LABUZA, T.P. (1973). *J. gen. Microbiol.,* **74**, 267

GOMEZ, R., TAKANO, M. and SINSKEY, A.J. (1973). *Cryobiology,* **10**, 308

GOULD, G.W. and DRING, G.J. (1974). *Adv. microbiol. Physiol.,* **11**, 137

GRAY, R.J.H., GASKE, M.A. and ORDAL, Z.J. (1974). *J. Food Sci.,* **39**, 844

GRAY, R.J.H., WITTER, L.D. and ORDAL, Z.J. (1973). *Appl. Microbiol.,* **26**, 78

GRIFFITHS, R.P. and HAIGHT, R.D. (1973). *Can. J. Microbiol.,* **19**, 557

HAMILTON, M.A. and BISSONNETTE, G.K. (1975). *J. Hyg.,* **74**, 149

HARTMAN, P.A., HARTMAN, P.S. and LANZ, W.W. (1975). *Appl. Microbiol.,* **29**, 537

HOADLEY, A.W. and CHENG, C.M. (1974). *J. appl. Bacteriol.,* **37**, 45

HORNER, K.J. and ANAGNOSTOPOULOS, G.D. (1975). *J. appl. Bacteriol.,* **38**, 9

HURST, A., COLLINS-THOMPSON, D.L. and KRUSE, H. (1973). *Can. J. Microbiol.,* **19**, 823

HURST, A., HUGHES, A., BEARE-ROGERS, J.L. and COLLINS-THOMPSON, D.L. (1973). *J. Bacteriol.,* **116**, 901

HURST, A., HUGHES, A. and COLLINS-THOMPSON, D.L. (1974). *Can. J. Microbiol.,* **20**, 765

JACKSON, H. (1974). *J. appl. Bacteriol.*, **37**, 59

JANSSEN, D.W. and BUSTA, F.F. (1973a). *Appl. Microbiol.*, **26**, 725

JANSSEN, D.W. and BUSTA, F.F. (1973b). *J. Milk Food Technol.*, **36**, 520

JANSSEN, D.W. and BUSTA, F.F. (1973c). *Cryobiology*, **10**, 386

KAPLAN, R. and APIRION, D. (1974). *J. biol. Chem.*, **249**, 149

KAPLAN, R. and APIRION, D. (1975). *J. biol. Chem.*, **250**, 1854

KLEIN, D.A. and WU, S.Y. (1974). *Appl. Microbiol.*, **27**, 429

LEE, A.C. and GOEPFERT, J.M. (1975). *J. Milk Food Technol.*, **38**, 195

MINOR, T.E. and MARTH, E.H. (1972). *J. Milk Food Technol.*, **35**, 548

MOATS, W.A. (1971). *J. Bacteriol.*, **105**, 165

MOATS, W.A., DABBAH, R. and EDWARDS, V.M. (1971). *Appl. Microbiol.*, **21**, 476

MORAN, J.W. and WITTER, L.D. (1976). *J. Food Sci.*, **41**, 165

MORICHI, T. and IRIE, R. (1973). *Cryobiology*, **10**, 393

MOSSEL, D.A.A. and RATTO, M.A. (1970). *Appl. Microbiol.*, **20**, 273

NAKAYAMA, H. and HANAWACT, P. (1975). *J. Bacteriol.*, **121**, 537

OKAMURA, S., MARUYAMA, H.B. and YANGGITA, T. (1973). *J. Biochem. (Tokyo)*, **73**, 915

PIERSON, M.D., PAYNE, S.L. and ADES, G.L. (1974). *Appl. Microbiol.*, **27**, 425

POSTGATE, J.R. (1967). *Adv. microb. Physiol.*, **1**, 1

PRENTICE, G.A. and CLEGG, L.F.L. (1974). *J. appl. Bacteriol.*, **37**, 501

RAY, B. and SPECK, M.L. (1973a). *Appl. Microbiol.*, **25**, 494

RAY, B. and SPECK, M.L. (1973b). *Appl. Microbiol.*, **25**, 499

RAY, B. and SPECK, M.L. (1973c). *C.R.C. Critical Rev., Clinical Laboratory Sciences*, p. 161

ROGERSON, A.C. and EZEKIEL, D.H. (1974). *J. Bacteriol.*, **117**, 987

ROSE, R.E., GELDREICH, E.E. and LITSKY, W. (1975). *Appl. Microbiol.*, **29**, 532

ROTH, L.A. and KEENAN, D. (1971). *Can. J. Microbiol.*, **17**, 1005

RUSSELL, A.D., MORRIS, A. and ALLWOOD, M.C. (1973). In *Methods in Microbiology*, vol. 8. Eds. Norris, J.R. and Ribbons, D.W. Academic Press, London

SEDGWICK, S.G. and BRIDGES, B.A. (1972). *J. gen. Microbiol.*, **71**, 191

SHIBASAKI, I. and TSUCHIDO, T. (1973). *Acta Alimentaria*, **2**, 327

SKALIY, P. and EAGON, R.G. (1972). *Appl. Microbiol.*, **24**, 763

SMITH, D.K., BENEDICT, C.D., BENEDICT, E.D. and WEINBERG, E.D. (1974). *Appl. Microbiol.*, **27**, 292

SMOLKA, L.R., NELSON, F.E. and KELLEY, L.M. (1974). *Appl. Microbiol.*, **27**, 443

SPECK, M.L., RAY, B. and READ, R.B., JR. (1975). *Appl. Microbiol.*, **29**, 549

STILES, M.E., ROTH, L.A. and CLEGG, L.F.L. (1973). *Can. Inst. Food Sci. Technol. J.*, **6**, 226

TANGUAY, A.E. and BOGERT, A.B. (1974). *Appl. Microbiol.*, **27**, 1175

TOMLINS, R.I. and ORDAL, Z.J. (1976). In *Inhibition and Inactivation of Vegetative Microbes.* Eds. Skinner, F.A. and Hugo, W.B. Academic Press, London

TOMLINS, R.I., VAALER, G.L. and ORDAL, Z.J. (1972). *Can. J. Microbiol.*, **18**, 1015

TRACI, P.A. and DUNCAN, C.L. (1974). *Appl. Microbiol.*, **28**, 815

TSUCHIDO, T., NAKAGAWA, Y., OKAZAKI, M. and SHIBASAKI, I. (1972). *J. Ferment. Technol.*, **50**, 93

WARSECK, M., RAY, B. and SPECK, M.L. (1973). *Appl. Microbiol.*, **26**, 919

WOODCOCK, E. and GRIGG, G.W. (1972). *Nature, New Biol.*, **237**, 76

WU, S.Y. and KLEIN, D.A. (1976). *Appl. environ. Microbiol.*, **31**, 216

10

STAPHYLOCOCCI IN CHEESE

A. SEAMAN
M. WOODBINE
Microbiological Unit, Department of Applied Biochemistry and Nutrition, University of Nottingham School of Agriculture, Sutton Bonington

Outbreaks of staphylococcal food poisoning due to contaminated cheese have been recorded but have greatly decreased since pasteurization of the milk before cheese-making has become a standard practice (Sharpe *et al.*, 1965). As sporadic cases are still reported, the origin of the staphylococci and the factors affecting their growth are of importance. Staphylococci in the milk tend to be concentrated in the curd at cheese-making (Takahashi and Johns, 1959) and increase until salting (Tuckey *et al.*, 1964). Pasteurization of the milk does not eliminate staphylococci from the cheese and Donnelly, Black and Lewis (1964) found that 22% of cheese made from pasteurized milk contained coagulase positive staphylococci of bovine phage type. Lyons and Mallman (1954) and Zottola and Jezeski (1963) had previously reported that there was much post-pasteurization contamination of cheese-making milk by staphyloccoci.

Food poisoning will only occur if these organisms grow in large numbers. Their growth is normally assumed to be inhibited by acid pH, but will also be affected by the extended lag phase which follows heat shock (Jackson and Woodbine, 1963) lactic acid *per se*, NaCl and the temperature at which the cheese is ripened. Toxin production is also affected by temperature and by the concentration of CO_2. *Staphylococcus aureus* is reported to grow in Cheddar cheese only over the range of 10–20°C (Abd-el-Malek and Gibson, 1951) but growth at 7.2°C has also been reported (Tuckey *et al.*, 1964). Enterotoxin production is slower than multiplication at lower temperatures and is reported to take three days at 18°C (Gastaldi, 1954). Since the upper limits of cheese ripening are 14.5°C for Stilton and 12.8°C for Cheddar, the temperature appears to control toxin production rather than numbers.

Modern selling techniques, with pre-packed cheese (where ripening has already reduced the acidity) in permeable or impermeable film and differing storage temperatures, may be affecting the balance of controlling factors. Over the last eleven years experiments in this laboratory have been investigating the relative value of these factors, firstly in laboratory media, then in cheese slurries, and finally by inoculating heat-shocked staphylococci into the cheese at manufacture.

Source of Staphylococci

Samples were taken from the milk reception and from the cheese on manufacture (in hoop) and during ripening, at a Stilton cheese factory which uses H.T.S.T. pasteurization. The initial load of staphylococci was established by plating on Baird-Parkers medium and counting after 26 h at 37°C. The results (*Table 10.1*)

Table 10.1 Incidence of staphylococci at Stilton factory

Source	N° X 10^5 g^{-1} or ml^{-1}	
Raw milk (10 samples)	0.39	2.1
	0.48	2.3
	0.50	3.2
	0.67	3.3
	1.50	7.4
Whey	0	
Fresh cheese (in hoop)	0.96	14.1
	1.00	19.7
	1.52	
1-Week cheese	1.0	9.1
	1.1	13.2
10-Day cheese	1.7	
2-Week cheese	0.1	2.6
	0.8	6.1
3-Week cheese	0.5	7.4
	1.4	

show a scattering ranging from 0.4 X 10^5 to 7 X 10^5 ml^{-1} in the milk and a maximum of 1.9 X 10^6 g^{-1} in the fresh cheese decreasing over 3 weeks to a minimum of 5 X 10^4 g^{-1}. This is in broad agreement with other workers (e.g. Sharpe *et al.*, 1965).

The phage typing of 75 colonies from these, using the international medical set of phages, gave only twelve typable strains and five of these were regarded as being of bovine origin. The 'bovine' strains came from both raw milk (three strains) and cheese (two strains). The low proportion typed by this set of phages is shown in *Figure 10.1*.

Subsequently, a bovine set of phages (Davidson, 1961) was used on the same isolates. Only three more strains were typable – all from cheese – but these, and the other eight typed with both this and the previous set of phages, were typable at RTD instead of the 1000 RTD when using the human set. Only two strains, both from milk, gave a 'human phage' pattern at RTD; three from milk and two from cheese did so at 1000 RTD.

Although the majority of strains remained untyped, all indications, from the numbers of strains and the strength of reaction, were that the majority of staphylococci were of bovine origin. The results were, however, not as clear-cut as those of Donnelly, Black and Lewis (1964) who identified 64 out of 89 food poisoning strains from cheese as being of the bovine type 42D. Stilton cheese is handled frequently in the early stages of ripening, but the source of the staphylococci, to judge from the fall in numbers and the phage typing, may be from

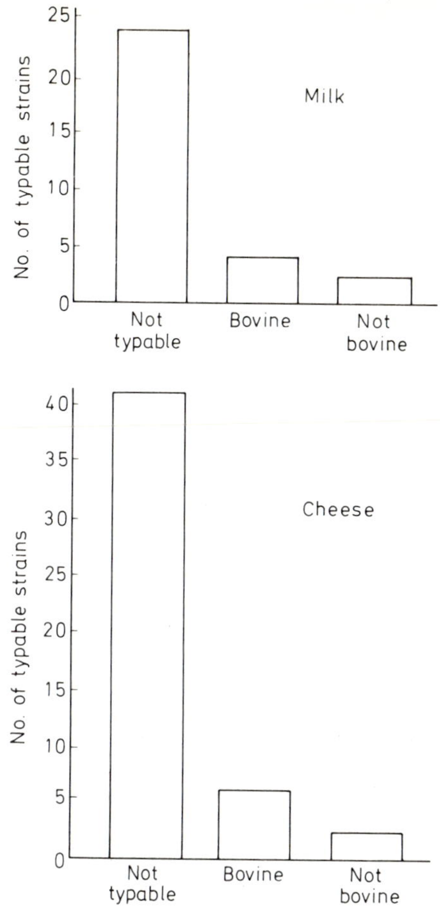

Figure 10.1 Histogram showing relation of all typable and non-typable staphylococci in milk and cheese

surviving organisms from the raw milk but is more likely to be due to recontamination from raw milk during the early stages of manufacture, since Hendricks, Belkropp and Chausler (1959) have found that the phage types isolated from food poisoning cheeses were the same as the phage types of the raw milk from which the cheese was made.

The Effect of pH

One of the main inhibitory factors in cheese is generally held to be the acid pH (Reiter *et al.*, 1964). The values determined by the British Standards method (Standard 770) for Stilton cheese obtained from one factory are shown in

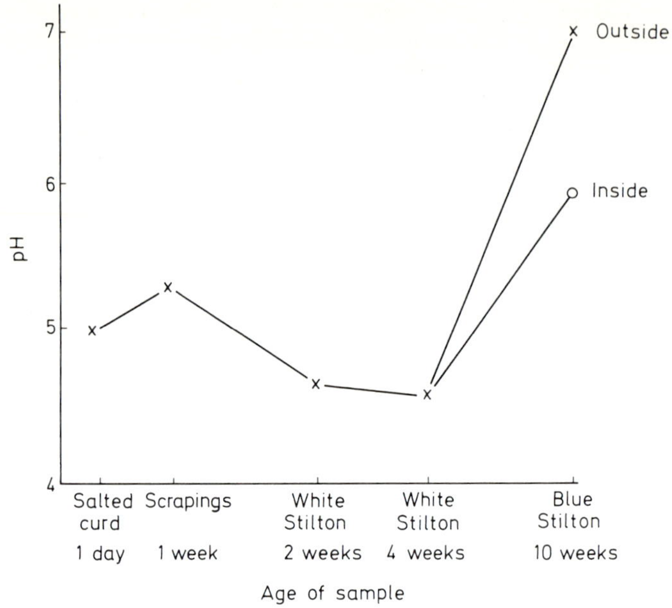

Figure 10.2 Graph of pH values of cheese samples during manufacture

Figure 10.2. The effect of these pH values on staphylococci has been followed in nutrient broth and in cheese slurries.

Staphylococcus aureus MF31 was incubated at 10°C in broth adjusted by HCl or NaOH to pH values between 3 and 7.5. The massive inoculation was of 10 ml of an 18-hour (37°C) culture into 300 ml of medium giving an initial level of approximately 3×10^7. A Miles-Misra plate count was performed after 1 and 2 weeks. The results (*Table 10.2*) showed that at pH 3.5 survival was below detectable values, at pH 4 and 4.5 there were survivors, but these were decreasing over the 2-week period. Above pH 4.5 the survival of the organisms did not seem adversely affected.

Table 10.2 The effect of pH on survival

pH	*Count ml*$^{-1}$ *(× 10*^{5}*)* *7 days*	*14 days*
3.0	0	0
3.5	0	0
4.0	0.18	0.03
4.5	0.72	0.6
5.0	7.1	13
5.5	217	165
6.0	224	270
6.5	270	270
7.0	141	330
7.5	111	106

The effect of pH on *Staph. aureus* in Stilton cheese slurries was measured indirectly by finding the heat resistance of six strains (all from food poisoning outbreaks) at various pHs.

Samples of 9 g of cheese curd (pH 5), white Stilton (pH 4.68) and blue Stilton (pH 6 and 7) were macerated with 90 ml Ringers solution and inoculated after reaching the experimental temperatures of 135, 140 and 145°F. Samples were withdrawn, cooled and plated at time intervals (usually six) and thermal death time curves established. These were linear, and statistical analysis showed there was no significant difference between the six strains ($P>0.05\%$). However, the pH was highly significant ($P<0.01$) in depressing the heat resistance as is shown in *Figure 10.3*, where the Z values are plotted against pH.

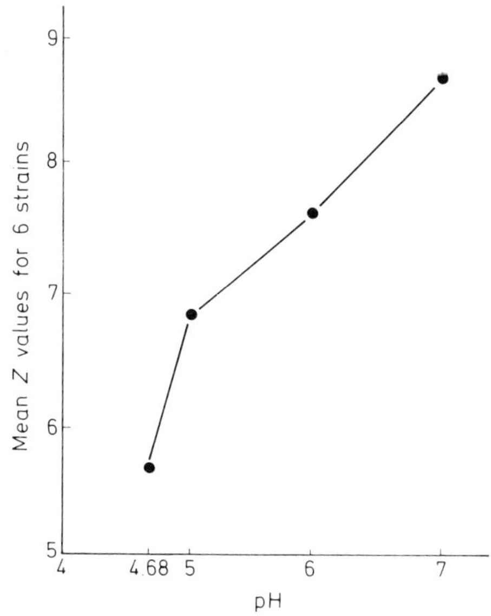

Figure 10.3 Graph relating Z values to pH of the cheese samples

It will be seen that there is a major difference between pH 4.68 and pH 5. This is in agreement with the work of Mattick, Neave and Chapman (1959), who found that the critical pH below which *Staph. aureus* was adversely affected was 5.2, and that differences of 0.1–0.3 units were significant. Sharpe, Neave and Reiter (1962) found a fast decline after a small initial multiplication when staphylococci were held in cheese at pH 5. The pH values during Stilton manufacture (*Figure 10.2*) mean that staphylococci are not held below this critical value for the first week, or again after the fourth week. The importance of this was shown accidentally in another series of experiments where staphylococci were inoculated into cheese slurries. A cottage cheese, slurried with phosphate buffer and inoculated with three strains of staphylococci at 10^4 ml^{-1} started at pH 4.6 and fell to pH 3.8 after 5 days. All three strains declined to undetectable numbers within 4 days (*Figure 10.4*).

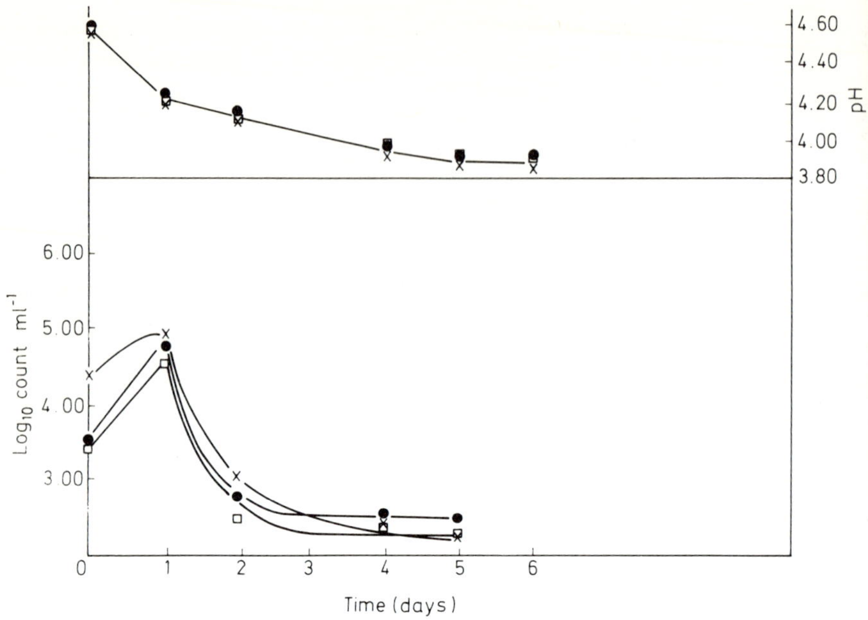

Figure 10.4 Relationship between nos. ml^{-1} of Staph. aureus *types 6/47 (X–X), 42D (□ – □) and 71 (● – ●) and pH and time in cottage cheese*

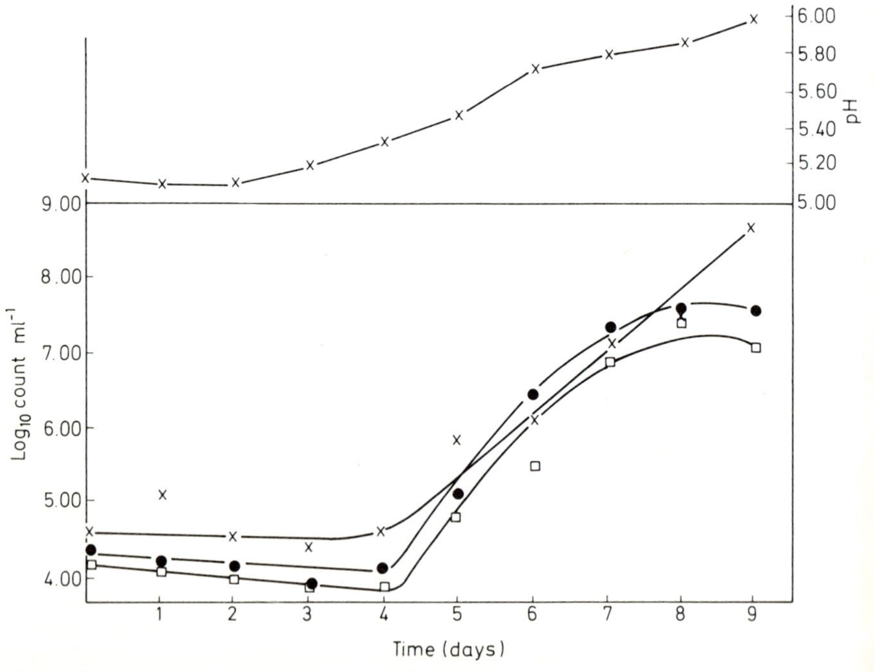

Figure 10.5 Relationship between nos. ml^{-1} of Staph. aureus *types 6/47 (X–X), 42D (□ – □) and 71 (● – ●) and pH and time in Cheddar cheese*

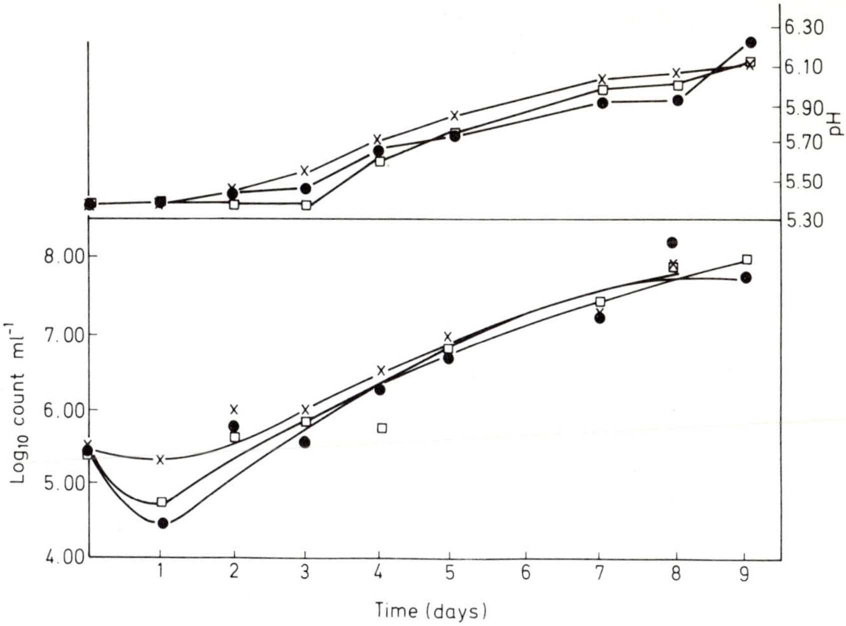

Figure 10.6 Relationship between nos. ml^{-1} of Staph. aureus *types 6/47 (X–X), 42D (□ – □) and 71 (● – ●) and pH and time in blue Stilton cheese*

Cheddar cheese and blue Stilton, slurried with a citrate buffer, were contaminated with a citrate-utilizing coliform. The Cheddar slurry (*Figure 10.5*) started at a pH of 5.1 and after 3 days this started to rise, reaching a pH of 6 after 9 days. The staphylococci started to increase after 4 days when the pH was approximately 5.3. The blue Stilton slurry (*Figure 10.6*) began at a pH of 5.3 and after 3 days this began to rise, reaching pH 6.3 after 9 days. The staphylococci, however, started to increase after 1 day, when the pH was 5.3. Both cheeses showed multiplication of the staphylococci at pH 5.3. McLeod, Roughley and Richards (1961) showed the persistence of the organism in cheese at pHs of 5.5–5.8.

The Effect of Caseolysis

The pH is affected not only by competitors but also by the staphylococci themselves which vary in their rate of acid production and in the ability to raise the pH by caseolysis.

The first effect of caseolysis seen in this series of experiments was with two strains (one isolated from a human carbuncle and one from bovine mastitis) which were grown in 10% reconstituted dried skim milk at 22°C for 6 days with an inoculum of 10^4 ml^{-1}. The milk was buffered with phosphate buffer over the range pH 5–6 in 0.2 unit steps. The results (*Table 10.3*) showed that the human strain produced a shift in pH, while the bovine one did not. The change in pH

Table 10.3 Changes in pH by staphylococci growth

Initial pH	*Change*		*Final pH*
	Human strain	*Bovine strain*	
5.0	0.6	0.2	5.6
5.2	0.6	0.1	5.8
5.4	0.9	–	6.3
5.6	0.5	0.0	6.1
5.8	0.6	0.0	6.4
6.0	0.3	–0.5	6.3

resulted in a final pH of approximately 6.3 for all initial pHs above 5.2. Counts performed during the 6 days showed an increase in numbers for all samples except those at pH 5.

When the growth of the two strains was compared on casein plates and in litmus milk it was apparent that the human strain was highly caseinolytic and fermented the lactose slowly while the bovine strain showed opposing characters (*Table 10.4*). This was confirmed when these strains, supplemented by another

Table 10.4 Caseolysis: acidity in litmus milk

Growth on casein plates:		*22°C*				*37°C*		
Strain	*Days:*	*1*	*2*	*3*		*1*	*2*	*3*	
Human		–	+	++		++	++	+++	
Bovine		–	–	–		–	–	–	
Acidity in Litmus milk:		*22°C*				*37°C*			
Strain	*Days:*	*1*	*2*	*3*	*4*	*1*	*2*	*3*	*4*
Human		–	–	–	–	–	±	+	++
Bovine		–	±	++	+++	++	++	+++	+++

caseolytic/non-caseolytic pair isolated from healthy humans were grown in unbuffered reconstituted dried skim milk at 22°C for 8 days. This resulted (*Figure 10.7*) in a change of pH from the initial 6.7 to 5.7–5.8 for the caseolytic strains and 5.3–5.4 for the non-caseolytic strains.

An attempt was made to follow differences between freshly isolated caseolytic and non-caseolytic strains of human and bovine origin. No caseolytic strains were found in 40 bovine isolates, so three strains were used to inoculate the surface of small blocks of Cheddar cheese in a technique described later. The cheese blocks were kept at 22°C.

The non-caseolytic strains of both human and bovine origin decreased rapidly in number (*Figure 10.8*). The caseolytic strain, however, maintained its numbers over 7 days. When blocks were stored at –8°C, 4°C and 22°C there were statistically significant differences in survival between strains at each temperature for

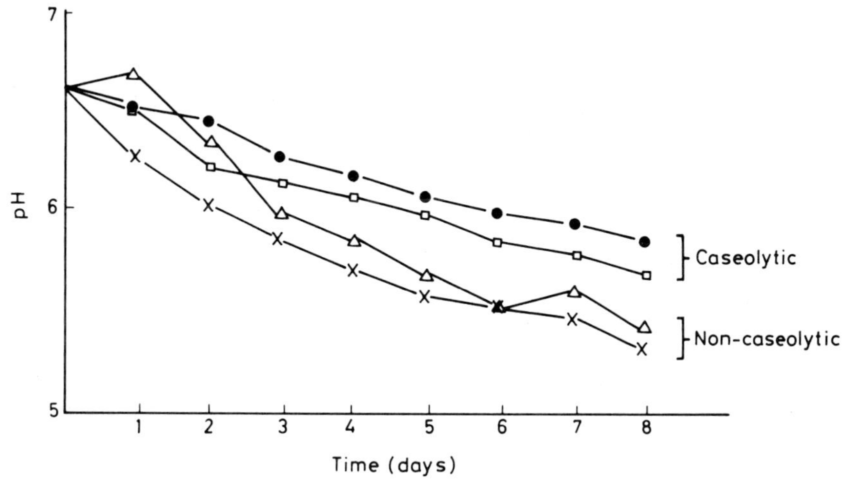

Figure 10.7 Changes in pH of skim milk during the growth of Staph. aureus

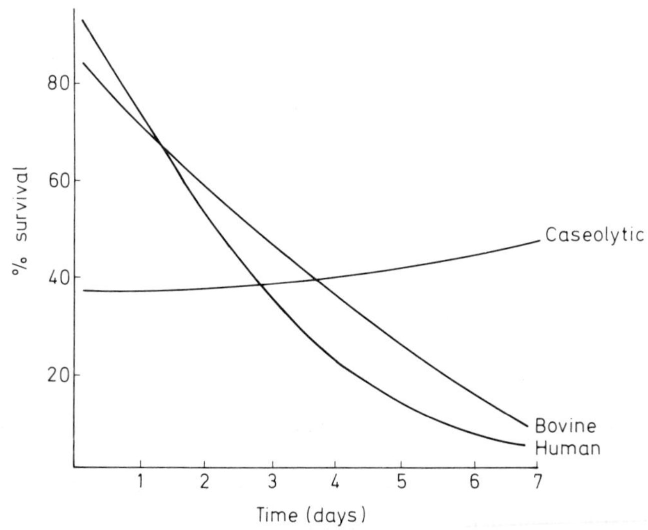

Figure 10.8 Survival of Staph. aureus *on Cheddar cheese surfaces*

Table 10.5 The effect of caseolysis on survival

Strain	% Survival at *−8°C*	*4°C*	*22°C*
Human non-caseolytic	25.7	34.0	7.7
Bovine non-caseolytic	74.7	59.8	7.2
Human caseolytic	21.3	10.8	37.3

Table 10.6 The relation of phage type to caseolysis

Phage group	*1*	*2*	*3*	*4*	*Miscellaneous*	*Untypable*	*Total*
No. in group	34	14	10	1	10	14	78
No. caseolytic	1	3	3	0	1	2	10

each strain. The only link with caseolytic ability appeared to be at 22°C (*Table 10.5*).

The caseolytic ability of staphylococcal strains needs further investigation but seems to be limited in range. Only 10 strains of 78 tested were caseolytic and this property was not limited to any one phage group (*Table 10.6*).

Lactic Acid

Lactic acid was reported by Nunheimer and Fabian (1940) to be the most active organic anion against *Staph. aureus*; this was confirmed by Minor and Marth (1972).

The effect of lactic acid is independent of the pH but the effect of the proportion of D- and L-isomers has not been reported. This was studied by a technique developed in this laboratory for inoculating the surface of standard cheese blocks. The cheese is cut to fit sterilized plastic cover slip boxes which normally store 18 × 18 mm microscope cover slips. After the top surface has been trimmed flush a standard depression is made by the pressure of a ball-bearing in an instrument designed for rheological studies on cheese.

The inoculum and any chemical for treatment is dropped by Pasteur pipette into this depression. If permeability is being studied the block is then covered with a plastic film before the lid of the box is replaced. After incubation the whole of the cheese block is slurried and counts made.

In these studies on lactic acid the hollows in the cheese surface were inoculated with *Staph. aureus* MF31 after 0.2 ml of lactic acid had been delivered with a Pasteur pipette and allowed to absorb into the cheese. Blue and white Stilton cheeses were used and incubated at 22°C.

Lactic acids were used at strengths of 10, 20, 30 and 40%. The effect on the pH of the cheese blocks is shown in *Table 10.7*. Even 40% lactic acid does not bring the pH of the blue Stilton to that of the untreated white Stilton. The pH

Table 10.7 Effect of lactic acids on pH of blue and white Stilton

Concentration		*Blue*	*White*
0%		6.8	5.55
	R	6.75	5.25
10%	D	6.7	5.5
	L	6.8	5.4
	R	6.6	5.1
20%	D	6.6	5.3
	L	6.65	5.2
	R	6.4	5.0
30%	D	6.5	5.2
	L	6.5	5.1
	R	6.25	4.8
40%	D	6.35	4.9
	L	6.45	5.0

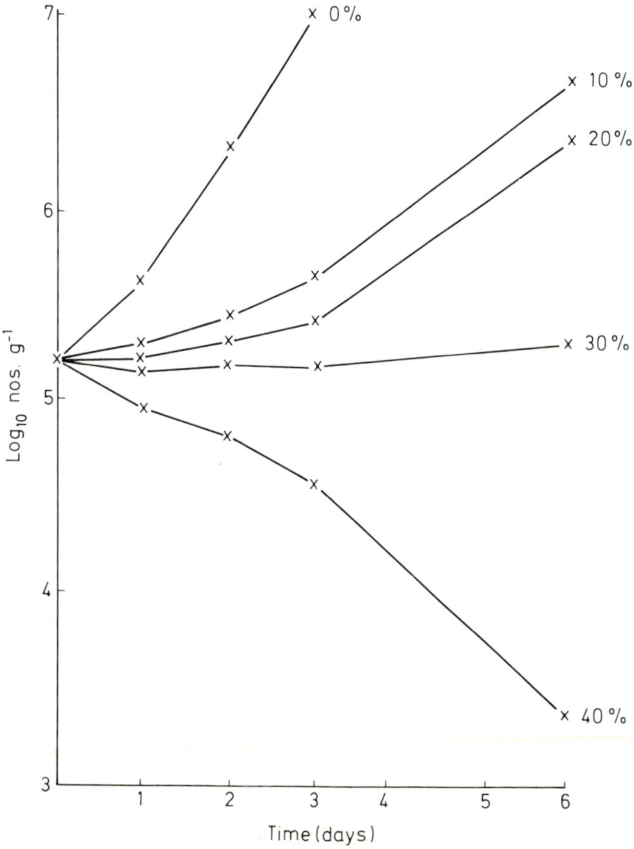

Figure 10.9 The effect of L(+) lactic acid on Staph. aureus *in blue Stilton*

of all blocks did not change significantly over the 7 days' incubation. The response of the staphylococci was similar for both blue and white cheese, in spite of the differences in pH (*Figure 10.9*). Forty per cent lactic acid was toxic under all conditions, while 10% lactic acid delayed growth to approximately the same extent. There were differences in response, however, to the forms of lactic acid at 20 and 30%. A typical example is shown in *Figure 10.10* where it is clear that

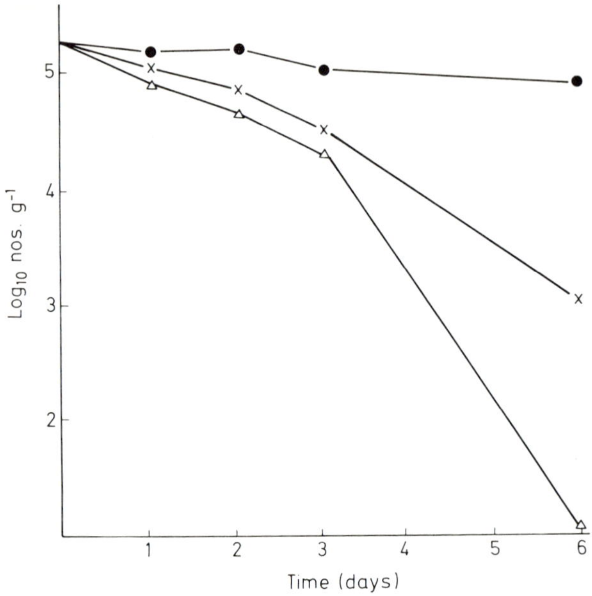

Figure 10.10 The effect of 20% lactic acid on Staph. aureus *in blue Stilton.* ●–● *= Racemic;* ×–× *= (+) isomer;* △–△ *= D (−) isomer*

the racemic form is the least inhibitory and the D-form the most. The difference in response to the isomers is marked but we have been able to trace little previous work on lactic acid racemase in staphylococci. Stockland and San Clemente (1969) record its identification in *Staph. aureus* and Stetter and Kandler (1973) characterize a racemase from several streptobacteria. Further work in this area is obviously indicated.

Salt

A single strain culture starter of *Str. lactis* was added as a 1% inoculum to fresh cheese curd to which NaCl had been added at concentrations of up to 25%. A culture of *Staph. aureus* MF31, which had been heat shocked at 52°C for 15 min, was then inoculated into the mixture. Counts were made over six days of incubation at 22°C. Without NaCl the staphylococci increased from 2×10^4 to 5×10^9 in 2 days and then decreased (*Figure 10.11*).

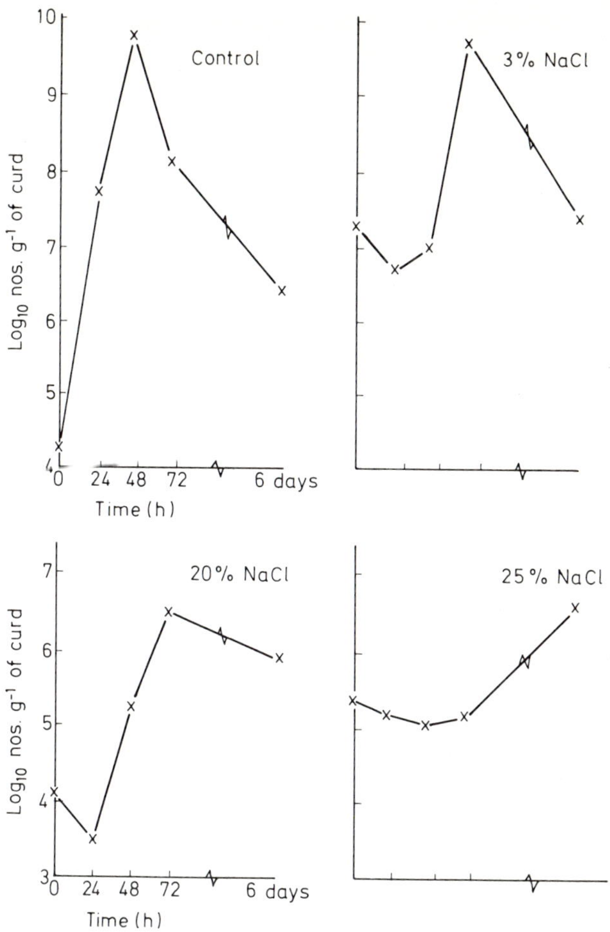

Figure 10.11 The effect of NaCl on the survival of Staph. aureus *in Cheddar cheese curd*

The effect of the salt was not obvious at concentrations of 3, 7.5, 9.5 or 15% although Iandolo, Ordal and Witter (1964) found that 8% NaCl was inhibitory for the same strain. At 20 and 25% the growth of the staphylococci was delayed and, once begun, was more gradual. There was no concentration found which prevented the final numbers of staphylococci being greater than the inoculum in spite of the fact that the cells had been heat shocked. Busta and Jezeski (1963) found that the same strain of staphylococci heated to 55°C for 15 min was unable to reproduce in the presence of 7.5% NaCl, but this has not been confirmed by the present study. Previous reports by Takahashi and Johns (1959) and Sharpe, Neave and Reiter (1962) that NaCl increased sensitivity to heat, were of experiments where exposure to the two stresses were simultaneous and not consecutive. The salt in a cheese is in the brine and in Cheddar, salting at 1.5% in a cheese of 40% H_2O results in a brine of 3.75% (Rammel, 1960). The higher levels of 2.25% NaCl and 37% H_2O result in a brine of 6.1% (Clark, 1971). The concentrations affecting the staphylococci were well in excess of those in cheese, even though the physical conditions were somewhat different.

Heat Shock

The effect of heat shock on numbers recovered by Mannitol Salt Agar was tested as a precursor to experimental contamination of Stilton cheese during manufacture, since both the agar and the cheese contain 7.5% NaCl. *Staphylococcus aureus* MF31 was heated in nutrient broth and plated on to M.S.A. The

Table 10.8 Survival after heat shock

Temperature (°C)	*% Survivors*	
	Heating for 10 min	*Heating for 13 min*
0	100	100
48	96	90
50	72	60
52	55	43
54	11	9
56	5	3

results (*Table 10.8*) show that 50% recovery was obtained by using a temperature of 52°C for 10 to 13 min and these two combinations were used to treat the cells used in the next experiment.

Survival in Blue Stilton Cheese

Milled and salted curd was obtained from a Stilton cheese factory and to each batch of curd, sufficient to make a 6 lb cheese, was added 7 × 10 ml aliquots of heat-treated *Staph. aureus* MF31. The curd was mixed at each addition and for a further 5 min after the last addition. The cheeses were then made in the normal fashion and matured at 15°C. Each type of cheese was made in duplicate. Needling was not considered necessary because of the small size of the cheeses. For counts, two 1 g samples were removed by corers and homogenized together in ¼ strength Ringers solution. The results (*Figure 10.12*) show an increase over the first three weeks to a level which was sustained for seven weeks for both the unheated staphylococci and those heated for 10 min. Those heated for 13 min increased slowly for four weeks and then declined. Since the staphylococci had been multiplying in the cheese for the whole of the normal ripening period, it was thought advisable to repeat the experiment with curd from a different factory. The heat-shocked staphylococci completely failed to establish themselves in these cheeses, and this was confirmed on a second attempt. The un-

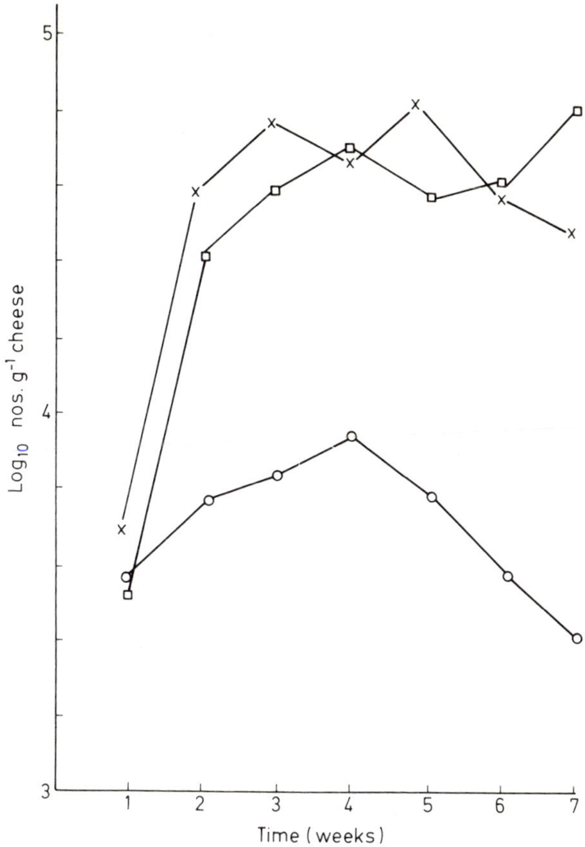

Figure 10.12 The survival of heat-treated Staph. aureus *in Stilton cheese.* □–□ *= Heated at 52°C for 10 min;* X–X *= unheated;* ○–○ *= heated at 52°C for 13 min*

heated cells (*Figure 10.13*) followed the growth pattern of the first factory cheeses for the first three weeks but then consistently declined. Two differences were noted in the curd from these factories. The curd from the second factory was closer-textured, and was machine-salted to a higher level than the hand-salting of the first.

Plastic Film

The final set of experiments concerned the effect of plastic wrapping on retail cheese. For these, Cheddar cheese was purchased locally. The technique used was that of surface depressions in cheese in plastic boxes described earlier. *Figure 10.14* shows that there was no difference in the decline of staphylococcal numbers under impermeable Saran, or permeable Cryovac, but that the decline was greater when no film was used. A more significant factor seemed to be the difference in pH between the two cheeses used. *Figure 10.15* shows the differ-

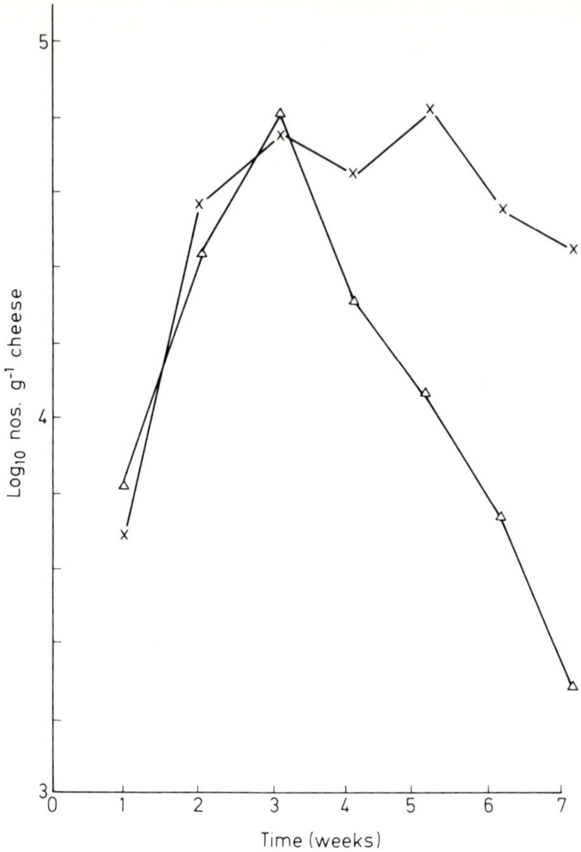

Figure 10.13 The survival of heat-treated Staph. aureus *in Stilton cheese of differing manufacture.* X–X *= factory 1;* △–△ *= factory 2*

ence between impermeable Saran and permeable Melinex to be greater. The effect was thought at first to be due to the rate of water loss but, as will be seen, the decline of numbers under Melinex is already greater before the difference in weight is observed. Although Soltys (1963) states that increase in CO_2 increases staphylococcal toxin production, the decline in staphylococcal numbers under the impermeable film indicates that this is not of practical importance in cheese wrapping. However, Cavett (1967) has warned that a misplaced trust in the hygienic and bacteriostatic effects of packing may cause a perishable product to be stored in unsuitable conditions.

Summary

This survey of factors affecting the numbers and growth of *Staph. aureus* in cheese confirms that the critical pH for controlling growth is 5.2 but, as the cells will survive lower pHs and for a large proportion of the ripening period the cheese

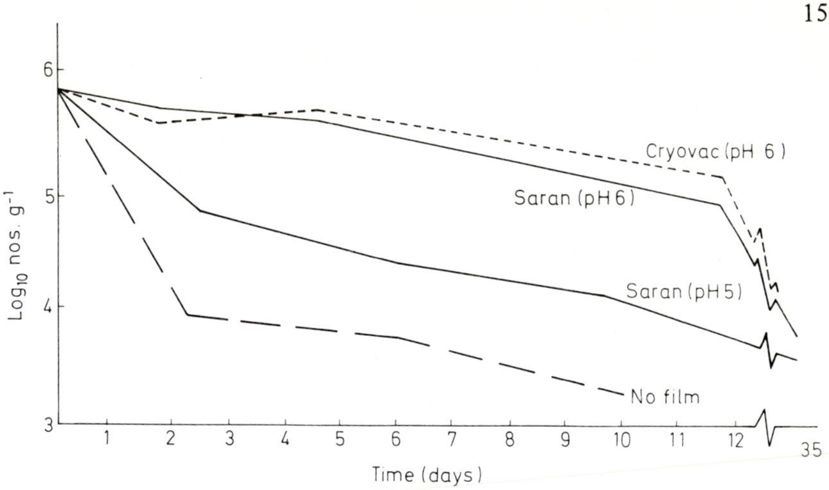

Figure 10.14 Effect of different plastic films on Staph. aureus *in Cheddar cheese*

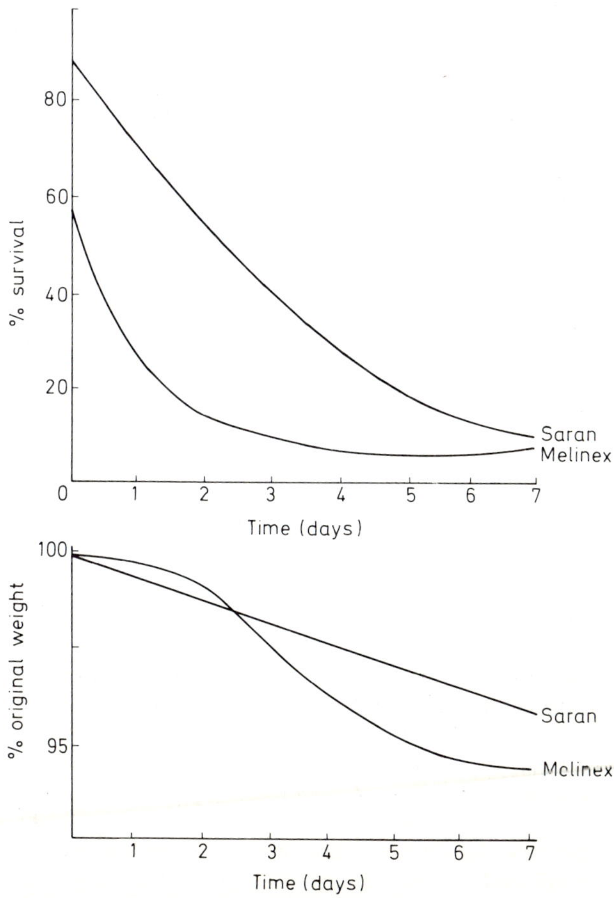

Figure 10.15 Effect of plastic films on weight loss and Staph. aureus *numbers in Cheddar cheese*

is above pH 5.2, other factors must interact. Points which need further investigation in particular are the role of caseolytic strains and the possible importance of the D- and L-forms of the lactic acid.

Even with the numbers of staphylococci found, toxin production at cheese temperatures is minimal, but modern production and sales practices may affect the complex interaction of pH, NaCl, lactic acid and heat damage which currently control food poisoning effects.

Acknowledgements

The work reported here was part of an undergraduate training programme and was performed by Marie Burton, J.A. Clark, Sally Higson, I.O. Holmes, M.J. Hurst, I.J. Sparham, W.R. Stevens, Valerie Stevenson and P.M. Tulloch. We are indebted to Dr. Davidson for the bovine phages and to Dr. Ordal for *Staph. aureus* MF31.

References

ABD-EL-MALEK, Y. and GIBSON, T. (1951). *Can. J. Microbiol.*, **3**, 203

BUSTA, F.F. and JEZESKI, J.J. (1963). *Appl. Microbiol.*, **11**, 404

CAVETT, J.J. (1967). *Prog. ind. Microbiol.*, **7**, 77

CLARK, J.A. (1971). Nottingham University dissertation

DAVIDSON, I. (1961). *Res. Vet. Sci.*, **2**, 396

DONNELLY, C.E., BLACK, C.A. and LEWIS, K.M. (1964). *Appl. Microbiol.*, **12**, 311

GASTALDI, C. (1954). *Riv. ital. Igiene,* **14**, 616

HENDRICKS, S.L., BELKROPP, R.A. and CHAUSLER, W.J. (1959). *J. Milk Fd Tech.*, **22**, 313

IANDOLO, J.J., ORDAL, Z.J. and WITTER, L.D. (1964). *Can. J. Microbiol.*, **10**, 808

JACKSON, H. and WOODBINE, M. (1963). *J. appl. Bact.*, **26**, 152

LYONS, P.H. and MALLMAN, W.L. (1954). *J. Milk Fd Tech.*, **17**, 372

MATTICK, A.T.R., NEAVE, F.K. and CHAPMAN, H.R. (1959). *XV Int. Dairy Congr.*, **3**, 1914

McLEOD, R.W., ROUGHLEY, R.J. and RICHARDS, T. (1961). *Aust. J. Dairy Tech.*, **17**, 54

MINOR, T.E. and MARTH, E.H. (1972). *J. Milk Fd. Tech.*, **35**, 191

NUNHEIMER, T.D. and FABIAN, F.W. (1940). *Amer. J. Publ. Hlth.*, **30**, 1040

RAMMEL, C.G. (1960). *J. Dairy Res.*, **27**, 341

REITER, B., FEWINS, G.B., FRYER, T.F. and SHARPE, M.E. (1964). *J. Dairy Res.*, **31**, 261

SHARPE, M.E., FEWINS, B.G., REITER, B. and CUTHBERT, W.A. (1965). *J. Dairy Res.* **32**, 403

SHARPE, M.E., NEAVE, F.K. and REITER, B. (1962). *J. appl. Bact.*, **25**, 403

SOLTYS, M.A. (1963). *Bacteria and Fungi Pathogenic to Man and Animals.* Balhiere, Tindall & Co, London

STETTER, K.O. and KANDLER, O. (1973). *Arch. Mikrobiol.*, **94**, 221

STOCKLAND, A.E. and SAN CLEMENTE, C.L. (1969). *J. Bact.*, **100**, 347

TAKAHASHI, I. and JOHNS, C.K. (1959). *J. Dairy Sci.*, **42**, 1032

TUCKEY, S.L., STILES, M.E., ORDAL, Z.J. and WITTER, L.D. (1964). *J. Dairy Sci.*, **47**, 604

ZOTTOLA, F. and JEZESKI, J. (1963). *J. Dairy Sci.*, **46**, 600

11

THE EFFECTS OF SO_2 AND CO_2 ON THE GROWTH OF *MICROBACTERIUM THERMOSPHACTUM*, A SPOILAGE ORGANISM FROM SAUSAGES

D. WELSBY*
A. SEAMAN
M. WOODBINE
Department of Applied Biochemistry and Nutrition, University of Nottingham, Sutton Bonington

Introduction

Microbacterium thermosphactum was first isolated – and so named – by McClean and Sulzbacher (1953) from pork sausages. The same organism has since been cited as an important component of the flora of sausages and of several other types of fresh and prepackaged meats (Rogers and McClesky, 1957; Gardner, Carson and Patton, 1967; Gardner and Carson, 1967; Dowdell and Board, 1968).

'The Preservatives in Food Regulations 1975' list 'sausages or sausage meat' as a specified food permitted to contain sulphur dioxide at a maximum level of 450 mg kg^{-1}. It is understood that this provision is made on the grounds that this concentration of sulphur dioxide suppresses the growth of salmonellae which are not infrequently found there (*see*, for example, Roberts *et al.,* 1975), and thus reduces the chance of salmonella food poisoning occurring.

Unpublished work by Leaton (1968) has indicated considerable resistance to sulphur dioxide by *M. thermosphactum,* and this corresponds with the reports of Dyett and Shelley (1966) and of Dowdell and Board (1967) concerning the effects of sulphiting on the flora of fresh sausages. According to these reports, the use of sulphur dioxide depresses the Gram-negative flora and results in the selection of a Gram-positive flora consisting of lactobacilli and *M. thermosphactum.*

The purpose of this work was to study the resistance of *M. thermosphactum* to sulphur dioxide and to investigate the possibility that carbon dioxide is implicated in this resistance. The work of Gardner, Carson and Patton (1967) indicated that high concentrations of carbon dioxide together with a depletion of oxygen selectively favours the growth of *M. thermosphactum* on pork stored under gas-impermeable films. Collins-Thompson, Witter and Ordal (1970) have more recently demonstrated that *M. thermosphactum* is in fact capable of fixing carbon dioxide into aspartate. Wrapped sausages containing sulphur dioxide

*Current address: Kerry Co-op. Creameries Ltd, Listowel, Eire.

preservative may, therefore, indeed provide a highly selective medium for the growth of *M. thermosphactum* and this possibility was a major consideration during this investigation.

Materials and Methods

Four strains of *M. thermosphactum* (from Dr. Dorothy Jones of the M.R.C. Unit, University of Leicester, designated G86, G100, G104 (type), and G107) were kept on nutrient agar slopes at about 5°C in the refrigerator and subcultured every 2 to 3 weeks. For the purposes of inoculation, 1 ml quantities of 18-hour cultures grown at 22°C in trypticase soy broth were used.

MEDIA AND CONDITIONS OF GROWTH

300 ml quantities of trypticase soy broth were inoculated with the standard inoculum of the appropriate strain.

250 ml quantities of broth were autoclaved at 15 lb for 15 min in 500 ml shaker flasks. An appropriate quantity of potassium metabisulphite (Analar grade) was added to 50 ml quantities of cooled, autoclaved broth and the resulting solution was filtered through a Sartorius membrane filter, pore size 0.45 μm, with a Sartorius glass-fibre pre-filter. This sulphited broth was then added aseptically to the 250 ml already in the shaker flask. Each of the flasks was duplicated and the sulphur dioxide concentration in each flask was measured before inoculation.

In experiments where the broth had to be both sulphited *and* carbonated, the procedure was as above, except that only 200 ml quantities of broth were added initially to the flasks. A further 50 ml was used to make up sulphited broth and membrane filtered as before, and to a further 50 ml was added solid sodium bicarbonate (Analar grade) and this carbonated broth was membrane-filtered separately. The two solutions were not mixed until they were in their diluted form to minimize the loss of carbon dioxide which occurred on mixing. The same concentration of bicarbonate (2.76 g^{-1}) was used in all the carbonated flasks, and this was calculated to produce an approximately 25% saturated solution of carbon dioxide at 25°C and pH 7. Flasks were placed in a Griffin orbital incubator at 22°C and continuously agitated during the period of growth-curve measurements.

SAMPLING AND TURBIDITY MEASUREMENTS

Samples were aseptically withdrawn at regular intervals after inoculation, and the optical density was measured in a 1 cm cell using a Unicam SP800 spectrophotometer at 600 nm. Duplicate samples were taken in each case.

SULPHUR DIOXIDE ESTIMATION

Sulphur dioxide concentrations in the broth were measured by direct iodometric titration, using a blank determination to allow for interfering substances,

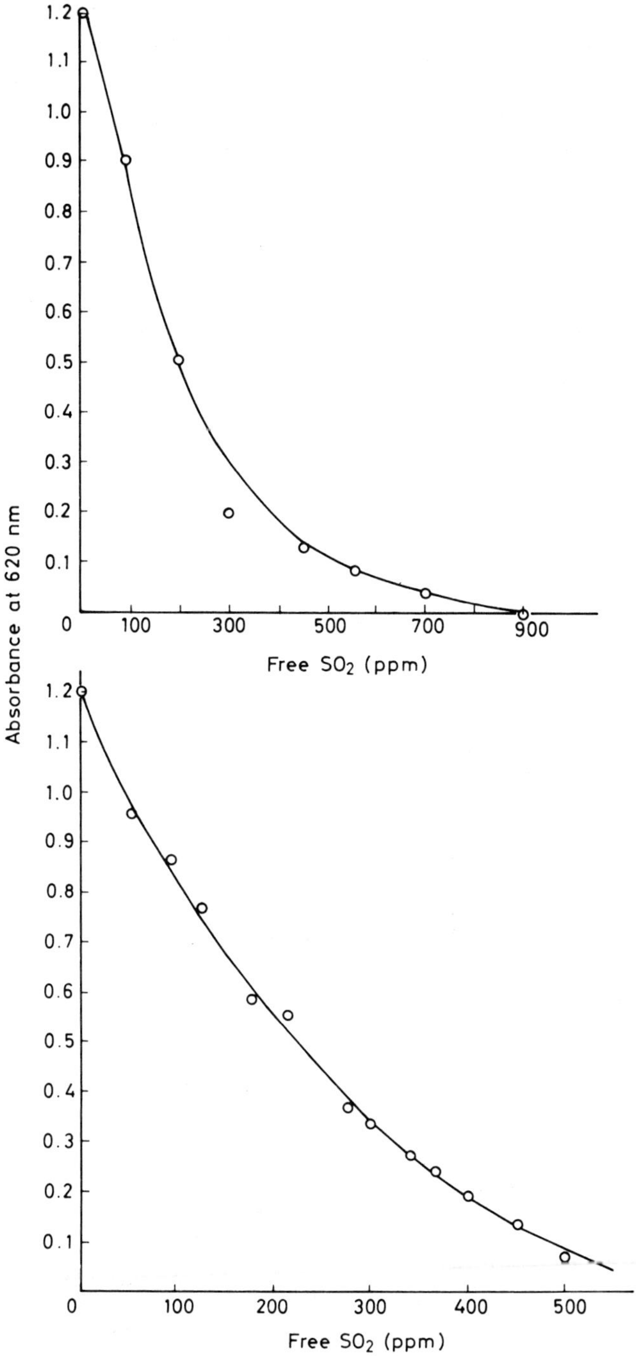

Figure 11.1 SO_2 calibration curve

or by a modified colourimetric procedure after Richter and Kny (1957). Malachite green is bleached by sulphur dioxide, and the degree of bleaching may be related to the free sulphur dioxide concentration. *Figure 11.1* shows the relationship between free sulphur dioxide concentration and absorbance at peak wavelength (620 nm). Towards the end of the log phase it became necessary to centrifuge off the cells to obtain a clear supernatant for sulphur dioxide determinations.

pH MEASUREMENTS

The pH was measured by immersing the glass electrode of a Pye pH meter into samples of broth withdrawn at the same time as samples for turbidity measurements.

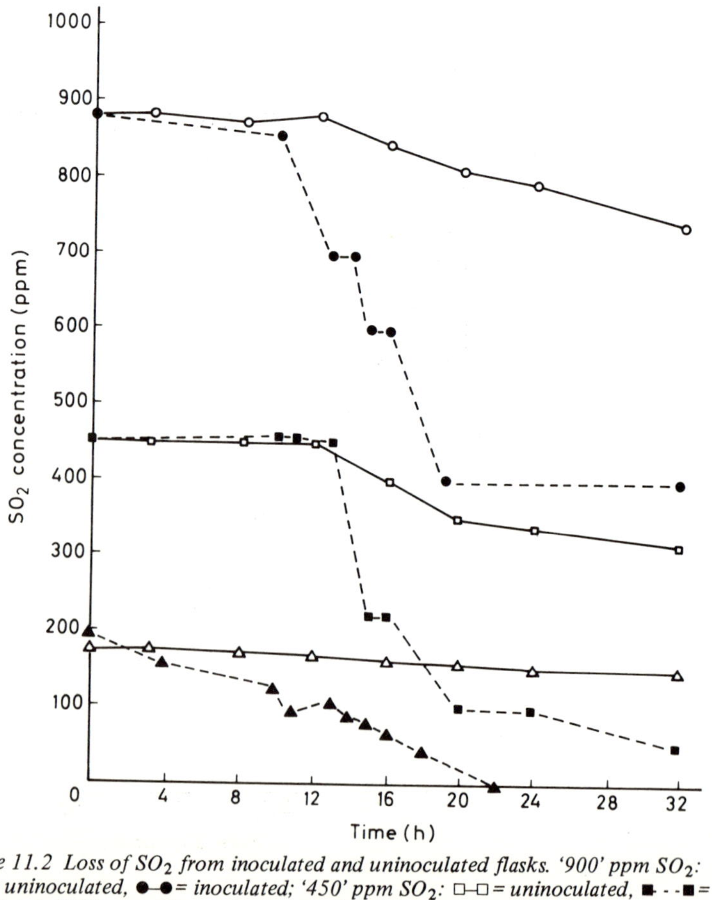

Figure 11.2 Loss of SO_2 from inoculated and uninoculated flasks. '900' ppm SO_2: ○–○ = uninoculated, ●–● = inoculated; '450' ppm SO_2: □–□ = uninoculated, ■- - -■ = inoculated; '200' ppm SO_2: △–△ = uninoculated, ▲- - -▲ = inoculated

Results

COMPARISON OF LOSS OF SULPHUR DIOXIDE FROM INOCULATED AND UNINOCULATED FLASKS

Figure 11.2 illustrates the fall in sulphur dioxide concentrations in uninoculated flasks and the averaged falls in sulphur dioxide for flasks inoculated with all four strains of *M. thermosphactum.* If potassium metabisulphite is added to give an initial concentration of 900 ppm sulphur dioxide, some 17% is lost from uninoculated flasks over a period of about 30 h. Some is presumably lost by binding with the carbonyl compounds present in the medium and some is undoubtedly lost by diffusion through the cotton-wool plugs of the flasks.

The growth of the organism increases the rate of loss and when the organisms enter their fastest phase of growth, the rate of loss of sulphur dioxide increased (*Figure 11.3*). This rapid loss of sulphur dioxide was most probably connected with the production of acid during carbohydrate metabolism, and the concomitant fall in pH (*Figure 11.5*). It is clear that only when potassium metabisulphite is added to give the highest concentrations of sulphur dioxide are there significant concentrations remaining after 30 h.

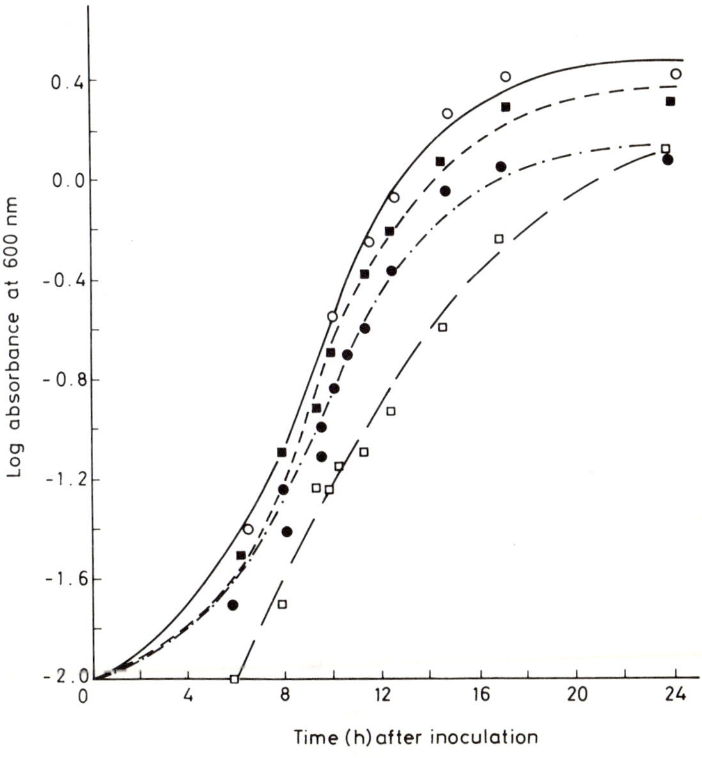

Figure 11.3 Growth of four strains of M. thermosphactum *in trypticase soy broth:* ○–○ = *G86;* ●–● = *G100;* ■---■ = *G104;* □---□ = *G107*

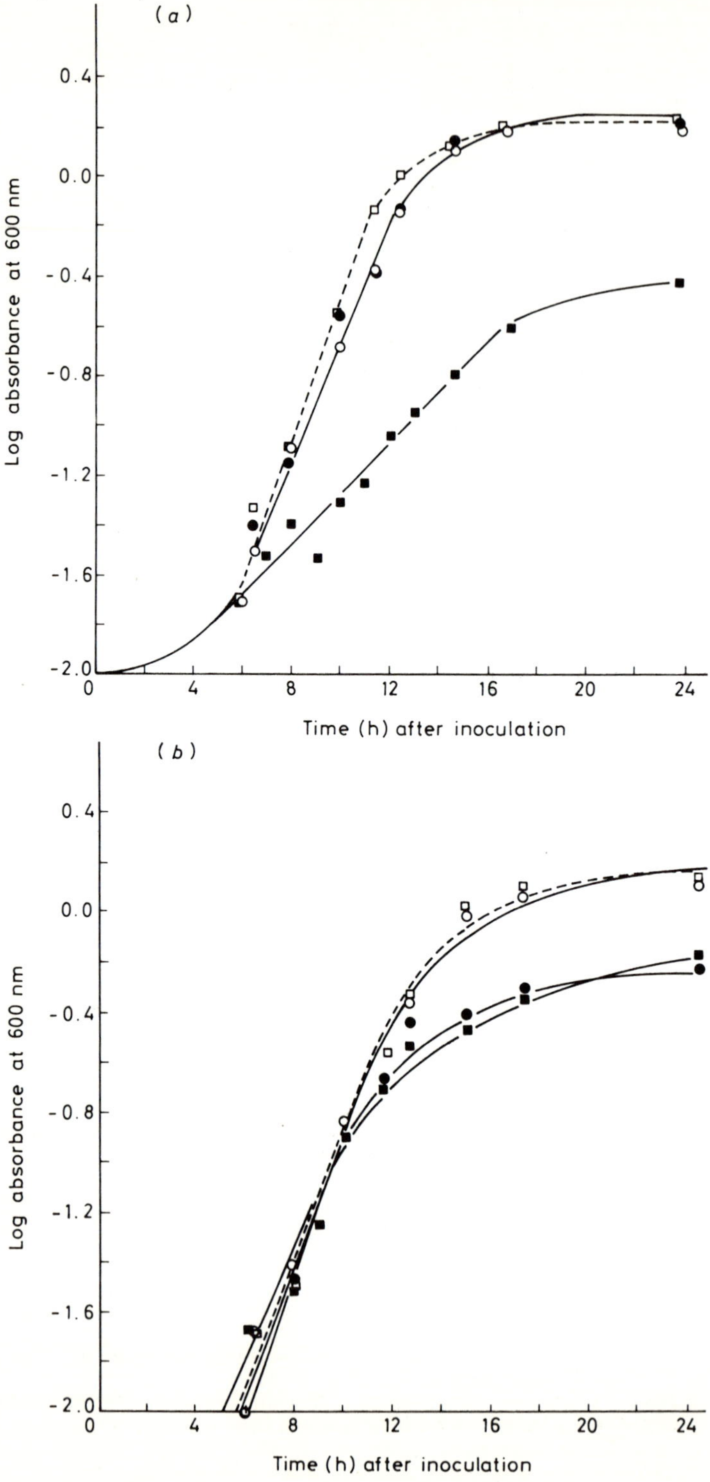
(a)
Log absorbance at 600 nm
0.4
0.0
-0.4
-0.8
-1.2
-1.6
-2.0
0
4
8
12
16
20
24
Time (h) after inoculation
(b)
Log absorbance at 600 nm
0.4
0.0
-0.4
-0.8
-1.2
-1.6
-2.0
0
4
8
12
16
20
24
Time (h) after inoculation

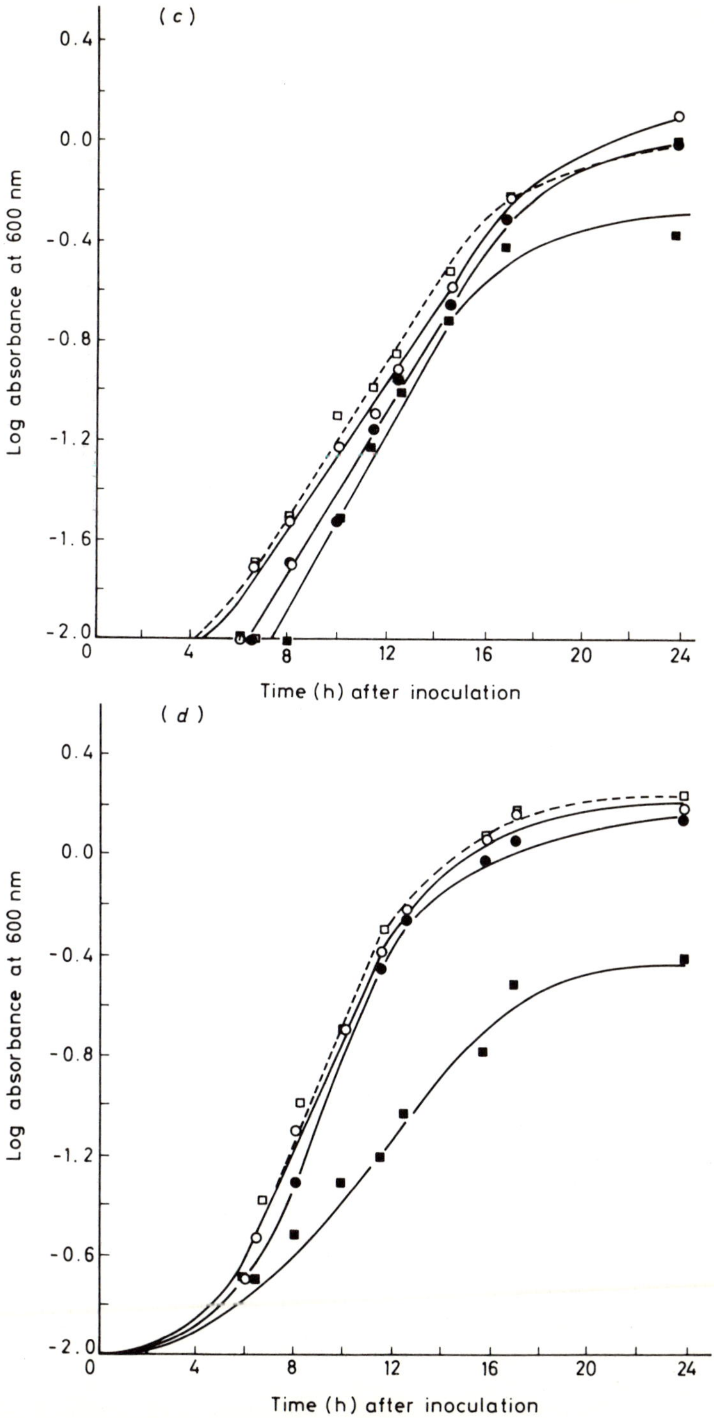

Figure 11.4 Effects of SO_2 on the growth of four strains of M. thermosphactum *in trypticase soy broth. (a) G86; (b) G100; (c) G104; (d) G107.* ○–○ = *Control;* □- - - □ = *'200' ppm SO_2;* ●–● = *'450' ppm SO_2;* ■–■ = *'900' ppm SO_2*

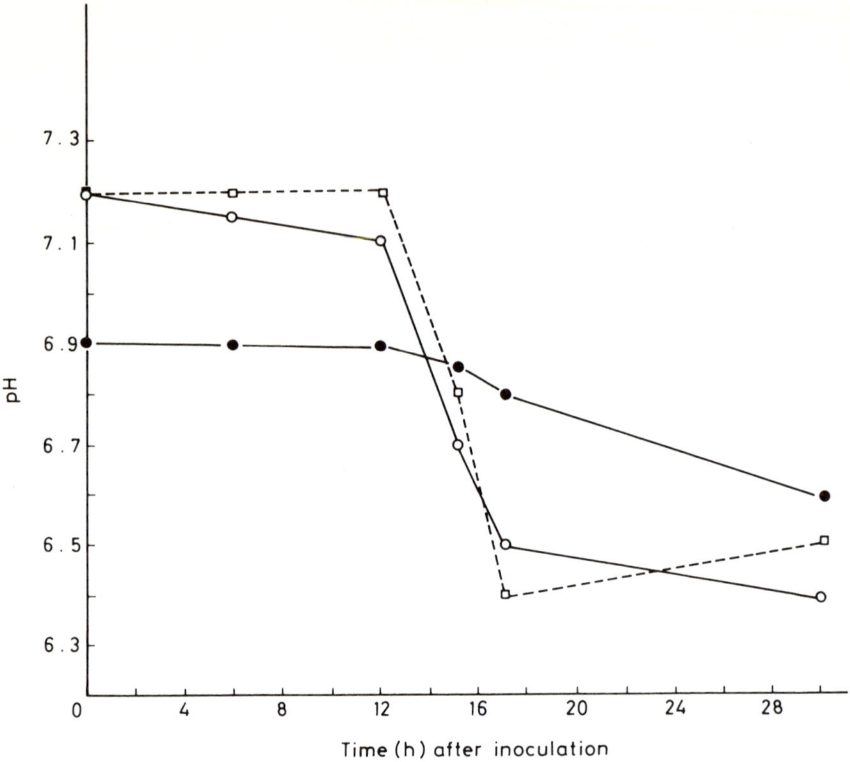

Figure 11.5 Changes in pH associated with the growth of M. thermosphactum *in the presence and absence of SO_2. ○—○ = Control; □- - - □ = '450' ppm SO_2; ●—● = '900' ppm SO_2*

GROWTH OF *M. THERMOSPHACTUM* AT DIFFERENT CONCENTRATIONS OF SULPHUR DIOXIDE

The rates of growth of strains G86, G100 and G107 were very similar in the absence of sulphur dioxide, having doubling times of 1½–2 h; strain G104 grew rather more slowly with a doubling time of about 3 h. The lag phases of all four strains were of approximately equal duration at about 6 h (*Figure 11.3*). *Figure 11.4* illustrates the effect of sulphur dioxide on the growth of all four strains when sulphur dioxide was present in the medium at initial concentrations of 200, 450 and 900 ppm. It is clear that only the highest concentrations of added sulphur dioxide have any *marked* effect on the growth curves of all four strains. There is some slender evidence that low concentrations of sulphur dioxide may even be slightly stimulatory.

COMBINED EFFECTS OF SULPHUR DIOXIDE AND CARBON DIOXIDE ON THE GROWTH OF *M. THERMOSPHACTUM*

In this experiment bicarbonate was added to both sulphited and non-sulphited broth, and growth curves were obtained as before. The two strains G86 and

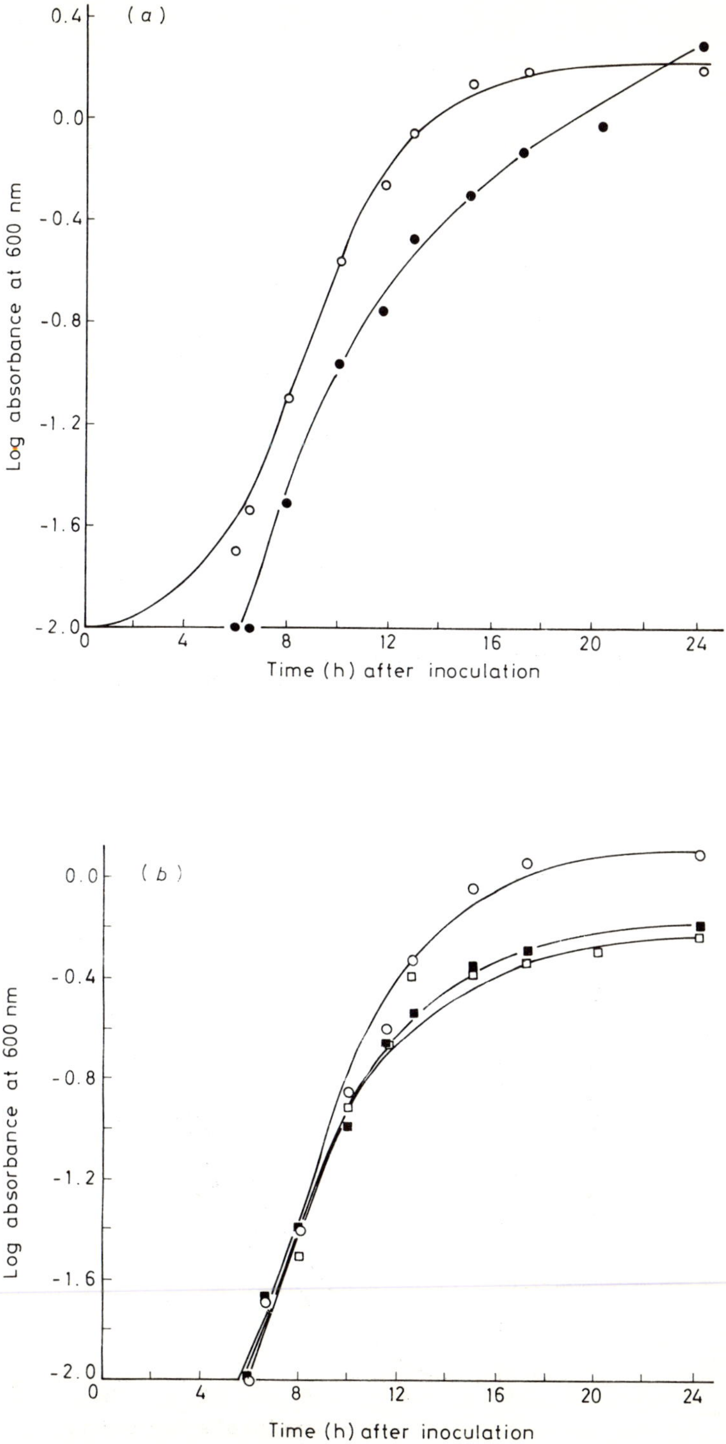
(a)
0.4
0.0
-0.4
-0.8
-1.2
-1.6
-2.0
Log absorbance at 600 nm
0
4
8
12
16
20
24
Time (h) after inoculation
(b)
0.0
-0.4
-0.8
-1.2
-1.6
-2.0
Log absorbance at 600 nm
0
4
8
12
16
20
24
Time (h) after inoculation

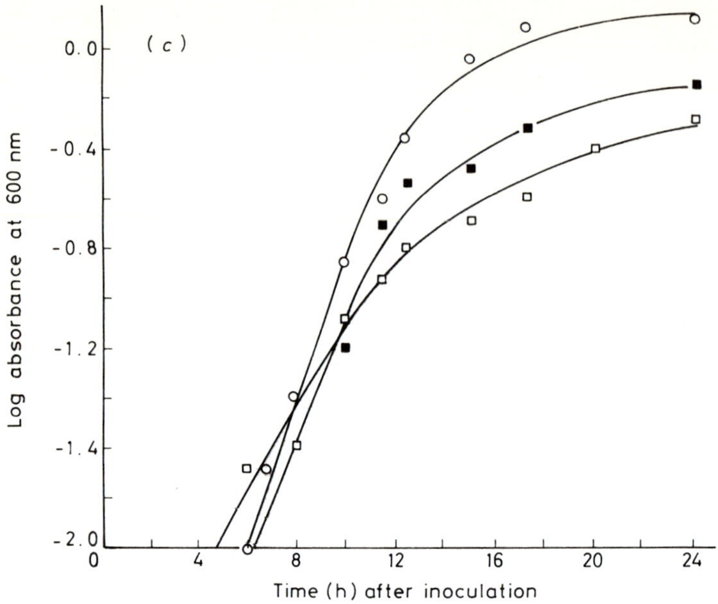

Figure 11.6 Effects of bicarbonate on the growth of strain G86 at various concentrations of SO_2. ○–○ = Control; □–□ = '900' ppm SO_2; ■–■ = '900' ppm SO_2 with added bicarbonate

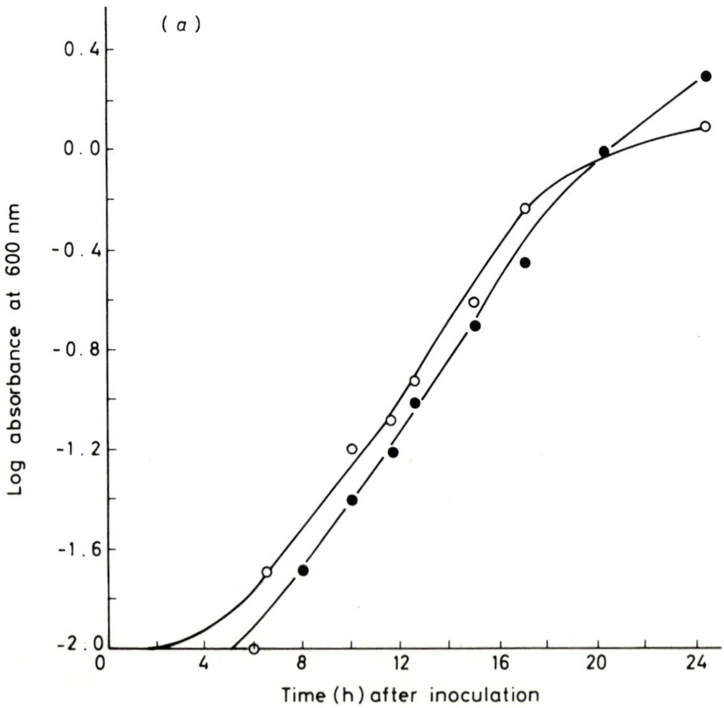

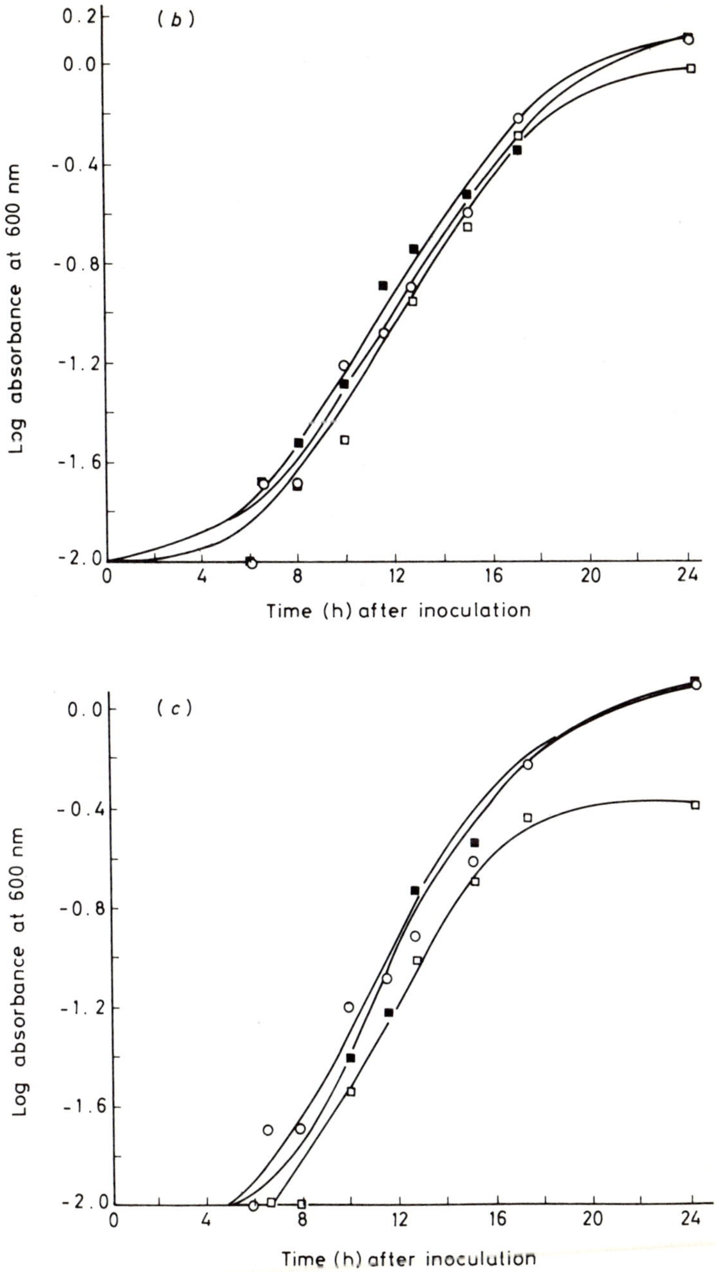

Figure 11.7 Effects of bicarbonate on the growth of strain G100 at various concentrations of SO_2. ○–○ = Control. (a) ●–● = bicarbonate added. (b) □–□ = '450' ppm SO_2; ■–■ = '450' ppm SO_2 with added bicarbonate. (c) □–□ = '900' ppm SO_2; ■–■ = '900' ppm SO_2 with added bicarbonate

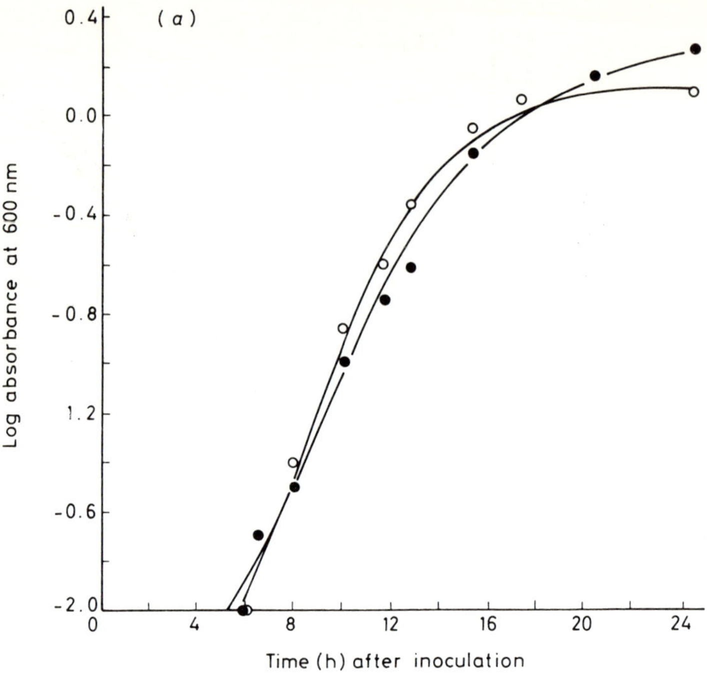
(a)
0.4
0.0
-0.4
-0.8
1.2
-0.6
-2.0
0
4
8
12
16
20
24
Log absorbance at 600 nm
Time (h) after inoculation

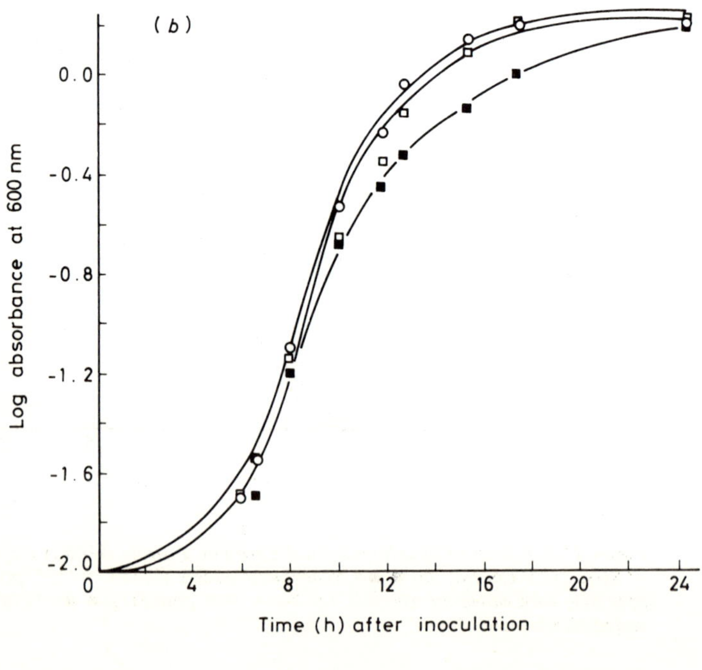
(b)
0.0
-0.4
-0.8
-1.2
-1.6
-2.0
0
4
8
12
16
20
24
Log absorbance at 600 nm
Time (h) after inoculation

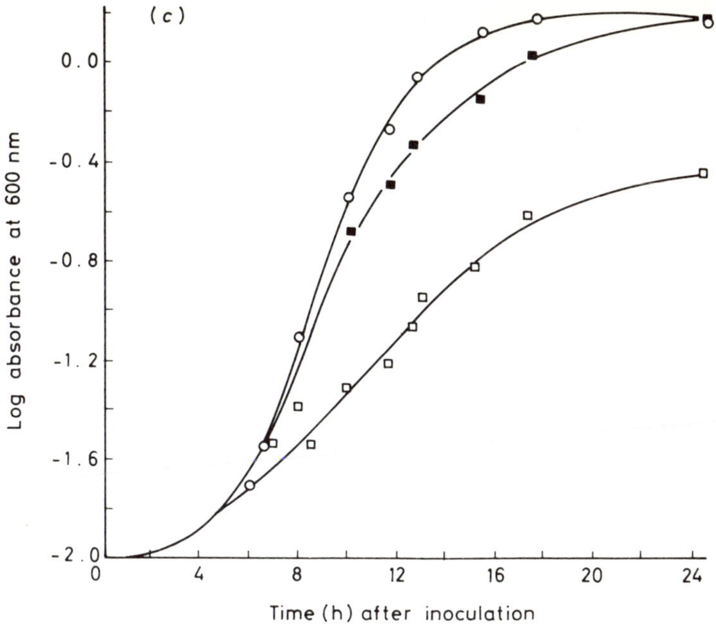

Figure 11.8 Effects of bicarbonate on the growth of strain G104 at various concentrations of SO_2. ○–○ = *Control. (a)* ●–● = *Bicarbonate added. (b)* □–□ = *'450' ppm* SO_2; ■–■ = *'450' ppm* SO_2 *with added bicarbonate. (c)* □–□ = *'900' ppm* SO_2; ■–■ = *'900' ppm* SO_2 *with added bicarbonate*

G107 showed a similar response to the presence of bicarbonate in the growth medium which was different from the response of the other two strains (*Figures 11.6* and *11.9*). G86 and G107 showed slightly increased lag phases over the controls, growth rates which were essentially similar to the controls, and then, after about 12 h for strain G86 and 15 h for G107, a slowing of the growth rates occurred. After 24 h no further decline in this new growth rate was apparent, and the cell numbers, as measured by optical density, showed no sign of levelling-off.

On strains G100 and G104, the effect of adding bicarbonate appeared to be the slight slowing down of the growth rate compared with the controls, and the onset of the stationary phase occurred later, and at a higher value of optical density than in the controls.

In general, flasks with added bicarbonate supported a heavier growth of *M. thermosphactum*, as measured by optical density, than the controls after 24 h.

The addition of bicarbonate to flasks containing 450 ppm sulphur dioxide depresses the growth of the organisms whereas sulphur dioxide alone has very little effect at this concentration (*Figures 11.6, 11.7* and *11.9*). Strain G104 provides an exception to this generalization, however (*Figure 11.8*). Here the addition of bicarbonate made only a slight difference to the rate of growth and to the optical density recorded after 24 h.

The addition of bicarbonate to those flasks containing broth with 900 ppm sulphur dioxide on the other hand, appeared in all respects to counteract the inhibitory effect exerted by sulphur dioxide alone at this concentration.

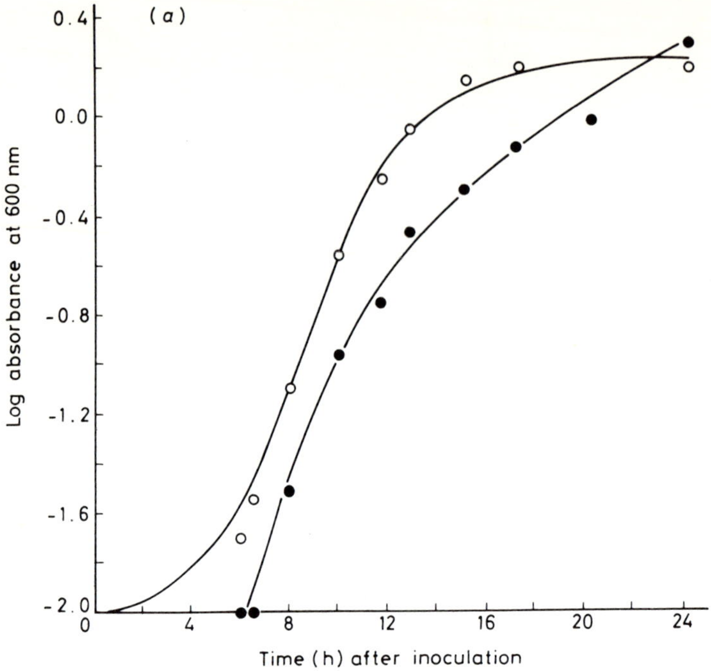
(a)
0.4
0.0
-0.4
-0.8
-1.2
-1.6
-2.0
Log absorbance at 600 nm
0
4
8
12
16
20
24
Time (h) after inoculation

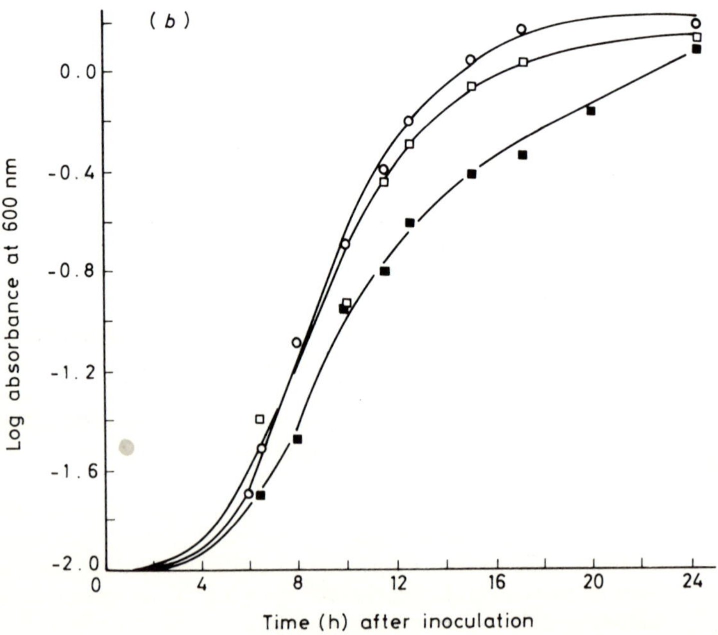
(b)
0.0
-0.4
-0.8
-1.2
-1.6
-2.0
Log absorbance at 600 nm
0
4
8
12
16
20
24
Time (h) after inoculation

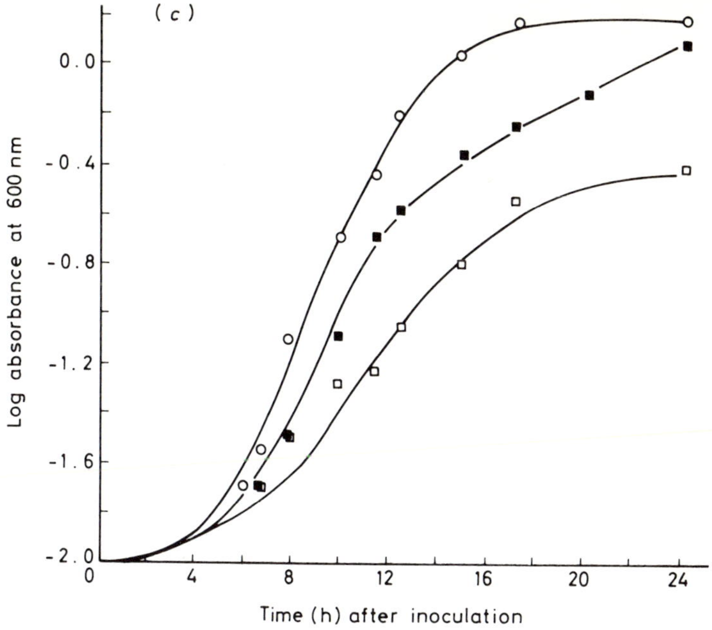

Figure 11.9 Effects of bicarbonate on the growth of strain G107 at various concentrations of SO_2. ○–○ = Control. (a) ●–● = Bicarbonate added. (b) □–□ = '450' ppm SO_2; ■–■ = '450' ppm SO_2 with added bicarbonate. (c) □–□ = '900' ppm SO_2; ■–■ = '900' ppm SO_2 with added bicarbonate

Discussion

Macris and Markakis (1974) have demonstrated that the reason for the extreme pH dependence of sulphur dioxide toxicity to *Saccharomyces cerevisiae* var *ellipsoideus* is attributable to the fact that it is molecular SO_2 which is the toxic agent and that molecules of SO_2 behave as though they are actively transported by enzyme-mediated reactions across the yeast cell membranes. Consequently, a fall in pH, which greatly increases the concentration of the toxic species in solution, greatly increases the rate of such active transport, and therefore the disruption caused inside the cell by this reactive moiety. However, although these findings concur with those of Rehm and Wittmann (1962), who reported that SO_2 is approximately 1000 times more effective than HSO_3^- in inhibiting *E. coli*, these workers did not exclude the toxicity of SO_3^{2-}. The importance of this observation lies in the fact that at the pH values of the broth used as a growth medium in these experiments (*Figures 11.5* and *11.10*), and indeed of most meats and meat products preserved with sulphur dioxide, the concentrations of free, molecular SO_2 are very low indeed. The toxic agent responsible for the observed changes in the flora of sausages preserved with sulphur dioxide is therefore likely to be a combination of HSO_3^- and SO_3^{2-}, and this combination does not have a great effect on the growth of *M. thermosphactum* at levels currently used to preserve sausages.

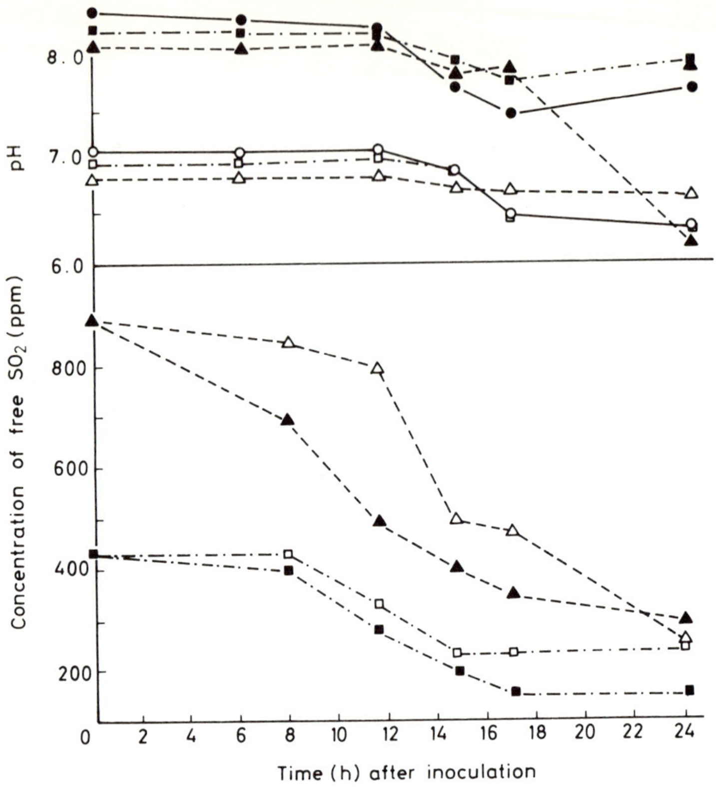

Figure 11.10 Changes in the pH and SO_2 concentrations associated with the growth of M. thermosphactum *in trypticase soy broth with and without bicarbonate.* ○–○ *= Control;* ●–● *= control with added bicarbonate;* □–□ *= '450' ppm SO_2;* ■–■ *= '450' ppm SO_2 with added bicarbonate;* △–△ *= '900' ppm SO_2;* ▲–▲ *= '900' ppm SO_2 with added bicarbonate*

Even at concentrations of sulphur dioxide around the 900 ppm level, rates of growth of *M. thermosphactum* strains G100 and G104 are not appreciably slowed, but the cultures grown in the presence of these high concentrations enter the stationary phase of growth at much lower absorbance values. This suggests that broth containing sulphur dioxide at these high levels supports a smaller number of organisms than the untreated broth. This phenomenon may perhaps be explained by the fact that carbohydrates in the broth are rendered unusable by the formation of hydroxysulphonate derivatives.

Presumably, if this supposition is correct, the organisms can overcome this growth-limiting factor if they are supplied with carbon from another source. Carbon dioxide supplied in the form of bicarbonate can act as such a source since the organisms can fix it into aspartate (Collins-Thompson, Witter and Ordal, 1970).

The implications of these data appear to be that sulphur dioxide is unlikely adversely to affect the growth of this particular spoilage organism at levels currently permitted in sausages. Increasing the concentration of carbon dioxide in the sausages by, for example, wrapping in a film which impedes the free diffusion of respiratory gases, probably further decreases the efficacy of sulphur dioxide as a preservative. Further, the growth of *M. thermosphactum* in sausages is in itself likely to reduce the concentration of sulphur dioxide to levels where it is no longer inhibitory to other organisms, either by the production of acid from carbohydrates (during growth) or possibly by producing substances that combine readily with sulphur dioxide.

References

COLLINS-THOMPSON, D.L., WITTER, L.D. and ORDAL, Z.J. (1970). *Biochem. Biophys. Res. Commun.*, **40**, 909

DOWDELL, M.J. and BOARD, R.G. (1967). *J. appl. Bact.*, **30**, ii

DOWDELL, M.J. and BOARD, R.G. (1968). *J. appl. Bact.*, **31**, 378

DYETT, E.J. and SHELLEY, D. (1966). *J. appl. Bact.*, **29**, 439

GARDNER, G.A. and CARSON, A.W. (1967). *J. appl. Bact.*, **30**, 500

GARDNER, G.A., CARSON, A.W. and PATTON, J. (1967). *J. appl. Bact.*, **30**, 321

LEATON, J. (1968). B.Sc. dissertation (Nottingham)

McLEAN, R.A. and SULZBACHER, W.L. (1953). *J. Bact.*, **65**, 428

MACRIS, B.J. and MARKAKIS, P. (1974). *J. Sci. Fd Agric.*, **25**, 21

THE PRESERVATIVES IN FOOD REGULATIONS (1975). S.I. 1487. H.M.S.O., London

REHM, H.J. and WITTMANN, H. (1962). *Z. Lebensmittunters. und Forsch.*, **118**, 413

RICHTER, J. and KNY, L. (1957). *Z. lebensmittunters. und Forsch.*, **106**, 337

ROBERTS, D., BOAG, K., HALL, M.L.M. and SHIPP, C.R. (1975). *J. Hyg., Camb.*, **75**, 173

ROGERS, R.E. and McCLESKEY, C.S. (1957). *Fd Tech., Champaign.*, **11**, 318

12

RECOVERY AND REVIVAL OF MICROBIAL CELLS, ESPECIALLY THOSE FROM ENVIRONMENTS CONTAINING ANTIBIOTICS

JANET E.L. CORRY
Metropolitan Police Forensic Science Laboratory, London

H. VAN DOORNE
Department of Pharmacy, University of Leiden, The Netherlands

D.A.A. MOSSEL
Department of Food Microbiology, University of Utrecht, The Netherlands

Introduction

An efficient method of isolating organisms is essential for almost any microbiological investigation, and when pathogenic or potentially pathogenic organisms are sought it is particularly important to have available reliable and sensitive methods for detection and enumeration of all the viable organisms present in the substrate to be examined. The sample could be from one of many sources – a human or animal feed, a pharmaceutical or cosmetic preparation, faeces or tissue, a swab from a drain or from a factory or slaughterhouse surface, or a sample of dust. In many situations the organisms present will have been exposed to one or more physical or chemical stresses, and the sample will contain cells sublethally damaged to various degrees of severity, in addition to dead and undamaged cells.

The rationale of attempting to isolate damaged organisms has been questioned. It is our opinion that this should always be done because there is evidence that sublethally damaged cells are still capable of causing infections, and that their pathogenicity after resuscitation is unaffected (Sorrels, Speck and Warren, 1970). However, *Salmonellae* after repeated sublethal heating have shown reduced pathogenicity, and similar treatment with gamma-radiation may show the same effect (Corry and Roberts, 1970; Epps and Idziak, 1970).

Cultural tests for the presence of microorganisms require that they are capable of multiplying, and consequently 'viability' is taken to be synonymous with the ability to form macroscopic colonies on agar, or visible growth in liquid medium after a limited period of incubation at a specified temperature. Whether or not a damaged organism appears viable depends very much on the conditions of cultivation; for instance, selective ingredients and even some nutrients in media which have no effect on undamaged cells may be lethal or at least inhibitory to damaged cells.

Although many publications over the last few decades have noted the importance of the conditions used for isolation and enumeration of 'damaged' or 'stressed' organisms (Curran and Evans, 1937; Nelson, 1943; Hartsell, 1951; Heather and Vanderzant, 1957; Sinskey *et al.,* 1964; Mossel, Jongerius and Koopman, 1965; Iandolo and Ordal, 1966; Corry, Kitchell and Roberts, 1969; Ienistea, Chitu and Roman, 1970; Mossel and Ratto, 1970; Caserio and Testa, 1971; Nelson, 1972; Raccach and Juven, 1973; Ray and Speck, 1973c; Stiles, Roth and Clegg, 1973; Gray, Gaske and Ordal, 1974; Barach, Flowers and Adams, 1975; Caserio, Turco and Gennari, 1975; Busta, 1976; Hurst *et al.,* 1976; Wilson and Davies, 1976), this aspect is frequently neglected during practical investigations. In addition, most studies to date have been carried out using bacteria damaged by physical factors, such as heating, freezing, drying or irradiating. This article will summarize information on the recovery ('resuscitation') of organisms damaged by chemicals and antibiotics, and will report some original investigations on resuscitation of microorganisms damaged by these agents.

Measurement of Inactivation

The effectiveness of antimicrobial compounds used to be tested by assessing the survival or death of a whole population only. More useful information can be obtained by determining numbers of survivors at intervals during treatment, and plotting $\log_{10}$ of the surviving fraction of organisms against the time of treatment, as is customarily done in examining the dynamics of death of populations of cells exposed to physical agents such as heating. When studying the death of antibiotic- or chemically treated cells it is particularly important to investigate the effect of possible neutralizing agents (e.g. proteins) in the stressing system, and the effect of varying the concentration of the antimicrobial agent and the initial numbers of microorganisms.

The survival curve obtained can be one of a number of different shapes including a straight line, but is often sigmoid with an initial 'shoulder' and a final 'tail'. The significance of the shapes has been discussed elsewhere (Sykes, 1965; Stumbo, 1965; Roberts and Hitchins, 1969; Brown and Melling, 1971). In some instances deviations from straight-line death curves can be caused by the experimental method employed, for instance 'shoulders' and 'tails' can be caused by clumps of organisms, but frequently no ready explanation can be found for the shape of a curve. This is hardly surprising considering that microbial death itself is likely to be caused by the interaction of numerous factors. However, the survival curve obtained usually has a portion where death is 'logarithmic' (exponential) and this can be used to calculate a decimal reduction time (D-value – the time, or with radiation, dose, under a given set of conditions, for the number of organisms to be reduced by 90%). To allow for deviations from linearity we have suggested that treatment should be expressed as the treatment required to give seven to twelve overall decimal reductions, which dispenses with the need to interpret multiphasic destruction curves – MPED (most probable effective destruction dose) – required to attain a given number of decimal reductions (Mossel, 1977). Methods of testing antimicrobial substances are discussed more fully elsewhere (Hugo, 1964; Crowshaw, 1976; Russell and Ditchett, 1976). Besides making allowance for sublethal damage when counting cells after treatment (discussed later), any residual chemical or antibiotic needs to be neutralized (*see* below). The resistance of organisms depends not only on the strain but on their history and their physiological state. For instance, rapidly multiplying cells (in the log phase of the growth cycle) are much less resistant than those in the lag phase or stationary phase of growth. Other factors that may affect resistance include the pretreatment growth medium, the composition, pH, redox potential and water activity of the suspending medium in which the cells are stressed, the initial population density, and the temperature of treatment (*see* later section on Resuscitation).

Neutralization of Inhibitors

Table 12.1 summarizes methods for neutralizing residual antibiotics or chemicals. Three main methods are used: enzymic inactivation, chemical inactivation and physical removal by dilution to a subinhibitory level, or washing (e.g. using a membrane filter). Enzymic inactivation has been used with success for several penicillins and cephalosporins (β-lactams), although care must be used to employ a β-lactamase that is active against the antibiotic in question. Lactamases are produced by a variety of bacteria. Resistance of bacteria to other antibiotics (e.g. chloramphenicol and some aminoglycosides such as streptomycin) may also be due to the production of degrading enzymes. These enzymes are, however, not widely employed as neutralizers, although Breeze and McAdam (1974) have suggested the use of chloramphenicol acetylase in the sterility testing of chloramphenicol. Understanding the mode of action of some other antibiotics has enabled effective neutralizers to be found; for instance, D-alanine neutralizes the action of D-cycloserine because of conformational similarity. Similarly, sulphonamides and sulphones compete with *p*-aminobenzoic acid during the biosynthesis of folic acid, and *p*-aminobenzoic acid is an effective neutralizer for sulphonamide- and sulphone-treated bacteria. The mechanism of action of neutralizers for other antibiotics cannot be so readily rationalized; divalent cations show some activity against tetracyclines (Newton, 1953; Weinberg, 1957; Hamburger, Carleton and Harcourt, 1957), which may be related to the tendency of tetracyclines to form chelation complexes with metal ions (Put, 1974). The use of recovery media containing sucrose and Mg^{++} ions prevents lysis of penicillin-induced spheroplasts, which may still be capable of multiplying and eventually revert to normal forms (Pennington and O'Grady, 1967; Bottone, Brandman and Schneierson, 1976). Similar media could be used for recovering organisms after treatment with other antibiotics that affect cell walls (e.g. bacitracin, D-cycloserine). For some chemicals and antibiotics, non-ionic surface active agents such as Tween or Lubrol-W have been found useful as neutralizers. Although some non-ionic surfactants may be toxic (Lamikanra and Allwood, 1976), they are sometimes used in combination with lecithin, or lecithin can be used alone. Lecithin is used for compounds which cause membrane damage (e.g. polymyxin, quaternary ammonium compounds and chlorhexidine), and its detoxifying action presumably depends on the high affinity of these agents for

Table 12.1 Neutralizing substances/methods for use in recovering antibiotic- or chemically stressed microorganisms

Agent	*Neutralizing substance/method*	*Reference*
Arsphenamines	Thioglycollate in meat medium	Sykes (1956, 1962) Russell and Gilbert (1964)
Sulphonamides, sulphones	*Para*-aminobenzoic acid (meat or serum-containing media)	Woods (1940), Vaichulis and Vedros (1966), Russell (1974b)
Sulphamethoxazole/ trimethoprim	Thymine	Anghern and Then (1973)
Chloramphenicol	Membrane filtration	Holdowsky (1957)
	Acetylase enzyme	Breeze and McAdam (1974)
Penicillins/ cephalosporins	Penicillinases (β-lactamases) or membrane filtration (0.33 M sucrose + 0.01 M Mg^{++} prevents lysis of spheroplasts)	Hugo and Russell (1961) Russell, Morris and Allwood (1973)
Cycloserine	D-alanine	Bondi, Kornblum and Forte (1957), Pittillo and Foster (1953)
Tetracyclines	Di-valent cations (Mg^{++}, Ca^{++}, Mn^{++}, Fe^{++}[+], Cu^{++}), membrane filtration	Weinberg (1954, 1957), Holdowsky (1957), Russell (1974c), Hamburger, Carleton and Harcourt (1957)
Streptomycin	Membrane filtration, cysteine	Sykes (1956), Holdowsky (1957)
Tobramycin	Mg^{++}	Russell (1974a)
Neomycin	Membrane filtration	Sykes and Hooper (1959)
Polymyxin	Lecithin, phosphatides, membrane filtration, Mg^{++}, Ca^{++}, Mn^{++}, Fe^{++}[+]	Bliss, Chandler and Schoenbach (1949), Russell (1974b), Newton (1953)
Quaternary ammonium compounds chlorhexidrine	Lubrol-W, Tween 80 ± lecithin	Hugo (1964), Russell and Gilbert (1964)
Bacitracin	Membrane filtration, ethylene diaminetetra-acetic acid (EDTA)	Holdowsky (1957), Weinberg (1959)
Mercury compounds	SH compounds (cysteine, thioglycollate)	Sykes (1956), Russell and Gilbert (1964)
Halogens	Nutrient medium, sodium thiosulphate	Russell (1974b), MacKinnon (1974), Hugo (1964)
Para-hydroxybenzoic acid esters	Tween 20 or 80	Patel and Kostenbauder (1958), Pisano and Kostenbauder (1959) Blaug and Ahsan (1961)
Phenols and cresols	Dilution, serum-containing media, Tween 80	Hugo (1964), Russell (1974b), MacKinnon (1974)
Formaldehyde	Morpholine + dimedone, dilution, nutrient broth, sodium metabisulphite	Hugo (1964), Russell (1974b), McKinnon (1974)
Glutaraldehyde	Glycine, thioglycollate, cystine, sodium bisulphite	Russell (1974c), Gorman and Scott (1976)

phospholipids. Most protein-containing media have some (non-specific) neutralizing effect against antibacterial agents in addition to their dilution effect. Serum or meat-containing media have been used especially for phenol- or cresol-treated cells, but this method would be ineffective for detecting low numbers or survivors. The most popular method at present, for examining pharmaceutical products containing antibiotics or other antimicrobial substances, is to use membrane filtration followed by rinsing.

The disadvantage of most of the above procedures is that they only remove residual free inhibitors; some antimicrobials bind firmly onto cells and would not be removed by dilution or filtration. Similarly, the inhibitors might not be available for chemical neutralization. An illustration of this is that serum is an efficient neutralizer of mercuric chloride if added before a microorganism, but inefficient if added after (Cook and Steel, 1959).

Another possibility is that the neutralizer can itself be toxic. This has been demonstrated for some organisms with thioglycollate, which is used as a neutralizer for arsphenamines and mercury compounds (Mossel and Beerens, 1968); D-alanine (Lark and Lark, 1959); for sodium thiosulphate and bisulphite, used for neutralization of halides and aldehydes respectively (MacKinnon, 1974); and for some non-ionic surfactants (Lamikanra and Allwood, 1976).

In practice, therefore, before attempting to isolate organisms from an environment containing microbial substances, it is necessary to try to ensure that (*a*) the inhibitor is completely removed or neutralized, and (*b*) that, if a neutralizer is used, it is not toxic to the organism(s) sought; it is difficult to be completely sure in either case, particularly (*b*). Complete inactivation of the antimicrobial agents present in the preparation can be checked by use of known sensitive strains; absence of toxicity from the neutralizer can be checked in essentially the same way. A wide variety of strains should be tested. It should be noted that neutralizers, as well as selective recovery media that are not inhibitory to healthy cells, may affect those sublethally damaged (*see* next section). While it is possible to check that a recovery method is non-toxic to undamaged organisms, it is not possible to do this in a system where organisms are damaged. This is because there is no way of counting absolute numbers of damaged cells. A recovery method can only be assessed relative to alternative methods investigated.

Resuscitation of Antibiotic- or Chemically-Damaged Cells

Table 12.2 summarizes the types of damage caused by a variety of agents – physical, chemical and antibiotic. Although one might imagine that there would be as many different types of lesion as damaging agents, different treatment frequently produces similar symptoms. Membrane damage is a particularly common lesion, which increases permeability, resulting in leakage of cell contents and sometimes increased uptake of antimicrobially active compounds. (Silver and Wendt, 1967). Membrane damage and cell wall damage may both be reasons for increased sensitivity to selective agents in recovery media.

Although most studies of the antimicrobial activity of chemicals (e.g. antiseptic testing) have not required the use of selective media, there has been a number of reports showing that some microorganisms sublethally damaged by

Table 12.2 Sites of sublethal damage caused by various antibiotic, chemical and physical agents

	Damage to:					
Stressing agent	*Cell wall or cell wall synthesis*	*Membrane (leakage)*	*Protein or protein synthesis*	*RNA (ribosomes) or RNA synthesis*	*DNA*	*References*
Penicillins Cephalosporins	+					
Phosphoromycin	+					
D-cycloserine	+					
Bacitracin	+	+				
Vancomycin	+	+				
Polyenes		+				
Chloramphenicol			+	+		
Tetracyclines		(+)	(+)	+		
Actinomycin-D			+	+	+	Gale *et al.* (1972) Franklin and Snow (1975)
Rifampicin				+	+	
Streptomycin		(+)		+		
Neomycin		(+)		+		
Kanamycin		(+)		+		
Erythromycin				+		
Tyrocidin		+				
Gramicidin		+				
Polymyxin		+				
Novobiocin		+			+	Morris and Russell (1971), Staudenbauer (1975)
Phenols	+	+				
Cationic detergents		+				
Chlorhexidine		+				Hugo (1967, 1976)
Salicilanilides carbanilides		+				
p-Aminohydroxy benzoic acid esters		+				Furr and Russell (1972a, b, 1973)
Heating		+	+	+	+	Allwood & Russell (1970), Tomlins (1976)
Freezing		+		+	[illegible]	MacLeod and Calcott (1976), Ray and Speck (1973a, b, c)
Drying	(+)	+		+	+	Maltman (1970), Stersky, Heldman & Hedrick (1972)

Table 12.2 (continued)

Stressing agent	*Damage to:* Cell wall or cell wall synthesis	*Membrane (leakage)*	*Protein or protein synthesis*	*RNA (ribosomes) or RNA synthesis*	*DNA*	*References*
Freeze-drying	+	+		+	+	Ray, Jezeski and Busta (1971), Sinskey & Silverman (1970), Ashwood-Smith & Grant (1976)
Gamma-irradiation	+	(+)	(+)	?	+	Bridges (1976) Davies (1976), Mitchel (1974)
Change of P_{O_2}		?+				Morris (1975, 1976)
Osmotic shock	+	+				Bayer (1967), Harrison & Morgan (1974), Birdsell & Cota-Robles (1967)
Senescence (Starvation)		+	?	+		Dawes and Large (1970), Fan and Rodwell (1975) Kaplan & Apirion (1974), Postgate (1967), Dawes (1976

*Higher (lethal) doses may produce other lesions (e.g. protein coagulation by heat and phenolics).

chemical agents are unable to grow on media containing selective agents that are non-toxic to undamaged cells (Harris and Whitefield, 1966; Walter and Jarvis, 1967; Maxey, 1970, 1975; Scheusner, Busta and Speck, 1971a, b; Braswell and Hoadley, 1974). In addition, various chemicals added to non-selective plating media increase apparent numbers of survivors (Heinmets, Taylor and Lehman, 1954; Jacobs and Harris, 1960; Thompson and De Voe, 1972). The latter may be acting either as neutralizing agents or by aiding repair mechanisms.

Methods for the isolation of pathogenic bacteria from non-sterile pharmaceutical preparations, as suggested recently by a working party of the Federation Internationale Pharmaceutique (Anon, 1976) include pre-enrichment steps for 24 h. The primary goal of this technique is to increase the sensitivity of the methods. Resuscitation of damaged cells and, later, multiplication occur. Sterility testing of pharmaceuticals does not require the use of selective media. However, a report by Gomez and Sinskey (1974) has shown that, as with heat-damaged salmonellae (Gomez *et al.*, 1973), rifampicin-damaged *Salmonella typhimurium* gave higher viable counts in a minimal (glucose/salts) medium than in a nutritionally rich non-selective medium. Further studies on the effect of non-selective recovery media, particularly on antibiotic-damaged cells are needed. An investigation of the effect of selective media on antibiotic- and chemically-damaged organisms is described in the last section of this paper.

Methods of Studying Resuscitation

The sequence of damage followed by resuscitation (repair) can be traced experimentally by use of the media that allow differentiation between damaged and undamaged cells. This is normally achieved by the use of a selective and non-selective solid and/or liquid medium to count the total of 'damaged' and 'damaged plus undamaged' cells respectively. The proportion of cells defined as damaged depends, of course, on the choice of media used for assessment (*see* below).

Figure 12.1 shows a typical graphical representation of the experimental damage/resuscitation sequence (Tomlins and Ordal, 1971; Stiles, Roth and Clegg, 1973). Log_{10} numbers of viable organisms are plotted versus time. The

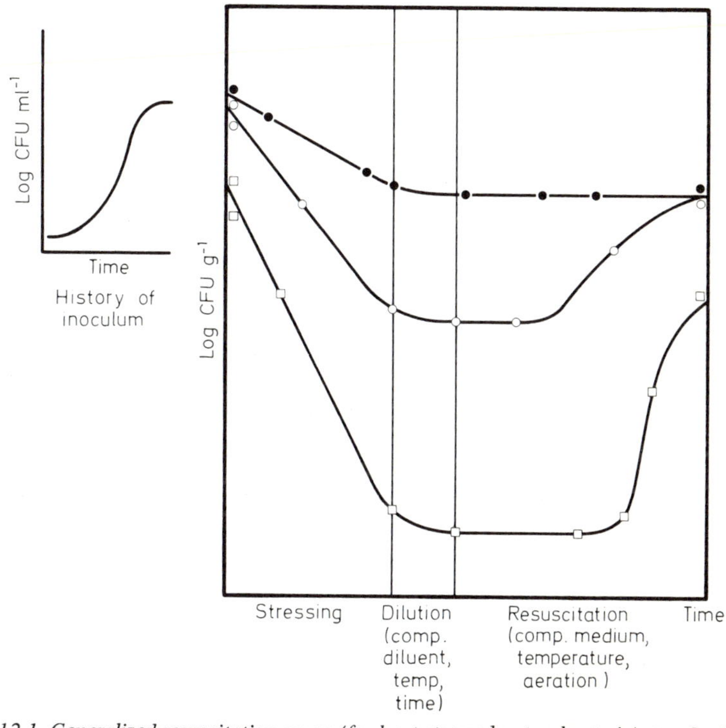

Figure 12.1 Generalized resuscitation curve (for heat-stressed enterobacteria). ● = Optimal non-selective medium; ○ = optimal selective medium; □ = suboptimal selective medium

characteristics of the figure obtained (and the optimum recovery conditions) vary according to the organism/damage combination being investigated. Results obtained using one strain cannot, unfortunately, necessarily be applied to other strains or to different types of damage. Important factors that influence the response of microorganisms to stress include the type of organism studied and the history of the organism before stress. For instance, the temperature and the medium of growth (Williams, 1929; Elliker and Frazier, 1938; Lechowich and

Ordal, 1962; Elliott and Heiniger, 1965; van Uden, Abranches and Cabenca-Silva, 1968; Corry, 1976) and the stage of growth (log, lag or stationary phase) can affect heat resistance (Lemke and White, 1959; Hurst, Hughes and Collins-Thompson, 1974). Rate of growth can affect susceptibility to cold shock, and the limiting nutrient can affect sensitivity to membrane active compounds or cold shock (Kenward, Brown and Fryer, 1976). Similar factors affect resistance to chemical agents (Russell, 1974b). The type and severity of stress and the conditions under which the stress is applied, but particularly the selective medium used to enumerate survivors, will greatly affect the results obtained (cf. *Figure 12.1*; Roth, Stiles and Clegg, 1973; Ray and Speck, 1973b, c; Scheusner, Busta and Speck, 1971b; Sinskey *et al.*, 1964).

The selective medium should be one that allows all unstressed organisms of the type required to grow, i.e. counts of undamaged organisms on selective and non-selective media should be equivalent; nevertheless differences sometimes do occur. Discrepancies between counts before deliberate stressing can result from at least two different mechanisms (Mossel, Harrewijn and Nesselrooy-van Zadelhof, 1974):

(1) Intrinsic toxicity of the selective medium to some strains of a particular organism under given conditions which seem very difficult to control.
(2) Fortuitous stressing, a more common phenomenon than is often supposed, since it has been observed that cells present in what, at first sight, might be considered optimal 'niches', such as fresh milk and meat, may show lesions (Gabis and Silliker, 1974; Edel and Kampelmacher, 1973).

If a diluent is used, it should be at such a temperature and of such composition that numbers of organisms are maintained (e.g. ice-cold diluent should not be used to dilute cells previously held at room temperature or above, and peptone-containing diluents rather than distilled or tap water, saline or 'quarter-strength Ringer's' should be used (Straka and Stokes, 1959; Jayne-Williams, 1963). The selective medium used affects the apparent numbers of damaged cells detected: for instance, brilliant green agar gives lower counts of damaged salmonellae than violet red bile glucose agar, and the time needed for resuscitation is apparently longer when the numbers are assessed on brilliant green agar (van Schothorst and Van Leusden, 1972). Differences of over one thousand-fold can be observed between selective media when heat-damaged salmonellae are plated directly (Corry, Kitchell and Roberts, 1969). The toxicity of bile-salt and brilliant green-containing media, in particular, should be checked for each batch (Read and Reyes, 1968; Mossel and Harrewijn, 1972; Northolt, 1972). The severity of the injury will also affect the recovery time.

Recommended isolation methods for organisms likely to be damaged involve resuscitating or 'pre-enriching' organisms in a liquid non-selective medium for between 5 and 24 h for *Salmonellae, Enterobacteriaceae, Staph. aureus* and *Pseudomonas aeruginosa* (Thatcher and Clark, 1968; Mossel and Ratto, 1970; British Pharmacopoeia, 1973; U.S. Pharmacopoeia, 1974; Gray, Gaske and Ordal 1974; Stiles and Clarke, 1974; Anon, 1976). It is likely that microorganisms in antibiotic-containing substrates would need similar methods for their isolation, particularly those in feeds and pharmaceuticals, which may additionally have been exposed to physical stresses such as drying, heating or irradiating.

Experimental Investigation of the Resuscitation of Antibiotic- or Chemically-Damaged Microorganisms

A literature survey revealed almost no information on resuscitation of antibiotic-damaged cells in particular, and a short report of our investigations follows.

MATERIALS AND METHODS

Resuscitation of three strains of bacteria (*Staphylococcus aureus, Escherichia coli* and *Aeromonas* sp.) was studied after exposure to Nipagin-M (methyl para-hydroxybenzoate) or oxytetracycline, and resuscitation of one strain of yeast (*Hansenula beyerinckii* CBS 2561) was followed after exposure to nystatin.

Inocula were prepared by washing log-phase cells from slopes of tryptone soy peptone agar (bacteria) or yeast extract dextrose agar (yeast) into sorbitol-phosphate solution (2.8% w/v sorbitol in 0.1 M phosphate buffer, pH 6). Sorbitol-phosphate treatment was carried out in order to simulate the physiological state of cells stored in Dutch-type lanette wax creams. One hundred ml quantities of the suspensions were incubated overnight at 30°C, shaking continuously, and the appropriate antimicrobial substances added to give final concentrations of 100 $\mu g\ ml^{-1}$ (nystatin and oxytetracycline) or 0.2% w/v (Nipagin-M). The two antibiotics were added as dry powders, and the Nipagin as a 20% solution in ethanol. Incubation was continued at 30°C, with shaking, for up to 2 h with the oxytetracycline and Nipagin, and for up to 24 h with the nystatin because the yeast was not very sensitive to this antibiotic. At the end of the treatment period the cell suspensions were diluted 1:20 in BHIT (brain heart infusion broth [Difco] + 0.1% w/v Tween 80) and repair allowed to proceed. The Tween 80 should neutralize any residual Nipagin. Divalent cations (50 mg 100 ml^{-1} $FeSO_4.7H_2O$) were added when required to the BHIT to test their neutralizing effect for bacteria damaged by oxytetracycline.

Viable surface counts of decimal dilutions in maintenance medium (0.9% w/v NaCl + 0.1% w/v peptone) were carried out in triplicate immediately before, during and after treatment with the antimicrobial agents, using non-selective and selective plating media. TSPA (tryptone soy peptone broth (Oxoid CM 129) + 15 $g\ l^{-1}$ agar) was used as the non-selective plating medium for the bacteria, and YDA (yeast extract 0.5% w/v; dextrose 2% w/v; agar 1.5% w/v) for the yeast. The selective media used were as follows:

H. beyerinckii	oxytetracycline-polymyxin agar (Nouws and Hymans, 1975) (OPA: YDA + 100 $\mu g\ ml^{-1}$ oxytetracycline and 100 $\mu g\ ml^{-1}$ polymyxin, added after sterilization)
S. aureus	(1) phenylethanol agar (Mossel *et al.*, 1977) (PEA: TSBA + 0.35% w/v 2-phenylethanol) (2) Vogel Johnson agar (VJ: Merck)
Aeromonas sp.	crystal violet agar (Mossel *et al.*, 1977) (CVA: TSBA + 2$\mu g\ ml^{-1}$ crystal violet, added after sterilization)

E. coli	(1) CVA (2) violet red bile dextrose agar (VRBG: Oxoid)

Incubation was at 30°C for 2 days for all media except OPA (22°C for 5 days) and VRBG (37°C).

RESULTS AND DISCUSSION

Figures 12.2–12.9 show the results obtained.

Counts of untreated cells

In some instances significant differences between counts on selective and non-selective plating media were observed before addition of the antibacterial agents (*Figures 12.3, 12.5* and *12.6*), which could have been due to the effect of the

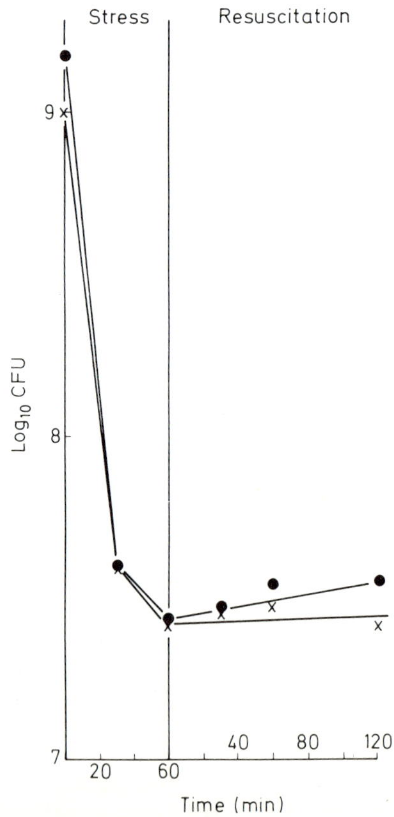

Figure 12.2 Resuscitation curve of Aeromonas *sp. exposed to Nipagin-M for 60 min, resuscitated in BHIT and counted on TSBA (•) and CVA (X)*

overnight incubation in sorbitol-phosphate medium since fresh log-phase cells gave similar counts on both types of media. In these cases the damage and resuscitation observed were therefore a combination of two effects, and cells could still be expected to give equivalent numbers on the two types of plating medium when resuscitation was complete.

Nipagin-M

No difference in counts of *Aeromonas*, and hence no evidence for sublethally-damaged cells, was observed with the plating media used (*Figure 12.2*). With *S. aureus* (*Figure 12.3*), however, some evidence of damage was observed with VJ (but not PEA). Damaged cells were able to form colonies on VJ after resuscitation for 80 min in BHIT.

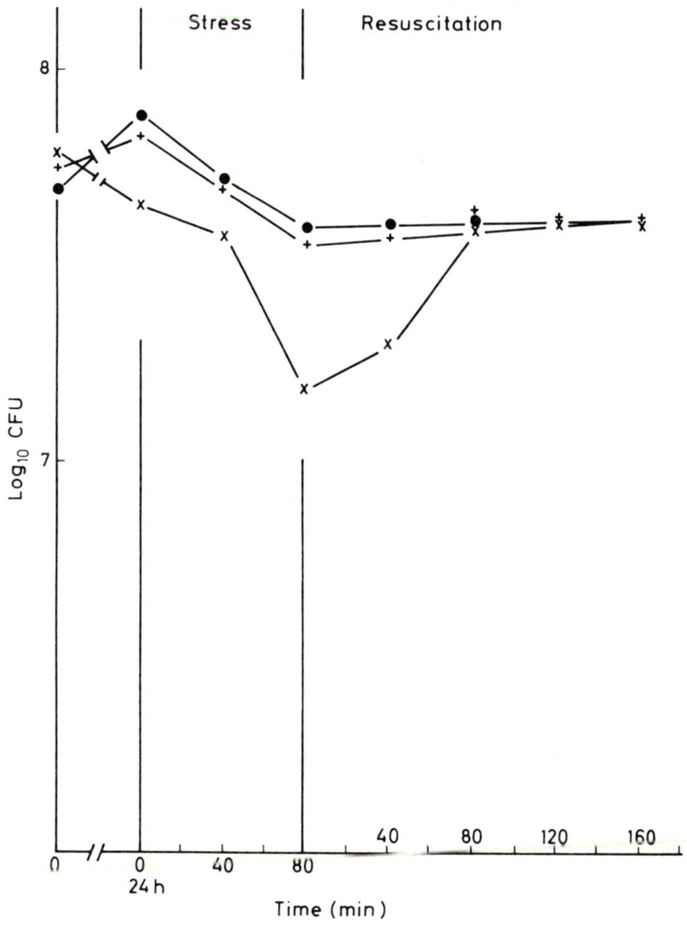

Figure 12.3 Resuscitation curve of Staphylococcus aureus *exposed to Nipagin-M for 80 min, resuscitated in BHIT and counted on TSBA (•), PEA (+) and VJ (×)*

E. coli (*Figure 12.4*) also showed slight, but significant, evidence of sublethal damage after exposure to Nipagin. Ability to form colonies on VRBG was restored after about two hours' incubation.

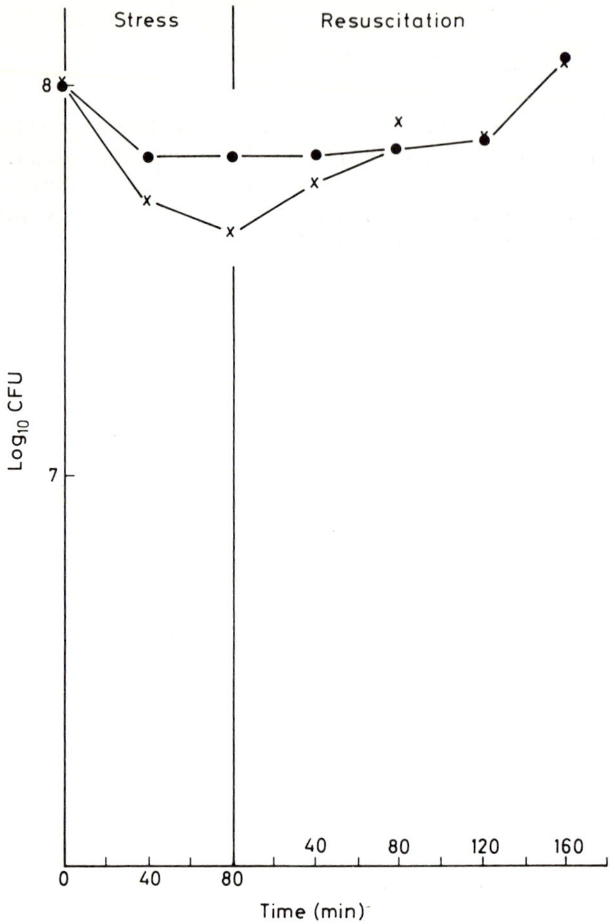

Figure 12.4 Resuscitation curve of Escherichia coli *exposed to Nipagin-M for 80 min, resuscitated in BHIT and counted on TSBA (•) and VRBG (X)*

Oxytetracycline

There was no evidence of damage caused by oxytetracycline to *Aeromonas* from comparison of the numbers counted on TSBA and CVA (*Figure 12.5*), although lack of added neutralizer may have been responsible for the fall in numbers on TSBA after dilution of the antibiotic.

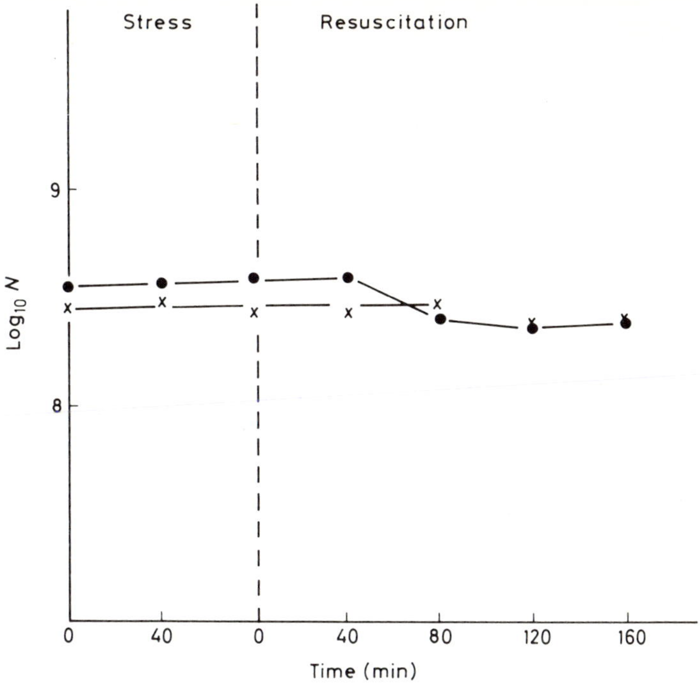

Figure 12.5 Resuscitation curve of Aeromonas *sp. exposed to oxytetracycline for 80 min, resuscitated in BHIT and counted on TSBA (•) and CVA (X)*

More extensive damage was evident after treatment of *S. aureus* (*Figure 12.6*); this was due to a combination of the overnight treatment and the antibiotic. As with Nipagin-treated *S. aureus*, more damaged cells were able to grow on PEA than on VJ agar. There was evidence of initial repair in BHIT followed by a fall in numbers, counted either on selective or non-selective medium. This may have been due to the presence of residual unneutralized antibiotic. The increasing difference in numbers of survivors counted on the different media after about 80 min resuscitation indicated that damage was still occurring. Many more oxytetracycline-damaged cells of *E. coli* were able to grow on VRBG than on CVA (*Figure 12.7*). Resuscitation was again apparently not complete within the time of the test (160 min after cessation of the antibiotic treatment). Addition of Fe^{++} ions to the resuscitation medium (*Figure 12.8*) increased the numbers of survivors detected on the non-selective medium, thus showing the necessity of inactivation, even when non-selective media are used. Resuscitation was complete within three hours.

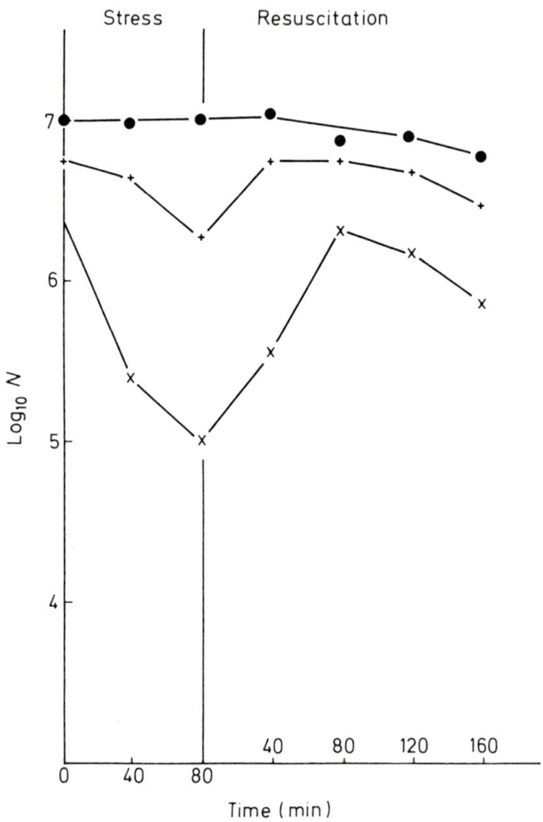

Figure 12.6 Resuscitation curve of Staphylococcus aureus *exposed to oxytetracycline for 80 min, resuscitated in BHIT and counted on TSBA (•), PEA (+) and VJ (X)*

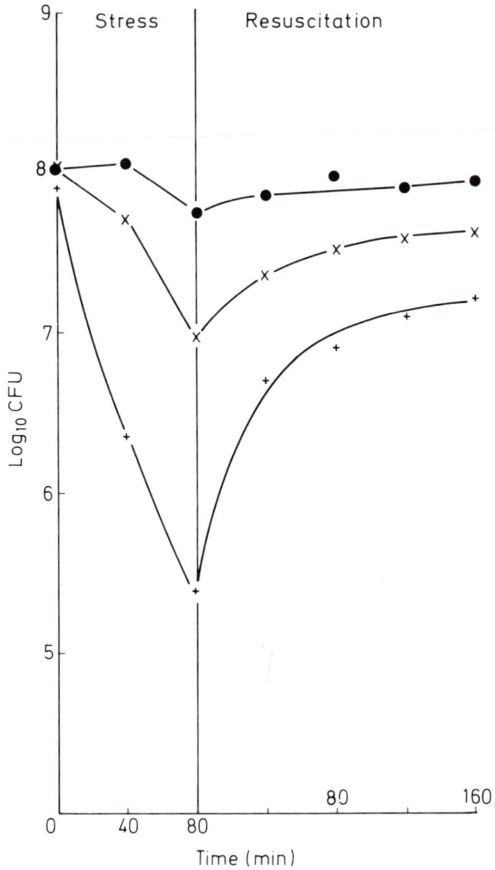

Figure 12.7 Resuscitation curve of Escherichia coli *exposed to oxytetracycline for 80 min, resuscitated in BHIT and counted on TSBA (•), VRBG (×) and CVA (+)*

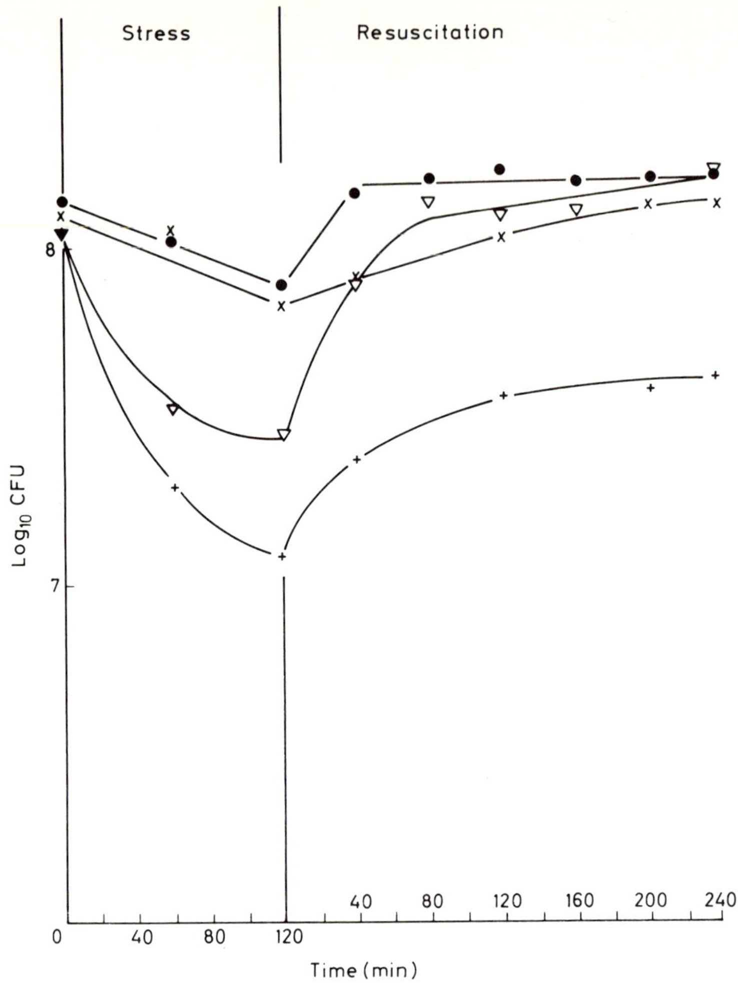

Figure 12.8 Resuscitation curve of Escherichia coli *exposed to oxytetracycline for 120 min, resuscitated in BHIT and counted on TSPA (×) and VRBG (+), or resuscitated in BHIT + $FeSO_4$ and counted on TSBA (●) and VRBG (▽)*

Nystatin

Numbers of surviving *H. beyerinckii* on YDA and OPA were similar (*Figure 12.9*).

The results illustrated here confirm that microorganisms treated with chemical agents can show evidence of sublethal damage and show that similar effects can occur with antibiotic-damaged cells, which, in common with the damage inflicted by physical agents, impairs their ability to grow on some selective media. This effect can be differentiated from that caused by residual chemicals

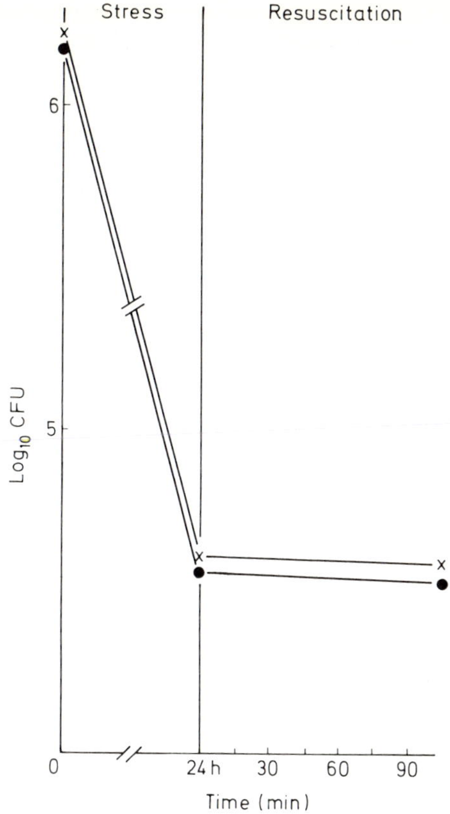

Figure 12.9 Resuscitation curve of Hansenula beyerinckii *exposed to nystatin for 24 h, resuscitated in BHIT and counted on YDA (•) and OPA (×)*

when a suitable neutralizer is available. It seems likely that when the appropriate media are used evidence of damage will be found in all systems.

The resuscitation time, defined as the time before numbers of viable organisms on selective and non-selective media are equivalent, was found to be between two and three hours for bacteria damaged by Nipagin or tetracycline. This is similar to the time required for the resuscitation of bacteria injured by other agents (Mossel and Ratto, 1970; Stiles, Roth and Clegg, 1973; Tomlins and Ordal, 1971; Gomez and Sinskey, 1974; Speck, Ray and Read, 1975).

General Conclusions

Recovery of microorganisms from environments containing antibiotics or other antimicrobial agents requires methods capable of allowing all sublethally damaged organisms to repair. In situations where specific organisms are being sought, selective media should be used only after use of a suitable resuscitation medium.

Further investigations to determine the most suitable non-selective resuscitation media are required with respect to both physically and chemically damaged microorganisms. In addition, effective methods of neutralizing residual anti-microbial agents are required. Better understanding of the nature and mechanism of damage and repair should help towards this aim.

Acknowledgment

We are grateful to Dr. A.D. Russell for helpful discussions during the preparation of this manuscript.

References

ALLWOOD, M.C. and RUSSELL, A.D. (1970). *Adv. appl. Microbiol.*, **17**, 89
ANGHERN, P. and THEN, R. (1977). *Chemotherapy*, **19**, 1
ANON (1976). *Pharm. Acta Helv.*, **51**, 33
ASHWOOD-SMITH, M.J. and GRANT, E. (1976). *Cryobiology*, **13**, 206
BARACH, J.T., FLOWERS, R.S. and ADAMS, D.M. (1975). *Appl. Microbiol.*, **30**, 873
BAYER, M.E. (1967). *J. Bact.*, **93**, 1104
BIRDSELL, D.C. and COTA-ROBLES, E.H. (1967). *J. Bact.*, **93**, 427
BLAUG, S.M. and AHSAN, S.S. (1961). *J. Pharm. Sci.*, **50**, 441
BLISS, E.A., CHANDLER, C.A. and SCHOENBACH, E.B. (1949). *Ann. N.Y. Acad. Sci.*, **51**, 944
BONDI, A., KORNBLUM, J. and FORTE, C. (1957). *Proc. Soc. exptl biol. Med.*, **96**, 270
BOTTONE, E.J., BRANDMAN, Z. and SCHNEIERSON, S.S. (1976). *Antimicrob. Agents Chemother.*, **9**, 327
BRASWELL, J.R. and HOADLEY, A.W. (1974). *Appl. Microbiol.*, **28**, 328
BREEZE, A.S. and McADAM, G.A. (1974). *J. Pharm. Pharmac.*, **26**, 122P
BRIDGES, B.A. (1976). In *Survival of Vegetative Microbes*, Society for General Microbiology Symposium, no. 26. Cambridge University Press
BRITISH PHARMACOPOEIA (1973). H.M.S.O., London
BROWN, M.R.W. and MELLING, J. (1971). In *Inhibition and Destruction of the Microbial Cell.* Ed. Hugo, W.B. Academic Press, London
BUSTA, F.F. (1976). *J. Milk Food Technol.*, **39**, 138
CASERIO, G. and TESTA, C. (1971). *Archs. vet. ital.*, **22**, 37
CASERIO, G., TURCO, G. and GENNARI, M. (1975). *Archs. vet. ital.*, **26**, 121
COOK, A.M. and STEEL, K.J. (1959). *J. Pharm. Pharmac.*, **11**, 666
CORRY, J.E.L. (1976). *J. appl. Bact.*, **40**, 269
CORRY, J.E.L., KITCHELL, A.G. and ROBERTS, T.A. (1969). *J. appl. Bact.*, **31**, 415
CORRY, J.E.L. and ROBERTS, T.A. (1970). *J. appl. Bact.*, **33**, 733
CROWSHAW, B. (1976). *J. Soc. Cosmet. Chem.* (in press)
CURRAN, H.R. and EVANS, F.R. (1937). *J. Bact.*, **34**, 179
DAVIES, R. (1976). In *Inhibition and Inactivation of Vegetative Microbes.* Ed. Skinner, F.A. and Carr, J.G., Soc. Appl. Bact. Symp. series, no. 5. Academic Press, London

DAWES, E.A. (1976). In *The Survival of Vegetative Microbes.* Society for General Microbiology Symposium, no. 26. Cambridge University Press

DAWES, E.A. and LARGE, P.J. (1970). *J. gen. Microbiol.,* **60**, 31

EDEL, W. and KAMPELMACHER, E.H. (1973). *Bull. World Hlth Organ.,* **48**, 167

ELLIKER, P.R. and FRAZIER, W.C. (1938). *J. Bact.,* **36**, 83

ELLIOTT, R.P. and HEINIGER, P.K. (1965). *Appl. Microbiol.,* **13**, 73

EPPS, N.A. and IDZIAK, E.S. (1970). *Appl. Microbiol.,* **19**, 338

FAN, C.L. and RODWELL, V.W. (1975). *J. Bact.,* **124**, 1302

FRANKLIN, T.J. and SNOW, G.A. (1975). *Biochemistry of Antimicrobial Action,* 2nd edn. Chapman and Hall, London

FURR, J.R. and RUSSELL, A.D. (1972a). *Microbios,* **5**, 189

FURR, J.R. and RUSSELL, A.D. (1972b). *Microbios,* **5**, 237

FURR, J.R. and RUSSELL, A.D. (1973). *Microbios,* **6**, 47

GABIS, D.A. and SILLIKER, J.H. (1974). *Can. J. Microbiol.,* **20**, 663

GALE, E.F., CUNDLIFFE, E., REYNOLDS, P.E., RICHMOND, M.H. and WARING, M.J. (1972). *The Molecular Basis of Antibiotic Action.* Wiley, London

GOMEZ, R.F. and SINSKEY, A.J. (1974). *Nature, Lond.,* **247**, 211

GOMEZ, R.F., SINSKEY, A.J., DAVIES, R. and LABUZA, T.P. (1973). *J. gen. Microbiol.,* **74**, 267

GORMAN, S.P. and SCOTT, E.M. (1976). *Microbios Letters,* **1**, 197

GRAY, R.J.H., GASKE, M.A. and ORDAL, Z.J. (1974). *J. Food Sci.,* **39**, 844

HAMBURGER, M., CARLETON, J. and HARCOURT, M. (1957). *Antibiotics Chemother.,* **7**, 274

HARRIS, N.D. and WHITEFIELD, M. (1966). *J. Pharm. Pharmacol.,* **18** (suppl.), 33S

HARRISON, A.P. and MORGAN, R.F. (1974). *Cryobiology,* **11**, 423

HARTSELL, S.E. (1951). *Am. J. publ. Hlth.,* **41**, 1072

HEATHER, C.D. and VANDERZANT, C. (1957). *J. Dairy Sci.,* **40**, 1079

HEINMETS, F., TAYLOR, W.W. and LEHMAN, J.J. (1954). *J. Bact.,* **67**, 5

HOLDOWSKY, S. (1957). *Antibiotics Chemother.,* **7**, 49

HUGO, W.B. (1964). In *Disinfection and Sterilisation.* Eds. Wittet, T.D. and Wilkinson, G.R. Heinemann Medical Books, London

HUGO, W.B. (1967). *J. appl. Bact.,* **30**, 17

HUGO, W.B. (1976). In *Inhibition and Inactivation of Vegetative Microbes.* Eds. Skinner, F.A. and Carr, J.G., Soc. Appl. Bact. Symp. series, no. 5. Academic Press, London

HUGO, W.B. and RUSSELL, A.D. (1961). *J. Bact.,* **82**, 411

HURST, A., HENDRY, G.S., HUGHES, A. and PALEY, B. (1976). *Can. J. Microbiol.,* **22**, 677

HURST, A., HUGHES, A. and COLLINS-THOMPSON, D.L. (1974). *Can. J. Microbiol.,* **20**, 765

IANDOLO, J.J. and ORDAL, Z.J. (1966). *J. Bact.,* **91**, 134

IENISTEA, C., CHITU, M. and ROMAN, A. (1970). *Zntbl. Bakt. Parasitk., Abt. 1 Orig.,* **215**, 173

JACOBS, S.E. and HARRIS, N.D. (1960). *J. appl. Bact.,* **23**, 294

JAYNE-WILLIAMS, D.J. (1963). *J. appl. Bact.,* **26**, 398

KAPLAN, R. and APIRION, D. (1974). *J. biol. Chem.,* **250**, 1854

KENWARD, M.A., BROWN, M.R.W. and FRYER, J.J. (1976). *Proc. Soc. gen. Microbiol.,* **3**, 83

LAMIKANRA, A. and ALLWOOD, M.C. (1976). *Microbios Lett.,* **1**, 97

LARK, C. and LARK, K.G. (1959). *Can. J. Microbiol.*, **5**, 369

LECHOWICH, R.V. and ORDAL, Z.J. (1962). *Can. J. Microbiol.*, **8**, 287

LEMKE, R.M. and WHITE, H.R. (1959). *J. appl. Bact.*, **22**, 193

MacLEOD, R.A. and CALCOTT, P.H. (1976). In *Survival of Vegetative Microbes*, Society for General Microbiology Symposium, no. 26. Cambridge University Press

MacKINNON, I.H. (1974). *J. Hyg., Camb.*, **73**, 189

MALTMAN, J.R. (1970). *Revue Hyg. Med. soc.*, **18**, 395

MAXCY, R.B. (1970). *J. Milk Food Technol.*, **33**, 445

MAXCY, R.B. (1975). *J. Milk Food Technol.*, **38**, 192

MITCHEL, R.E.J. (1974). *Fed. Proc.*, **33**, 1242

MORRIS, A. and RUSSELL, A.D. (1971). *Progr. med. Chem.*, **8**, 39

MORRIS, J.G. (1975). *Adv. microb. Physiol.*, **12**, 169

MORRIS, J.G. (1976). *J. appl. Bact.*, **40**, 229

MOSSEL, D.A.A. (1977). *Microbiology of Foods*, 2nd edn. University of Utrecht

MOSSEL, D.A.A. and BEERENS, H. (1968). *J. Hyg. (Camb.)*, **66**, 269

MOSSELL, D.A.A., DOORNE, H. VAN, EELDERINK, I. and VOR, H.DE. (1977). *Pharm. Weekbl. Ned.*, **112**, 41

MOSSEL, D.A.A. and HARREWIJN, G.A. (1972). *Alimenta*, **11**, 29

MOSSEL, D.A.A., HARREWIJN, G.A. and NESSELROOY-VAN ZADELHOFF, C.F.M. (1974). *Health Lab. Sci.*, **11**, 260

MOSSEL, D.A.A., JONGERIUS, E. and KOOPMAN, M.J. (1965). *Ann. Inst. Pasteur, Lille*, **16**, 119

MOSSEL, D.A. and RATTO, M.A. (1970). *Appl. Microbiol.*, **20**, 273

NELSON, F.E. (1943). *J. Bact.*, **45**, 395

NELSON, F.E. (1972). *Appl. Microbiol.*, **25**, 499

NEWTON, B.A. (1953). *Nature, Lond.*, **172**, 160

NORTHOLT, M.D. (1972). *Antonie van Leeuwenhoek*, **38**, 632

NOUWS, J.F.M. and HYMANS, P.G. (1975). *Arch. Lebensm. Hyg.*, **26**, 175

PATEL, N.K. and KOSTENBAUDER, H.B. (1958). *J. Am. Pharm. Ass. Sci. Ed.*, **47**, 289

PENNINGTON, J.H. and O'GRADY, F. (1967). *Nature, Lond.*, **213**, 34

PISANO, F.D. and KOSTENBAUDER, H.B. (1959). *J. Am. Pharm. Ass. Sci. Ed.*, **48**, 310

PITTILLO, R.F. and FOSTER, J.W. (1953). *J. Bact.*, **67**, 53

POSTGATE, J.R. (1967). *Adv. microb. Physiol.*, **1**, 1

PUT, H.M.C. (1974). *Arch. Lebensmittel hyg.*, **25**, 73

RACCACH, M. and JUVEN, B. (1973). *J. Food Technol.*, **8**, 211

RAY, B., JEZESKI, J.J. and BUSTA, F.F. (1971). *Appl. Microbiol.*, **22**, 401

RAY, B. and SPECK, M.L. (1973a). *C.R.C. Crit. Rev. Clin. Lab. Sci.*, **4**, 161

RAY, B. and SPECK, M.L. (1973b). *Appl. Microbiol.*, **25**, 494

RAY, B. and SPECK, M.L. (1973c). *Appl. Microbiol.*, **25**, 499

RAY, B., SPECK, M.L. and DOBROGOSZ, W.J. (1976). *Cryobiology*, **13**, 153

READ, R.B. and REYES, A.L. (1968). *Appl. Microbiol.*, **16**, 746

ROBERTS, T.A. and HITCHINS, A.D. (1969). In *The Bacterial Spore*. Eds. Gould, G.W. and Hurst, A. Academic Press, London

ROTH, L.A., STILES, M.E. and CLEGG, L.F.L. (1973). *Can. Inst. Food Sci. Technol., J.*, **6**, 235

RUSSELL, A.D. (1974a). *Microbios*, **11**, 193

RUSSELL, A.D. (1974b). *Microbios,* **10**, 151

RUSSELL, A.D. (1974c). *Manufacturing Chemist and Aerosol News* (September) p. 28

RUSSELL, A.D. and DITCHETT, P.J. (1976). In *Encyclopaedia of Environmental Science and Engineering.* Eds. Pfafflin, J.R. and Ziegler, E.N. Gordon and Breach, London (in press)

RUSSELL, A.D. and GILBERT, R.J. (1964). *Manufacturing Chemist,* **35**, 42

RUSSELL, A.D., MORRIS, A. and ALLWOOD, M.C. (1973). In *Methods in Microbiology,* vol. 8. Eds. Norris, J.R. and Ribbons, D.W. Academic Press, London

SCHEUSNER, D.L., BUSTA, F.F. and SPECK, M.L. (1971a). *Appl. Microbiol.,* **21**, 41

SCHEUSNER, D.L., BUSTA, F.F. and SPECK, M.L. (1971b). *Appl. Microbiol.,* **21**, 46

SILVER, S. and WENDT, L. (1967). *J. Bact.,* **93**, 560

SINSKEY, A.J., McINTOSH, A.H., PABLO, I.S., SILVERMAN, G.J. and GOLDBLITH, S.A. (1964). *Health Lab. Sci.,* **1**, 297

SINSKEY, A.J. and SILVERMAN, G.J. (1970). *J. Bact.,* **101**, 429

SORRELS, K.M., SPECK, M.L. and WARREN, J.A. (1970). *Appl. Microbiol.,* **19**, 39

SPECK, M.L., RAY, R. and READ, R.B. (1975). *Appl. Microbiol.,* **29**, 549

STAUDENBAUER, W.L. (1975). *J. molec. Biol.,* **96**, 201

STERSKY, A.K., HELDMAN, D.R. and HEDRICK, T.I. (1972). *J. Milk Food Technol.,* **35**, 528

STILES, M.E. and CLARK, P.C. (1974). *Can. J. Microbiol.,* **20**, 1735

STILES, M.E., ROTH, L.A. and CLEGG, L.F.L. (1973). *Can. Inst. Food Sci. Technol. J.,* **6**, 226

STRAKA, R.P. and STOKES, J.L. (1959). *J. Bact.,* **78**, 181

STUMBO, C.R. (ed.) (1965). *Thermobacteriology in Food Processing.* Academic Press, London

SYKES, G. (1956). *J. Pharm. Pharmac.,* **8**, 561

SYKES, G. (1965). *Disinfection and Sterilisation.* Spon, London

SYKES, G. (1962). *J. appl. Bact.,* **25**, 1

SYKES, G. and HOOPER, M.C. (1959). *J. Pharm. Pharmac., Suppl.,* **11**, 235T

THATCHER, F.S. and CLARK, D.S. (1968). *Microorganisms in Food.* University of Toronto Press, Canada

THOMPSON, J. and DE VOE, I.W. (1972). *Can. J. Microbiol.,* **18**, 841

TOMLINS, R.I. (1976). In *Inhibition and Inactivation of Vegetative Microbes.* Eds. Skinner, F.A. and Carr, J.G., Soc. Appl. Bact. Symp. series, no. 5. Academic Press, London (in press)

TOMLINS, R.I. and ORDAL, Z.J. (1971). *J. Bact.,* **107**, 134

U.S. PHARMACOPOEIA (1974). 19th revision. Mack Publishing Co., Easton, Pa.

VAICHULIS, E.M.K. and VEDROS, N.A. (1966). *Chemotherapia,* **11**, 315

VAN SCHOTHORST, M. and VAN LEUSDEN, F.M. (1972). *Zntbl. Bakt Hyg. I Abt. Orig.,* **22**, 19

VAN UDEN, N., ABRANCHES, P. and CABENCA-SILVA, C. (1968). *Arch. Mikrobiol.,* **61**, 381

WALTER, G. and JARVIS, S. (1967). *Soap and Chem. Specialities,* **43** (3), 45

WEINBERG, E.D. (1954). *J. infect. Dis.,* **95**, 291

WEINBERG, E.D. (1957). *Bact. Rev.,* **21**, 46

WEINBERG, E.D. (1959). In *Antibiotics Annual 1958–1959,* p. 924. Medical Encyclopedia Inc., New York

WILLIAMS, O.B. (1929). *J. infect. Dis.,* **44**, 421

WILSON, J.M. and DAVIES, R. (1976). *J. appl. Bact.*, **40**, 365
WOODS, D.D. (1940). *Brit. J. exp. Path.*, **21**, 74
WRIGHT, J.H. (1917). *J. Bact.*, **2**, 315

IV

ANTIBIOTICS, ANTIBIOSIS AND ANIMALS

13

THE USE OF ANTIBIOTICS IN THE VETERINARY FIELD IN IN THE 1970s

G.C. BRANDER
Beecham Pharmaceuticals, Tadworth

Since the last symposium in 1962, many changes have taken place in our attitude to the use of antibiotics, both for therapy and as 'growth promoters', and the most significant event in the assessment of antibiotic therapy was the publication of the Swann Report in 1969.

This report made a number of recommendations which have influenced the thinking of animal health administrators in Europe and the U.S.A. Implementation of the recommendations has been slow, but regulations now agreed in Brussels should lead to a general acceptance of the 'Swann concept' on the use of therapeutic drugs and antibacterial feed additives.

The Swann report recommended that antibacterials suitable for addition to animal feeds without prescription should be restricted to:

(1) Those that are of economic value in livestock production.
(2) Those that have little or no application as therapeutic agents in man or animals.
(3) Those that will not impair the efficacy of a prescribed therapeutic antibiotic or antibiotics through the development of resistant strains or organisms.

In a contribution to Advances in Veterinary Science and Comparative Medicine (1971), Dr. Williams Smith, when discussing the future of antibacterials said:

'Antibacterial drugs have now been used for a sufficiently long time for the treatment and prevention of disease and as growth promoters in animals to enable conclusions to be drawn as to the extent drug-resistant strains of bacteria are likely to minimize the beneficial effect of drugs.

'As far as important pathogens like *Streptococcus agalactiae* and most other streptoccoci, pasteurellae, *Erysipelothrix rhusiopathiae*, and *Corynebacterium pyogenes* are concerned, it is probable that resistant strains are unlikely to emerge and complicate the therapy of diseases caused by these organisms; it is reasonable to assume they would have arisen by now if they were going to.

'The position with regard to important causal organisms of animal disease such as *Staphylococcus aureus*, salmonellae, pathogenic serotypes of *Escherichia coli* and, possibly *Mycoplasma gallisepticum*, is quite different. Not only single-resistant but also multiple-resistant strains of these organisms are progressing towards dominance, and it is probable that the chemotherapy of the diseases they cause will increase in complexity unless the present policies on the use of antibacterial drugs are subjected to considerable modification.

'The increasing incidence of drug resistance is also of some significance from the viewpoint of human health.'

He therefore presses the necessity for a reconsideration of the methods of use of antibacterial drugs. It seems appropriate therefore that in this paper I should put forward for your consideration some suggestions on how we might use antibacterials in the animal health field to the best advantage. I would like therefore to discuss the control of animal diseases in terms of their relationship to animal production, rather than as separate entities which occur in individual animals and require individual treatment.

Penny in a paper presented to the British Veterinary Congress in 1975 indicated that the annual loss of potential food through disease in U.S. livestock and poultry production amounted to 10–15% of the total production. In Iowa alone, a major pig producing area, there was estimated to be an annual loss due to disease of 155 million dollars. Apart from atrophic rhinitis and reproductive failure, the major sources of loss were due to diarrhoea, pneumonia and Swine dysentery – all diseases in which bacteria can play an important part.

In the monthly reports of the Veterinary Investigation Services for 1975 and early 1976, certain disease syndromes play a dominant role. These are: salmonellosis, mastitis, pneumonia, bovine abortion, diseases due to *Erysipelothrix rhusiopathiae,* pasteurellosis and psittacosis. Although psittacosis, because of its importance as a zoonosis is mentioned specially, the reports indicate that certain infectious entities do dominate animal production. In a study of post mortem reports from V.I. Centres in England and Wales reported in 1971, the incidence of various bacteria at different times in the life of a calf are reported (*see Table 13.1*). It will be seen that *E. coli* and *Salmonella* are the dominant bacterial infections.

Table 13.1 Diagnosis of infectious diseases (V.I. Centres U.K., 1971)

Bacteria recovered diseases considered infectious	*Gram +ve or −ve*	*0–7 weeks*	*2–4 months*	*5–8 months*	*Total*	*Percentage*
Clostridia	+	17	22	15	54	3
Corynebacteria	+	56	21	6	83	4
Escherichia coli	−	912	54	13	979	50
Pasteurella	−	76	59	25	160	8
Salmonella	−	543	133	16	692	35

In Tables *13.2* to *13.5* I have indicated a number of key disease entities, and the bacteria which are frequently associated with these infections. Additional infections of importance are the agalactiae syndrome and Swine dysentery in pigs. In practically every case the cause of clinical disease may be of multiple origin, but bacteria usually play a part at some stage in the infection.

Table 13.2 Bacterial infections of domestic animals: cattle

Disease	*Bacteria involved*
Calf scours and pneumonia	*E. coli* Staphylococci *Pasteurella* species
Calf enteritis and septicaemia	*Salmonella* species
Mastitis	Staphylococci Streptococci *E. coli* *Pseudomonas*
Metritis	*E. coli* Staphylococci *Streptococcus faecalis* *Proteus* species
Pyelonephritis	*Corynebacterium renale*

Table 13.3 Bacterial infections of domestic animals: pigs

Disease	*Bacteria involved*
Enteritis and pneumonia	*E. coli* *Salmonella* *Pasteurella* species
Erysipelas	*Erysipelothrix rhusiopathiae*
Metritis	*E. coli* Staphylococci

Table 13.4 Bacterial infections of domestic animals: horses

Disease	*Bacteria involved*
Enteritis and septicaemia in the young foal	*E. coli* *Proteus* Staphylococci
Metritis	*E. coli* Staphylococci
Pneumonia	Staphylococci *Pasteurella* species
Strangles	*Streptococcus equi*

Table 13.5 Bacterial infections of domestic animals: dogs

Disease	*Bacteria involved*
Enteritis	*E. coli*
Ear infections	Staphylococci Streptococci *E. coli* *Pseudomonas*
Leptospirosis	*Leptospira canicola*
Respiratory infections	Staphylococci Streptococci

In *Figure 13.1* is shown a diagrammatic impression of the sequence of infections which can occur in the respiratory tract of pigs. Although the sequence of events may not be replicated on every occasion, it is clear that in a large pig unit, the herd are at risk from infections throughout their lives and that the maintenance of reasonable health is dependent on effective control of the different organisms involved in disease.

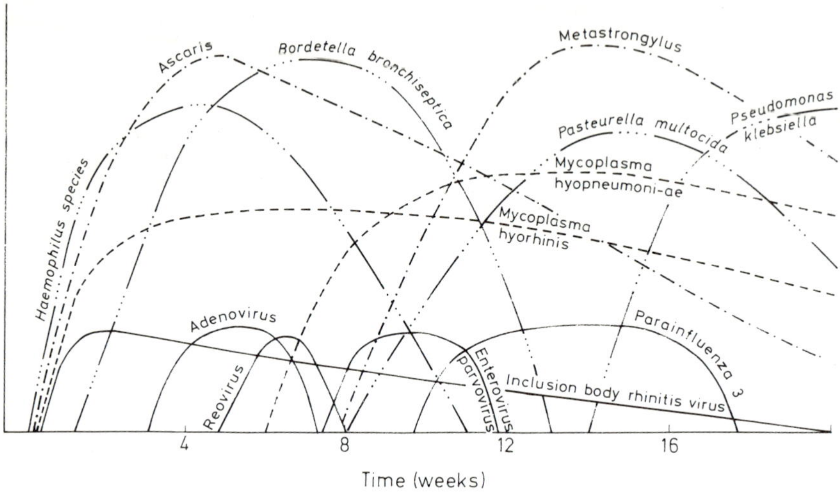

Figure 13.1 Diagram showing a possible sequence of infections occurring in the upper respiratory tract of pigs. —·— = Helminths; – = viruses; — — — = mycoplasmas; — - - - — = bacteria (from Vet. Res. *[1975]*, **96**, *25, 543)*

In the second report of the Joint Consultative Organization of R & D in Agriculture and Food, certain problems were identified as of key importance in animal production and two of them are significant in the field which we are discussing:

(1) death of the newborn;
(2) enteric and respiratory diseases.

In addition to bacteria, mycoplasmas and viruses can play a key role in the production of disease, but in the context of this paper the part played by antibacterials in disease control is considered.

Antibacterials

In *Table 13.6* is given a list of the major antibacterials used for the therapy of animal disease, differentiated according to their area of activity. i.e. Gram-positive, Gram-negative or broad spectrum. All these antibiotics are of considerable value in animal therapy, but their effectiveness will depend on a proper diagnosis being made, and the antibiotic formulation being applied for the right period.

Table 13.6 Antibacterial agents used in animal therapy

Gram-positive	*Gram-negative*	*Broad spectrum*
Penicillin	*Framycetin	Ampicillin
Erythromycin	*Neomycin	Cephalosporin
Lincomycin	Polymyxin	Chloramphenicol
Tylosin	*Streptomycin	Furazolidone
		Sulphonamides
		Sulphonamide/ trimethorpim
		Tetracyclines

*Some Gram-positive activity.

In veterinary medicine, as in human therapy outside the hospital, drugs are administered at least initially without a full knowledge of the bacteria involved or their sensitivity to the drug used. It is important, therefore, that the veterinary practitioner does have a good understanding of the range of antibiotics available to him and, where possible, the type of infections present on the farms he is advising.

Tables 13.7 and *13.8* give a comparison between the range of activity of penicillin G and the semi-synthetic penicillin ampicillin, and I think they highlight the importance of knowing both the activity and range of antibiotics before therapy is applied.

Table 13.7

Strain	*Penicillin G* ($\mu g\ ml^{-1}$)	*Ampicillin* ($\mu g\ ml^{-1}$)
*Staph. aureus**	0.03	0.05
Strep. agalactiae	0.018	0.07
Strep. dysgalactiae	0.02	0.02
Strep. uberis	0.035	0.018
C. pyogenes	0.02	0.20
C. bovis	0.10	0.40
B. anthracis	0.008	0.06
Cl. welchii (perfringens)	0.06	0.025

*Sensitive strains.

Table 13.8

Strain	*Penicillin G* ($\mu g\ ml^{-1}$)	*Ampicillin* ($\mu g\ ml^{-1}$)
Strep. faecalis	1.25–12.5	1.25–5
Pasteurella spp.	0.3	0.3
Salmonella spp.	8	1.25
Klebsiella Spp.*	250	1.25
E. coli	64	5
Proteus mirabilis	32	4

*Sensitive strains.

Since the Swann Report a number of antibacterials have come to be described as 'growth promoters' and these are listed below.

Carbadox
Emtryl
Flavomycin
Nitrovin (Payzone)
Virginiamycin
Zinc Bacitracin

All these drugs conform to the Swann criteria, and can be added to the feed or water supply by the farmer without veterinary supervision. I think it is important that all farmers who use 'growth promoters' should be aware of their limitations, and should not look on them merely as a means of covering a bad system of animal production, as it is possible to mask a more serious virus or mycoplasma infection by continual use of growth promoters.

Before discussing therapy, I would like to stress a number of aspects of the formulation of antibacterials which can influence their efficacy in disease entities.

Intramammaries

Figure 13.2 shows the difference in release rate between a formulation suitable for therapy during lactation, and that now used for treatment during the dry period.

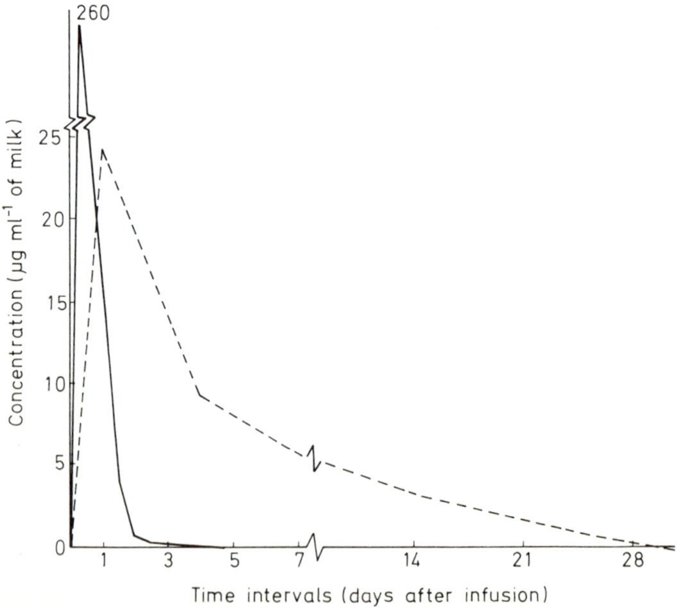

Figure 13.2 The persistence of antibiotic in udder secretion following the infusion of two cloxacillin products. — = A cloxacillin product in a quick release base; - - - = a cloxacillin product in a slow release (dry cow) base

It was demonstrated by Smith *et al.* (1967) that using benzathine cloxacillin, a relatively insoluble salt in a long acting base during the dry period, it was possible to achieve persistence of the drug and to increase the bacteriological control of staphylococcal infections from 50 to 70%. This finding has established that two different types of formulations are necessary for mastitis control:

(1) A short acting formulation for lactation therapy which will be active against streptococci, staphylococci and *E. coli* and will milk out readily. The bacteriological activity of this formulation will be variable against staphylococcal infections, but will give a clinical cure in over 90% of infections.

(2) A long acting formulation for treating the cow at the start of the dry period. The aim of this formulation is to deal with both clinical and sub-clinical staphylococcal infections which may not have responded to therapy during lactation. The formulation should also deal with streptococcal and Gram-negative infections.

Formulations for Oral Use

A range of formulations are now available for animal therapy and they consist of capsules, tablets, powders suitable for addition to the food or water, and oral dosers (which are generally used for dosing baby pigs.) The formulations are usually broad spectrum antibiotics, with the exception of certain antibiotics which have antimycoplasma activity, and are used mainly for the control of enteric infections.

Formulations for Injection

There are solutions or suspensions which are given intramuscularly, subcutaneously or intravenously and are suitable for the treatment of acute, clinical conditions. It is possible to obtain rapid significant blood levels, which ensure adequate antibiotic levels at the site of infection.

Animal Production and Disease Control

When antibacterials were first developed for animal treatment, they were thought of and investigated to a certain extent as an extension of human therapy, and treatment was related to the individual diseased animal. Then in the late 1950s and early 60s with the development of intensive methods of animal management, particularly in the pig and poultry field, antibacterials were added to the feed for prolonged periods to control or prevent the development of clinical disease. This led to the development of high levels of resistant organisms both in the gut of treated animals and in their environment, so that as a result of the findings of the Swann Report and the comments on bacteria mentioned by Dr. Williams Smith, it is now appropriate to look again at animal therapy so that systems of treatment can be evolved which will minimize the risk of perpetuating resistant strains.

The economic importance of disease in animal production units has been emphasized by Morris and Ellis in the case of mastitis, and Govier in a paper in the *Pig Farmer* produced evidence to show that losses due to bacterial and other infections in a 1000-sow unit can be very significant. He lists:

Losses	£
Stillbirths, neonatal scours, etc. over a 6 week period	9 070
Swine dysentery – 5 week period	21 000
Enzootic pneumonia	37 000

I propose, therefore, to discuss a number of disease problems in animal production and to suggest how antibacterials can be used at therapeutic levels as a key aspect of the control of disease.

Mastitis

Since penicillin was first used to treat mastitis due to *Strep. agalactiae,* the place of antibiotics in mastitis therapy has been studied by dairy scientists throughout the world, and their conclusions on their value have been influenced by the incidence of disease, the size of the herds, and the individual national policy employed for disease control. The studies carried out at the N.I.R.D. and the Central Veterinary Laboratory in the U.K. during the 1960s and at Cornell University in the U.S.A. culminated in a series of papers which described a mastitis control programme involving the use of teat dipping, milking machine maintenance, and antibiotic therapy. Therapy has to be carried out in two ways, during lactation to destroy bacteria and to remove clinical symptoms, and during the dry period to eliminate the majority of infections which are present at the end of lactation.

Table 13.9 Efficiency of treatment

		Average bacteriological cure			
Time	*Reason for*	*Strep. infections*	*Staph. infections*	*Other infections*	*Milk loss*
Lactation	50% cases recognized by the farmer	75% 1253*	30% 1204*	65% 310*	5 Days
Dry period	Mastitis control	95% 625*	72% 663*	70% 20*	Nil

*Infections.

Tables 13.9 and *13.10* show the difference in therapeutic response that one can expect when using lactation and dry cow formulations.

Table 13.10

Dry cow treatment

(1) It is possible to treat all cows at a known period
(2) Therapy is more effective
(3) There is no loss of milk
(4) The system is complementary to dairy hygiene during lactation

Lactation therapy

(1) Clinical disease has to be recognized
(2) Difficult to control length and effectiveness of therapy
(3) Milk has to be discarded (time varies)
(4) Infected cow has to be segregated
(5) Treatment relatively ineffective in 'Staph. infections'

Dry cow therapy is now accepted as an integral part of a mastitis control programme. It has the merit that it provides a means of applying antibiotic in the udder at a time when it is likely to achieve the maximum bacterial cure, and is more convenient to the farmer. In addition, it eliminates the likelihood of antibiotic residues in the milk following therapy.

Enteritis in Pigs

Because of the present system of housing pigs, it is inevitable that the level of bacteria, viruses, mycoplasma, etc., to which pigs of all ages are exposed will fluctuate, so that outbreaks of infectious disease are an integral part of any production process. Govier has indicated the financial loss that can follow outbreaks of disease at all ages, so that effective therapy must play an important part in any system of management.

Neonatal Scours

Scouring usually due to pathogenic *E. coli* can occur within 12 h of birth in some litters and, if it is not treated, death may follow within 48 h.

Studies with amoxycillin and ampicillin against both natural and artificially induced coliform scours have shown that early oral therapy can prevent losses. Affected piglets should be dosed once or twice daily for three days. Similar results have been reported for other broad spectrum antibiotics.

Weaning and Adult Scours

Outbreaks of enteritis in pigs can occur at weaning (from 3 to 8 weeks) and occasionally up to 16 weeks of age. The symptoms can be associated with *E. coli, Salmonella,* or Swine dysentery due to *Treponema hyodysenteria.* Svendsen *et al.* (1974) reported on post-weaning *E. coli* diarrhoea in three herds and found 25% mortality and high morbidity among untreated pigs. The disease usually occurred during the first two weeks after weaning.

Treatment with an antibiotic either in the drinking water or feed for up to 5 days will reduce mortality and morbidity. Where there is evidence of a bacteraemia, parenteral therapy plus oral therapy is necessary to control the infection. *Salmonella* infections in pigs usually occur sporadically and can be a serious problem in hysterectomy-produced herds, when infection may be introduced via contaminated feed. Heard *et al.* (1965) reported an outbreak of *Salmonella typhimurium* in which 10-week old and in-pig gilts were affected with acute salmonellosis; there was a morbidity of about 30%. Treatment with both chloramphenicol and ampicillin given parenterally was carried out and 94% of the animals treated with antibiotic recovered. The use of an antibiotic is valuable in that it will prevent unnecessary losses. It has to be remembered that therapy, whilst effective in reducing loss, may not eliminate the carrier state, so that in the event of an outbreak, control measures in addition to antibiotic therapy must involve the investigation of the cause of the outbreak, total disinfection of the premises and the removal of carriers where necessary. It is also necessary under the Zoonosis Order to report the presence of *Salmonella* on the affected farm.

Swine dysentery is now a well recognized entity and is due to *Treponema hyodysenteriae* alone or in association with *E. coli* and other enterobacteria and can be induced by feeding cultures of the major organism. In the field the disease is usually recognized after weaning from eight weeks onwards and must be differentiated from *E. coli* scours. The scours are usually mucohaemorrhagic and progressive.

Antibacterials at high dosage will control swine dysentery but Emtryl (dimetridazole) given in the ration at 0.01 to 0.015% will prevent the appearance of clinical symptoms.

Pneumonia

Bille *et al.* (1974) carried out a study in 17 Danish sow herds to determine the typical bacteria found on post mortems in cases of pneumonia. They recorded Streptococci groups C and L and other serotypes in 25% of cases, *Haemophilus parahaemolyticus* in 24.5%, *Pasteurella* sp. 11.4%, *C. pyogenes* 6.0%, *E. coli* 6.8%. *Haemophilus parahaemolyticus* had a definite herd predilection probably related to the indoor climate.

Although pneumonia in pigs can be of mixed mycoplasma, viral, bacterial origin, parenteral antibiotic therapy with a drug effective against the common bacterial pathogens is of value when carried out early in the infection.

The disease entities described here vary in their significance according to the management system employed on the farm, but in the foreseeable future antibiotic therapy applied in association with other control measures will prevent the perpetual scours and pneumonias seen on many farms.

The pig unit has been chosen to illustrate the relationship between bacterial infections and the other disease entities which occur on the modern farm. In a similar way in the calf unit 'scouring' and pneumonia are related to a variety of management practices, and bacteria form part of the infection pattern. Control of the bacteria by the use of therapeutic doses of an antibiotic is frequently successful in a high percentage of outbreaks, but successful long-term control is related to a detailed appreciation by the farmer and his veterinary surgeon of the interrelated pattern of infections occurring on a specific farm. Intensive methods have meant that the disease problem can vary from farm to farm.

Conclusion

Antibiotic therapy is likely to remain an integral part of disease control in all animal units, and its successful use is related to a detailed understanding of the management practices on the individual farm.

References

BILLE, N., NIELSEN, N.C., SVENDSEN, J. and RIISING, H.J. (1974). *Report of 3rd International Pig Veterinary Congress,* Lyons, France, June 12–14. ESPIC, Toulouse

HEARD, T.W., LINTON, A.H., PENNY, R.H.C. and WILSON, M.R. (1965). *Vet. Rec.,* **77**, 44

SMITH, A., WESTGARTH, D.R., JONES, M.R., NEAVE, F.K., DODD, F.H. and BRANDER, G.C. (1967). *Vet. Rec.,* **81**, 504

SVENDSEN, J., LARSEN, J.L., BILLE, N. and NIELSEN, N.C. (1974). *Report of 3rd International Pig Veterinary Congress,* Lyons, France, June 12–14. ESPIC, Toulouse

WILLIAMS-SMITH, H. (1971). *Advances in Veterinary Science and Comparative Medicine,* Vol. 15, pp. 67–100. Academic Press, London and New York

14

FARM ANIMAL DISEASE: VETERINARIAN AND ANTIBIOTICS

B. MARTIN
Kilmarnock, Scotland

I am pleased to have been invited to this important Symposium as a representative of the practising sector of the Veterinary Profession and to have the opportunity to offer you an account of the disease situations which confront the veterinarian in the field, and as they relate to the use of antimicrobial substances for the maintenance of health and productivity of farm livestock. In practice I am concerned with dairy cattle in Ayrshire in South West Scotland and my remarks are confined largely to that species in that area, although the disease situations and the principles involved in the use of antibiotics seem likely to have general veterinary application.

The Disease Situation

No one is likely to dispute the economic and other justifications for the emergence of present day systems of intensive livestock husbandry which have resulted in an improvement in whole-farm efficiency and productivity. The very nature of these systems and not least their inherent high stocking rates, however, present environmental conditions which expose their animal populations to a variety of diseases of infectious nature, and which require careful supervision and control if they are not to threaten the benefits for which intensive systems were first designed.

A major factor which contributes to the occurrence and spread of infectious disease among intensively managed cattle of all ages is the difficulty of maintaining satisfactory environmental hygiene in every sense. Dense stocking rates signify high levels of pollution of the animals' environment and the presence of intensive populations through which rapid and widespread contagion may occur. Consequently, the practising veterinarian finds himself confronted by a variety of environmental infectious diseases represented by coliform mastitis, infectious abortion, infectious foot disease, the complex of contagious pneumonias and upper respiratory disease, and enteric conditions caused by viral agents, coliform and *Salmonella* bacteria.

The veterinary profession and our colleagues sharing allied interests in the health and productivity of farm livestock, are much aware of the part which environmental factors play in the occurrence of these diseases which may present a major economic problem in intensively managed herds. These are by no means new disease entities. They have occurred in more tolerable form in less intensive times, but their prevalence and clinical severity have increased in the latest man-made animal environments. The veterinary aims for the prevention and control of diseases of intensively managed livestock are quite clear. It is only through precise understanding of the multitude of epidemiological factors that the events of infection, disease process and subsequent lateral spread may be interrupted and disease prevented or controlled. We require detailed knowledge of environmental features, the ecology of pathogenic bacteria and viruses which pollute the environment, factors influencing the immune status and immune response of exposed animals, disease heritability, and the interplay of all of these and many other factors involved in the onset and spread of infectious disease.

This is a challenge which has not been disregarded. It has been well identified and accepted and already we are committed to a multi-disciplinary approach to methods of disease investigation and control, but the necessary studies are of a long-term and ongoing nature. Systems for disease control are already in existence and, particularly in the case of many metabolic and parasitic diseases, have been shown to be highly effective if applied conscientiously. In the case of infectious diseases, however, the interplay of environmental factors and the ecology of infectious agents and their animal hosts is more complex and often less well understood. Control measures are not likely to be totally effective when they are based on knowledge which is yet incomplete and in some areas our knowledge may be so lacking as to offer little opportunity to devise worthwhile control systems at this time.

The effect of these circumstances for the livestock owner and the veterinary surgeon are quite similar. As far as the farmer is concerned, an effective or partly effective system for control of a specific infectious disease or complex may or may not exist. If it does not exist, infectious disease will occur. If it does exist, it is unlikely to be always wholly effective however well the necessary programme is applied, if at all, and again, infectious disease will continue to occur at some level. More often than not, animal environments are created first and disease follows as a result of unforeseen faults in the new environment or shortcomings in management which, themselves, may arise in part from imperfections in the design of the livestock system.

It is seldom a simple matter to remedy environmental faults in accommodation which has been erected at some expense and around which the entire livestock system is already operating, so that disease occurrence may become accepted by the farmer as an inherent part of the whole and to be controlled by the regular use of antibiotics. However undesirable the situation may be, it is sadly a matter of fact that, for the farmer, it is often more convenient though seldom less expensive in the long term, to rely on antibiotics for the treatment and control of infectious disease, as a substitute for improving the environment or correcting shortcomings in management. Antibiotics, therefore, may remain an indispensable means of protecting the productivity and profitability of many a livestock enterprise.

As far as the veterinary profession is concerned, we accept that the therapeutic use of antimicrobial substances is unlikely ever to be replaced by systems of management which will result in disease-free populations of farm livestock.

Already there are major advances in systems of disease control and prevention but these and those to come cannot be expected to be always totally effective or universally implemented. Disease occurrences will always be part of the livestock scene and antibiotics a major contribution to veterinary therapeutics.

At the same time, we in the veterinary profession support and endorse the conclusions and recommendations of the 1969 Report of the Swann Committee on the use of Antibiotics in Animal Husbandry and Veterinary Medicine. That report, while recognizing the continuing need for the use of antibiotics for therapeutic purposes and of non-therapeutic antibiotics for the promotion of growth in farm livestock, emphasizes the dangers to man arising from the administration of antibiotics to animals and the hazards of antibiotic resistance to man and animals alike, and the need for the judicious use of antibiotics is underlined. We agree also, that while the need for the therapeutic use of antibiotics continues, 'more attention should be paid to other possible ways of modifying the environmental flora of animals' and 'that there is a need for research into the consequences of influencing the bacterial environment by higher standards of hygiene and other means'.

In practice, therefore, the veterinary profession has a dual responsibility. We are much aware of the continuing need to promote and establish further programmes for disease prevention and control where our epidemiological knowledge and farm conditions allow us to do so. At the same time we accept that with or without control programmes, infectious disease occurs and will continue to occur and our responsibility then concerns how best and how prudently we may use antimicrobial substances for the improvement of animal health and productivity and always mindful of the need to protect the health of the human consumer.

Veterinary Use of Antibiotics

The essential action of microbials is to interfere with the vital structures or metabolic processes of microorganisms so that they are killed or their multiplication inhibited, and it is this bactericidal or bacteriostatic effect which we utilize in our efforts to obtain a rapid and satisfactory return to health and productivity of an infected animal. To achieve this result a suitable antibiotic must be administered at an effective therapeutic dose rate. Ideally, the choice of antibiotic should be based on the identification and known sensitivity of the causal organism, since treatment, to be successful, must be aimed at the microorganism responsible for the disease process (Garrod and O'Grady, 1971). In veterinary practice, however, a number of factors seldom permit such an ideal approach to the selection of an antibiotic. Not least of the problems is the clinical severity of disease in an acutely ill animal, which does not allow for the collection of material for laboratory culture and sensitivity testing, prior to the institution of specific therapy. Likewise, the commercial demand for a rapid return to health of an infected animal and its contribution to herd production does not accept delay in commencing treatment. An example of these circumstances is offered by the high yielding dairy cow experiencing an episode of acute mastitis. No clinical features of such a case offer the opportunity to surmise what the causal organism might be and mastitis of that type may be due to one or several of a variety of Gram-positive or Gram-negative bacteria. The need for laboratory identification of the organism and its sensitivity to antibiotics might seem to be a prerequisite to treatment, but in practice the postponement of therapy pending laboratory reports would be generally unacceptable, since undue loss of mild yield, permanent damage to the udder or death of the animal may result.

In contrast, and in the case of the occurrence of a specific disease likely to have only one microbial cause, such as calf diarrhoea due to *E. coli* infection, it may be thought that the selection of an antibiotic generally known to be effective against Gram-negative organisms, is likely to be straightforward and not requiring laboratory knowledge of sensitivity. In this case, however, the causal organism is well known at times to exhibit resistance to a number of antibiotics usually effective against Gram-negatives, and indeed the need for sensitivity testing is really no less than in the case of mastitis. Again, however, the affected calf is frequently in a state of collapse following enteric infection and its systemic consequences, and delay in instituting therapy would be considered intolerable in normal clinical and commercial circumstances.

The demand on the veterinary surgeon is to commence antibiotic treatment as soon as clinical examination confirms or suggests the nature of the disease which is presented. At the same time, where the location of the disease process allows the collection of material for laboratory investigation, this is normally carried out routinely so that subsequent treatment may be altered to conform with laboratory reports, if the response to initial treatment proves to be unsatisfactory. The initial choice of antibiotic is therefore largely empirical but nevertheless judicious, as we shall see, and when specimens are taken in the meantime for laboratory investigation, the value of the ultimate report is greatest when the primary treatment has failed to bring about the expected clinical improvement. Also, pertinent information is then available for any further cases of the same disease which may occur soon after the first, and in intensive animal groups this is more likely to happen than not.

The selection of antibiotic for virtually all cases, therefore, requires to be made at the time of the first examination of the animal, to be followed later by precise laboratory information, except when the location or nature of the disease process does not permit collection of specimen material. In effect, these circumstances present no more of a problem to the veterinary clinician than the everyday need to reach an instant diagnosis on the clinical signs to be found by the totally objective examination of a diseased animal. The choice of antibiotic for the case in hand is based on a variety of factors within the clinician's appreciation of that case and of its environment, his knowledge of the spectrum of activity and mode of action of available antibiotics, knowledge of the nature of the known or suspected pathogen, and not least, and without apology, on his clinical experience.

Naturally, the known spectrum of antibacterial activity of antibiotics is a priority consideration when initial treatment is being selected. Where a specific disease entity such as *Fusiformis* diphtheria or *Actinobacillosis* is diagnosed, an appropriate antimicrobial such as penicillin or streptomycin, respectively, may be used since these bacteria are generally known to be sensitive to these preparations. Where the identity of the organism is unknown or uncertain, or where a variety of bacteria are known to be capable of causing the clinical condition which has been identified, it is established practice to select a preparation which has a broad spectrum of activity and in veterinary medicine members of the tetracycline group are widely used in these circumstances. Alternatively, combinations of antibiotics may be selected and it is in this connection that the question of synergism in veterinary therapeutics arises. While the combination of two bactericidal antibiotics such as penicillin and streptomycin, or of two bacteriostats such as trimethoprim and sulphadoxine, potentiates the antibacterial activity of both substances, it is not generally for this specific reason that these are used in combination. Rather, it is the relatively broad spectrum of the combination which receives the greater consideration and which results in their common usage in situations where the identity of causal organisms is unknown or uncertain, although it may be that the range of their combined spectrum is due in part to their synergic partnership.

The mode of action of antibiotics may influence the selection of treatment. It is not normal practice to use a bacteriostatic preparation in conjunction with a bactericidal, where the former may antagonize the action of the latter, and while a bactericidal effect seems likely to be more effective than a bacteriostatic mode of action, the range of bactericidal antibiotics in large-animal veterinary medicine is restricted to penicillin, streptomycin, and neomycin. Choice on this basis, therefore, is not wide and the priority for the treatment of cattle tends to be generally in favour of a preparation of suitable spectrum to be given at generous therapeutic dose rates.

Clinical experience is not to be disregarded as one of the less important or less acceptable factors influencing the selection of antibiotics for veterinary use. It bears significantly in the initial establishment of treatment where factors such as local knowledge of the nature of epidemics or experience of recent circumstances on certain farms, are applicable to current disease situations. From previous experience and investigation, the regular practitioner may be aware that a specific infectious disease on one farm may normally respond to sulphonamides, while on other premises causes of the same specific disease may not respond unless tetracyclines are employed. Experience of up-to-date circumstances on any one farm may be critically important for the emergency treatment of conditions such as enteric colibacillosis of calves, when the antibiotic sensitivity of resident pathogens may vary almost from week-to-week during an intensive winter or spring calving period, and where regular monitoring of sensitivity has been carried out in the recent past.

Notwithstanding the constant demand for the establishment of antibiotic therapy at the time of first examination of a diseased animal, the importance and usefulness of sensitivity testing is widely appreciated in veterinary practice. Following initial treatment and while laboratory reports on sensitivity are awaited, response of the patient to early therapy is assessed by further clinical appraisal as required. Where clinical response is unsatisfactory, it is normal practice to introduce a change of antibiotic such that the spectrum of antibacterial effect is altered. Experience has shown that the first choice of antibiotic, or any subsequent necessary alteration on clinical grounds, is usually proved to be consistent with ultimate laboratory reports on the sensitivity of organisms cultured from specimen materials. Nevertheless, it is still routine practice to investigate the bacteriological and sensitivity nature of specimen materials where appropriate. While a later sensitivity report consistent with the treatment chosen for the now recuperating animal is perhaps little more than reassuring, bacteriological details are often an epidemiological guide to the source of the original disease, particularly in the case of mastitis.

The value of sensitivity testing in cattle disease is restricted largely to mammary and enteric infections from which specimen materials can be readily collected. In the case of pneumonias, where a wide variety of bacteria, viruses, and mycoplasmas may be isolated from the naso-pharynx, their pathogenic or commensal nature cannot be readily determined and sampling is not commonly practised.

In mastitis it is by no means always the case that satisfactory clinical results follow treatment which conforms with laboratory observations on the sensitivity of what has appeared to be the causal organism. This is particularly true in cases of severe acute forms of the disease. In the case of enteric infections, however, laboratory observations on the antibiotic sensitivity of isolated organisms are of high value and often essential for the satisfactory and continuing control of enteric colibacillosis in young calves. This is a complex which offers an outstanding example of a disease problem whose control can be greatly frustrated by rapidly changing antibiotic resistance. During an intensive calving period the virulence of coliform organisms often appears to be stepped up, presumably in part due to the increasing number of hosts available for passage of infection, and assisted by conditions of overcrowding and progressive deterioration of hygiene. Numerous other epidemiological factors are no doubt involved, not least the immune status of the neonate relative to the intensity of the challenge. Whatever the epidemiological complexities may be, when bacterial diarrhoea commences and spreads rapidly in these conditions, many animals may require antibiotic by the oral route. The susceptibility pattern of resident or imported serotypes of *E. coli* in these circumstances may alter so frequently and so rapidly that any suspicion of the onset of inferior clinical response in new cases must be followed at once by further sensitivity testing if serious losses are to be avoided.

Frequent laboratory investigation of specimen materials from infected animals requiring treatment or of post-mortem specimens, do not suggest that resistance of the common pathogens of farm livestock to much of the range of available antibiotics is a feature of the veterinary scene. This is still the case after many years of widespread antibiotic usage, and it is an unusual laboratory report which does not offer the clinician a number of antibiotics which show *in vitro* activity against pathogens from field cases, dead or alive.

In such an otherwise acceptable situation, it is a source of disappointment to the veterinary clinician that many cases of two of the most commonly occurring disease conditions to afflict present day livestock, so often fail to respond to any of the antibiotics indicated by *in vitro* sensitivity tests. In field practice the failure of cases of severe acute mastitis in cows and to a lesser extent of pneumonias in young cattle, to respond to antibiotics is well known. In the case of mastitis the lack of clinical response to an initially chosen antibiotic or combination given by intramammary and parenteral routes is often confounded by a later laboratory report which reveals an *in vitro* susceptibility of the apparent causal organism to the same antibiotics which have failed to effect even a clinical improvement. In the case of pneumonias, sensitivity testing of specimen materials from the live animal is not commonly carried out for reasons which have been explained, although reports may be obtained from examination of post-mortem material taken from dead representatives of a group incident of pneumonia. In any case, large doses of broad-spectrum antibiotics, rotated with others as necessary, and given by the intravenous route and maintained by the same or the intramuscular route, frequently fail to relieve the clinical distress in severe acute cases and mortality rates may be quite high in some outbreaks.

It may be that the nature of the lesion in these two disease processes does not permit effective penetration of antimicrobials to the site of bacterial invasion, and the gross cellular proliferation which is a dominant feature of their pathology may be a factor. The early lesions of the contagious pneumonias of young cattle are almost always associated with a variety of respiratory viruses and mycoplasmas against which the common antibiotics have little activity, but it has been shown experimentally that the majority of these agents *per se* seldom cause clinical respiratory disease and it is generally accepted that it is the secondary bacterial bronchopneumonia which produces the field syndrome. It seems likely that this is the reason for the response of the majority of field cases to antibiotic therapy, but totally refractory cases are not uncommon.

Further and successful research into the *in vivo* behaviour of antibiotics relative to the nature of pathological processes in mammary and pulmonary tissues, with a view to improving antibacterial effect in these locations would be a major advance and is awaited with some impatience by veterinary clinicians and no doubt by the livestock industry, whom they serve.

In conclusion, the veterinary surgeon appreciates the instrumental importance of antibiotics in controlling the bacterial environment of man and his domestic livestock, and he employs them for the treatment of animal disease along with other means of chemotherapy and supportive treatment which are often no less important. We see them, often as a poor but necessary substitute for disease prevention and good management which reduce but seldom remove their need. It is to be hoped that their long-term usefulness will be protected and their potential hazards to man and animals reduced, if they are used with the discretion and control which they surely demand.

References

GARROD, L.P. and O'GRADY, F. (1971). In *Antibiotic and Chemotherapy,* 3rd edn. Livingstone, London

REPORT OF THE JOINT COMMITTEE on the use of *Antibiotics in Animal Husbandry and Veterinary Medicine,* (1969). Cmnd. 4190

15

INTRAMAMMARY THERAPY: ITS ACHIEVEMENTS AND LIMITATIONS

J.K.L. PEARSON
Government of Northern Ireland, Department of Agriculture, Veterinary Research Laboratories, Stormont, Belfast, U.K.

Summary

The principal achievements of intramammary therapy in the control of udder infections in cattle during the past 30 years are summarized, together with some of the problems and possible hazards which have arisen in parallel.

The paper discusses the situation under five different themes (1) Elimination of udder infection from herds, (2) Lactation and dry cow therapy, (3) The evaluation of intramammary formulae, (4) The changing pattern of bacteria following antibiotic therapy and (5) Inhibitory substance residues in milk. Recent reviews and the results of others are discussed as relevant in each area from a veterinary and medical viewpoint and some recommendations are put forward for consideration.

Introduction

In approaches towards the control of bovine mastitis, the introduction of antibiotics into intramammary formulae over thirty years ago was welcomed with great enthusiasm and anticipation.

Many thousands of papers have since been written on the use of intramammary products, and the object of this paper is to piece together some of the many benefits which have accrued during these years and to summarize some of the problems which have arisen and which still confront us. Plommet and Le Louedec (1975) recently discussed therapy during lactation, referring to the optimism of earlier years followed by the changing pattern of bacterial flora, the antibiotic residue problem and the varied success of many workers in obtaining bacteriological cures. Some of these points will be considered more fully in this paper in relationship to the role of lactation therapy.

In the late 'forties, different bases were used for penicillins and other products and I took a considerable interest in the use of a slow-release based penicillin formulae for the prevention of the so-called 'summer mastitis' of dry cows (Pearson, 1950, 1951) a disease commonly associated with *C. pyogenes.*

Following the observations of Neave, Dodd and Henriques (1950) in their studies on new infections during the dry period, it was natural that consideration should be given to the use of dry cow therapy on a wider basis, and its value in this respect has been studied by many workers throughout the world for 25 years. Schultze gave an excellent review of the situation in 1975, summarizing the approaches using different drugs and formulae, their therapeutic efficiency, the design of trials, the problems of the pharmaceutical chemist and many other aspects of the dry cow therapy story, areas of controversy and future research.

There is little merit in duplicating the references of the above American and French workers; instead the principal achievements obtained from lactation and dry cow therapy will be highlighted here, and some of the problems and shortcomings which accompany them at the present time will be discussed.

Lovell (1962) and Edwards (1962) focused mainly on the benefits which had been achieved at that time, but even so Lovell made reference to the emergence of resistant strains of staphylococci, *E. coli* and salmonellae; while Edwards referred to the serious problems arising from antibiotic residues in market milk, and the possible hazards to man and animals through increased numbers of antibiotic resistant strains or allergies (Barber, 1960). At the same time, Smith (1962) recorded that Wilson (1961) had noted that resistant bovine staphylococci had increased from 40% in 1955, to 62% in 1958 and 70% in 1961 in the United Kingdom.

It was not unexpected, therefore, that a Government White Paper was produced in 1963 on the use of 'Antibiotics in Milk in Great Britain' to consider the position and to recommend courses of action through legislation, milk producers' contracts, and the control, sale and use of intramammary products.

Perhaps the most suitable way of commenting on these various themes is to discuss some of the more important of them briefly, and then put forward some recommendations for discussion.

Elimination of Udder Infections from Herds

Edwards (1962) made a bold statement in relation to the obligatory pathogen *Str. agalactiae* when he said that 'today this organism is relatively unimportant'. He assumed from his own work and that of others that penicillin intramammary products were rapidly eradicating the organism in the national herd, but although the Danes have reduced the herd incidence to about 1% in an intensive campaign, the United Kingdom still has a high level of infected herds considering the quantity of antibiotics which have been used for therapy during the past 25 years.

No national surveys to my knowledge have been carried out recently in Britain in this respect, but from personal contact with veterinarians in Scotland, *Str. agalactiae* is still said to be a wide-spread herd pathogen, while the incidence in herds in Northern Ireland (in both churn and bulk tank producers) was recently found to be 37% (Greer and Pearson, 1973; Pearson, Greer and Pollock, 1976). In many parts of the United States and Europe the organism is still very prevalent – 90% of herds in some areas – but much of this continues because of the common practice of interchange of stock. In France, Plommet and Le Louedec (1975) put much of the blame on lack of follow-up, poor hygiene, apathy, and the erratic use of therapeutic measures.

Newbould (1975) also stressed the need for a conscientious and constructive approach, but perhaps because of the absence of an immediate financial incentive, and in some cases the existence of a high initial cost, the problem is still a major one in many countries. The same writer refers to the possibilities of eradicating other udder infections, but it is even clearer in his comments here that lactation therapy is only a *part* of a control programme and this is a view commonly held by most research workers.

The contribution made by dry cow therapy preparations is also considerable in the elimination of udder infections, and reviews by Schultze (1975) and Dodd and Griffin (1975) should be closely studied. As with lactation treatment, however, it is only *part* of a mastitis control system and during the past decade we have observed that there is far too much reliance on dry cow therapy on its own – many farmers making little progress whatsoever. In one such study of 25 high incidence herds and 25 low incidence herds (Pearson *et al.*, 1972), 68% of herds in each group used automatic dry cow therapy, but 48% of the high incidence herds had *Str. agalactiae* infection and annual mean cell counts remained at over 1 million cells ml^{-1}.

Many milk producers have come to depend too much on dry cow therapy and, in consequence, methods of drying off cows efficiently have been relaxed in some herds and other husbandry standards have deteriorated, with the result that often little overall reduction in the herd incidence is achieved.

Lactation Therapy and Dry Cow Therapy

The primary object of lactation therapy is to treat existing and new infections with a view to eliminating them. Successful clinical response may be achieved, but in many such cases the infection recurs – especially where coagulase positive staphylococci are responsible; indeed, many observers consider that a response rate of 40% is encouraging. The response to therapy depends largely on the severity of pathological reaction and in acute cases resulting from *E. coli* and *C. pyogenes* it may be nil, unless systemic therapeutic support is also given.

Treatment of infections during lactation may not be confined to clinical cases, but may also be applied to subclinically affected quarters confirmed by indirect tests and usually laboratory support. Danish workers have invested in a comprehensive system of this type since 1955, but few countries have injected so much veterinary effort and financial capital into a similar type of mastitis control programme to compare costs and the resulting benefits they quote (Olsen, 1975). They overcome the antibiotic residue problem which can arise from lactation therapy, in the same way as the Dutch, by strict legislation on the use of intramammary products by veterinarians and by the application of severe penalties for contaminated milk.

Dry cow therapy in the prophylaxis of *C. pyogenes* infection in cows has stood the test of time for 25 years and I would still insist that, until someone proves otherwise, a comparatively cheap antibiotic such as penicillin in a slow release base, will be as effective as any of the newer and more expensive synthetic products.

The extension of dry cow therapy on a wider scale is, however, another matter and has now been widely studied throughout the world since the initial work of

Smith *et al.* (1967). Despite the great pressure emanating from some workers in Britain and America that it is an essential part of every control programme, it is of interest to see how many people have reservations about it, some who wish to use it selectively and others who do not wish to use it at all. The reasons for these varying opinions are clear in some cases, but many arise from the results obtained in poorly designed experimental trials.

Schultze (1975) refers to 'the first of a series of large-scale field experiments' (Dodd and Neave, 1970) but if this work is closely studied, it is seen that no adequate control herds were kept, and even the definition of 'infections' cleared would by today's standards be strongly challenged by workers in Scandinavia, New Zealand, and by many pathologists. Schultze suggests that we might have expected to see better uniformity with dry cow therapy in field application and comments on the possible influence of variable penetration of udder tissue. Certainly Bratlie (1973), Uvarov *et al.* (1967), and Pearson and Wright (1969) would agree with this being an important factor.

We must also ask ourselves why dry cow therapy is not recommended by such a progressive country as Denmark, as the only reasons they give is that the prolonged use of sub-therapeutic doses of antibiotic might accelerate the development of resistant strains (Olsen, 1975). Resistant strains did, however, appear in many other countries long before dry cow treatment became popular, so this may not be particularly good reasoning. Many herds in the United Kingdom and elsewhere have benefited from the use of dry cow therapy, and most farmers who have adopted the routine would not abandon it whatever the arguments, and there is always the added bonus of minimal risk from antibiotic milk residues.

Many of the more recent papers on dry cow therapy however are either against its use in blanket form (Morse, 1975; Plommet and Le Louedec, 1975) or favour its use selectively (Serieys and Roguinsky, 1975), or, like Funke (1975) and myself, suggest that we should not be so reliant on it as an artificial masking replacement for good husbandry.

The Evaluation of Intramammary Formulae

This is not an area in which I have any specialist knowledge, but clearly in the minds of all who look at their application in the field, two factors are of outstanding relevance:

(1) The product ultimately available commercially must be evaluated properly in field trials and not, as is often the case, be based solely on *in vitro* assessments.

(2) It must be economically acceptable.

As Uvarov (1971) stated, the product must be formulated for the benefit of two groups of people: the users and the legislators, taking into account tolerance, excretion rates and therapeutic efficiency. The pharmaceutical organizations are primarily responsible for the formulation which the veterinarian uses and the optimistic *in vitro* story is often misleading in view of the sensitivity patterns obtained against specific pathogens. It requires little imagination for the clinician to understand why a chronic fibrosed staphylococcal or an acutely affected *C. pyogenes* udder will not respond to cloxacillin or penicillin respectively, despite the *in vitro* sensitivity patterns. If a laboratory is simply asked to test isolates and pathogens for sensitivity in relation to particular cases, is the procedure of any realistic value to the practitioner?

In human medicine Steigbigel, Greenman and Remington (1975) state that *in vitro* studies correlate with some aspects of *in vivo* results but conflict quite clearly with others. In veterinary medicine the pharmaceutical chemist has an enormous task in unravelling this problem, primarily because of the high cost of animal studies. At best, a new formulation can only be screened, and the research worker must follow the manufacturer with adequately designed trials, including control herds, animals or half-udders, and ensure that the standards of diagnosis, definition, cure, failure, etc. will attract international respect.

Intramammary formulae are numerous and on the whole good, but even more testing headaches confront the industry as more is learnt and demanded in relation to drug absorption, distribution, metabolism and excretion. Along with many others, Ziv (1975) has extensively studied the pharmacokinetics of antibiotics of dry cow and lactation therapy, and visualizes more economical and quicker ways of evaluating new formulae than existed previously. In view of the massive worldwide use of intramammary products – many of them used blindly, automatically and irrationally – one must hope that this approach will be helpful.

Drug combinations in veterinary medicine are numerous and make evaluation of the final product more difficult, Swidler (1971) recording that a list of no fewer than 1300 drug interactions existed at that time. More recently, Parker (1976) outlined some of the advantages and disadvantages of fixed-dose combinations in veterinary medicine, and although on the credit side he comments on the values of synergism where they exist and the convenience of multiple drug therapy to the clinician, together with their lower cost, he considers that they encourage careless diagnosis and foster the use of more than one drug when only one may be required.

The Changing Pattern of Bacteria following Antibiotic Therapy

Reference has already been made to Wilson's observations in Britain (1961) that the incidence of penicillin-resistant bovine staphylococci rose from 40% to 70% within a period of 6 years. In Northern Ireland we test 500 isolates each year and during the past 10 years the incidence has varied between 80% and 90%. In 1963 Nyhan found 34% of bovine staphylococci in the Republic of Ireland to be penicillin-resistant.

Why the situation has not changed in Denmark is difficult to understand. They may have a different phage type of staphylococcus; it is difficult to believe that the situation exists simply because antibiotics are more rigidly controlled than in the United Kingdom, nor that their lack of favour with dry-cow therapy can contribute.

An important point made by Pedersen (1975) in this respect is the lack of uniformity which exists between countries in classifying strains as resistant. This varies from inhibitory levels of 1–16 i.u. penicillin ml^{-1}, now often referred to in micrograms, and the unification of techniques used is also far from standard. In Northern Ireland a disc containing a concentration of 1.5 i.u. is used, while in Germany and Austria the concentration used is 10 i.u. and in the Netherlands and Denmark it is 1.0 i.u. ml^{-1}.

The incidence of staphylococci resistant to streptomycin has also increased and according to Wilson (personal communication, 1976) appears to fluctuate in direct relation to its popularity and use.

Other changes occurring are in the proportion of staphylococci to streptococci and in the ratio of Gram-negative organisms to Gram-positives. In the early 'fifties we observed that staphylococci took the place of *Str. agalactiae* following blitz therapy of specific herds, and I was strongly reprimanded by higher authority for allowing this unwelcome change to arise. Edwards (1962) may have received similar advice and perhaps the Danes (Madsen *et al.*, 1975) are also wondering what they have achieved following the reduction of B, C, G and L streptococci, coupled with an increase of *Staph. aureus* from 25% in 1955 to 50% in 1972 – whatever their resistance pattern.

In the medical world there are many references to the shift of bacteriological ecology equilibrium and the majority of these quote that Gram-negative infections are becoming increasingly prevalent at the expense of those which are Gram-positive. The theme is similar to that of Parker (1976) who comments on the veterinary application of antibiotics, and Simmons and Stolley (1974) are especially critical about the use of antibiotics in a prophylactic role in humans. They quote the observations of Finland (1970) and Altemeier, Todd and Inge (1967) on the seriousness of this shift in hospital practice and more recent American observers (Kunin, Tupasi and Craig, 1973; Jackson, 1974; Aronson, 1975) state that antibiotics are overused – particularly in blanket therapy and prophylactic use – and more than half of them are not needed. Common to them all and many others, is their concern about the increasing prevalence of nosocominal Gram-negative infections, and it is interesting to see that both Aronson (1975) and Kagan, Fannin and Bardie (1973) feel that in this 'antibiotic era' insufficient attention is given to the role of host resistance and to the optimum nutritional factors which are of prime importance in maintaining animal and human health.

In bovine mastitis Howell (1972) drew attention to the changing pattern of infections found in the clinical form of the disease, the possible source of many Gram-negative environmental bacteria and made reference to Schalm's (1968) hypothesis about the risks of very low cell counts. She mentioned that the use of automatic dry cow therapy may be contributory in changing the pattern of future infections and there is no doubt that many observers consider this to be occurring now. Wilson and Birn (1966) warned that rapidly growing acid-fast organisms might follow dry cow treatment, although this was probably a result of bad technique; but more significant was the observation of Wilson *et al.* (1971) that L forms of *Str. agalactiae* appeared in a large herd following dry cow therapy and they suggested that 'the practice of treating all cows as they go dry with synthetic penicillin might have to be reconsidered'.

Even more significant, however, is the Gram-negative story and why it has apparently become more important during the past six years. Schultze (1975) quotes that no evidence has been found that dry cow therapy is a predisposing factor. Neither do Brander (1975) or Keefe (1975), but it is significant that the National Mastitis Council in America set up a special Coliform Mastitis Research Committee in 1974 to study this field anew, and we await with interest the results of intensified research at present being undertaken by NIRD workers and others.

An interesting but disturbing phenomenon in relation to coliform mastitis was seen by us in field studies with Northern Ireland veterinary surgeons during the past two winters, both of which were mild but very wet. The incidence of acute *clinical* cases in cows after calving was very much higher than usual, and the majority of these were in well managed herds with low mean cell counts. Automatic dry cow therapy and teat dipping or spraying were practised, a situation observed by Faull and Gillett (1973) who found *Str. uberis* and *E.coli* to be responsible for large numbers of clinical cases occurring in a herd with a mean cell count of 300×10^3 cells ml^{-1} during a two-year study.

Clearly, the balance between environment and host is complex and a fuller understanding is required of the role antibiotics play in altering this balance, particularly when they are used for prophylaxis.

In France (Plommet and Le Louedec, 1975) it was observed in 1970 that 1000 kg of antibiotic per year were estimated to be used for intramammary treatment of the country's 10 million cows, and in other parts of the world where there is even less rigid control of sales, there must be even greater use and waste.

In Northern Ireland one wholesaler, who distributes to veterinary surgeons only, issued 347 000 intramammary tubes in 1975, and sales through other channels would, with little difficulty, bring the total number used to over 2 million tubes for the 230 000 dairy cows in the province. If the average quantity of antibiotic per tube is 500 mg, the amount of antibiotic infused into udders during one year would be 1000 kg – 40 times more per cow in the national herd than estimated by Plommet to be used in France.

Inhibitory Substance Residues in Milk

Before considering the contribution made to antibiotic residues in milk through the use of intramammary tubes, it is worth re-emphasizing that the systemic treatment of animals for many diseases may also lead to milk residues of considerable significance, and veterinarians and other users must always be aware of this.

The most widespread problem however arises from lactation therapy and the principal residue detected is penicillin. The laboratory tests used are numerous: Galesloot and Hassing, TTC, Disc-assay, Intertest, Delvotest, Brilliant Black dye reduction and, more recently, gas chromatography, and their sensitivity in detection often varies according to technique.

Edwards (1962) discussed the residue problem which existed at that time, quoting a survey in England and Wales which showed that 16% of churn samples were positive and he referred to the potential hazards to human health, the emergence of resistant strains and the problem confronting manufacturers of cheese. Following the Government White Paper of 1963 the situation in the United Kingdom was reviewed in 1967 on behalf of the Milk Marketing Boards in the United Kingdom by Green *et al.* (1967), and clearly progress was seen to have been made.

At a level of 0.05 i.u. ml^{-1} or greater the incidence of penicillin in milk in England and Wales had fallen from 6% in 1961 to 1.5% in 1966; in Northern Ireland to less than 2% in 1966 at the same level; while the Scottish Boards opted for a level of 0.02% i.u. ml^{-1} and in one survey observed a failure rate of

3.43%. Contracts with milk producers had been drawn up to include penalties for persistant offenders, and the British Veterinary Association and the British Pharmaceutical Industry were involved in playing their part through advice and the clear labelling of products used for therapy.

At about the same time Kelly and Collins (1967) found much to be desired as far as incidence of penicillin in milk was concerned in the Republic of Ireland, supplies positive in one case being 12.5%. O'Reilly reviewed the situation in the same area at a later date (1972) and found 8.2% of ex-farm milk and 5.7% of pasteurized samples to be antibiotic positive.

Some stabilization in the situation may have occurred in the United Kingdom during the past 10 years, but I am still a little concerned about existing levels in Northern Ireland as shown by two recent surveys and other data presented here.

The 0.05 i.u. ml^{-1} level was used as the lowest detectable level in the first two surveys (Greer and Pearson, 1973; Pearson, Greer and Pollock, 1976) and in the former 1.73% of the 4221 herd samples were found at some time to be positive, the incidence in the 379 herds studied (tested monthly for one year) being 13.46%. In the second survey 526 smaller herds throughout the province were studied and in contrast showed a sample and herd residue incidence of 0.71% and 7.6% respectively.

Continuous monitoring of bulk tank herds in the Belfast area has been carried out since 1969 in respect of somatic cell counts, *Str. agalactiae* and inhibitory substance residues, and in 1974 we raised our standards to cover IHS levels down to 0.01 i.u. ml^{-1} using the Galesloot and Hassing method.

Table 15.1 shows the results obtained in 6737 samples from 561 herds tested during the twelve-month period ending February 1976, and it is of interest to

Table 15.1 Number of samples positive for inhibitory substance (IHS) in 6737 samples tested from 561 herds in 12 months

No. of samples tested	*No. IHS positive*	*No. positive at* 0.05 i.u. *or above*	*No. positive* 0.01–0.04 i.u.
6737	249 (3.7%)	110 (1.6%)	139 (2.1%)

see that the inclusion of the number of residues detected below 0.05 i.u. more than doubles the total positive; Green found an almost identical situation in 1967. *Figure 15.1* illustrates the situation more clearly together with the seasonal winter peaks which are commonly found elsewhere. The number of producers positive – tested monthly for a year – was 170 (30%); 115 (67.6%) of these being positive once, 41 (24%) twice, 9 (5.3%) three times, while 5 (3%) others were positive on 4 occasions or more.

More severe penalties have recently been introduced by the North of Ireland Milk Marketing Board to discourage milk producers from submitting positive residue milk, but we still have a long way to go to emulate the situation achieved by countries such as Denmark and the Netherlands – two EEC countries where the national residue incidence is well below 1%, and at detection levels of 0.01 i.u. ml^{-1}. Olsen (1976) states that 'milk shall be free from antibiotic' and this should be our aim, but at the same time we should consider the economics of

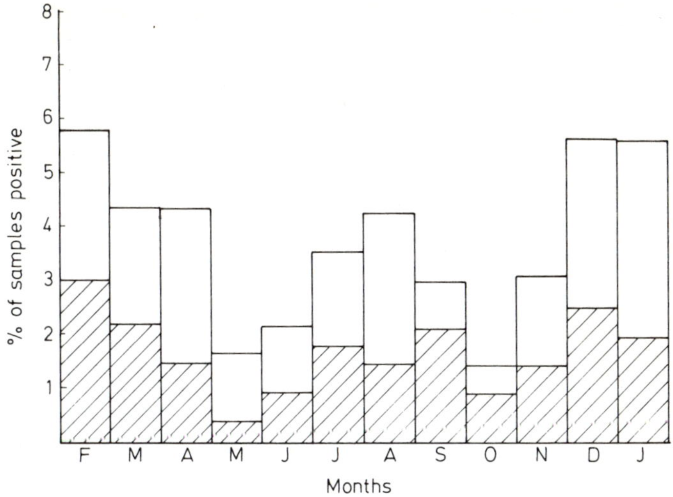

Figure 15.1 Seasonal distribution of inhibitory substances (IHS) in 6 737 bulk tank milk Samples (February 1975–January 1976). Unshaded area = 0.01–0.04 i.u.; shaded area = 0.05 i.u. and above

testing systems, the optimum frequency of applying tests and the practical advantages of testing below 0.02 i.u. from the manufacturers viewpoint and even that of human health.

Discussion and Conclusions

In the present paper only a few of more important points relating to the application of intramammary therapy in bovine mastitis have been covered. The area is vast and I have purposely avoided discussing the merits of one particular antibiotic against another in view of the large number of these available and the confusion which arises from assessing the value of drug combinations, dose frequency and the influence of bases.

Some discussion could also have usefully been made on antibiotics which readily combine with tissue and protein, as the antibiotic residue problem is still largely considered to be one associated with penicillin G, the principal residue detected by existing tests in milk. How important is it, however, from a public health point of view, or that of the manufacturer of milk products, that we should seek more sophisticated and expensive tests to detect residues bound to protein?

The five themes selected in this paper are perhaps sufficient to promote a useful discussion on our overall achievements and future research, and on the first of these I have often wondered how beneficial it would be to initiate a national *Str. agalactiae* eradication scheme in the United Kingdom. Many individual herds have achieved clearance, some acquiring new and more stubborn infections while others have not, and a random national survey of the existing situation is thus desirable. This should be followed by a frank discussion on the cost and practicability of an eradication programme in relation to the economic benefits likely to accrue, and we must look for the principal reasons why it has not been achieved to date.

On the theme of lactation and dry cow therapy we have still many gaps in our knowledge and application. Veterinarians have become poorer diagnosticians as a result of their use, possibly for economic reasons arising from minimal laboratory support and some way of overcoming this should be sought to enable clinicians to use drugs more selectively. The prophylactic use of dry cow therapy is, in the eyes of some workers, beginning to present us with new problems and must be closely watched. Medical workers consider that the prophylactic use of antibiotics is giving us a false sense of security and that we are paying too little attention to our physiological function, resistance and optimum nutrition. Perhaps this is happening in the animal world also, as often indicated by lowered standards of husbandry and through metabolic profiles.

The third point discussed was that of the evaluation of intramammary formulae and clearly the pharmaceutical chemist has far too much responsibility here. One of the greater difficulties in adequate assessment is the enormous cost of *in vivo* trials and it is to be hoped that research workers of the future, with help from newer pharmacokinetic studies, will be able to assist the pharmaceutical industry in the testing of new products and cutting down their ultimate cost to the user.

The changing pattern of intramammary infections is clearly illustrated in many countries, although the reasons for the changes are far from clear. Maybe the evolution of new bacterial populations will never be fully understood, but it might be a little easier if international workers adopted more uniform bacteriological standards and tests for resistance as far as possible. Even in the area of diagnosing udder infection itself there is still disagreement between workers, although this situation may never be resolved between the pathologist and bacteriologist.

Finally, the problem of antibiotic residue in milk is still with us in some measure and requires the attention of advisers, legislators and users. The entry of the United Kingdom into the European Common Market stimulates us once more to take action to reduce it and to detect it at lower levels. With penicillin this should be relatively easy, but to the academic, at least, the detection of other antibiotics much more commonly used for intramammary therapy is perhaps a greater headache.

References

ALTEMEIER, W.A., TODD, J.C. and INGE, W.W. (1967). *Ann. Surg.*, **166**, 530

ANTIBIOTICS IN MILK in Great Britain (1963). Report of the Milk Hygiene Sub-Committee of the Milk and Milk Products Technical Advisory Committee, H.M.S.O., London

ARONSON, A.L. (1975). *Mod. vet. Pract.*, **56**, 383

BARBER, M. (1960). *Rpt. Inst. Biol.*, 89

BRANDER, G.C. (1975). *14th Ann. Meet., Nat. Mastitis Council (U.S.A.)*, p. 69

BRATLIE, O.(1973). *Vet. Rec.*, **93**, 430

DODD, F.H. and GRIFFIN, T.K. (1975). *Proc. IDF Seminar on Mastitis Control, Doc.*, **85**, 282
DODD, F.H. and NEAVE, F.K. (1970). *Bienn. Rev. Natl. Inst. Res. Dairy.*, **p. 21**
EDWARDS, S.J. (1962). In *Antibiotics in Agriculture*, p. 43. Ed. Woodbine, M. (Proc. Univ. of Nottingham. 9th Easter School in Agric. Sci.)
FAULL, W.B. and GILLETT, A. (1973). *Vet. Rec.*, **93**, 447
FINLAND, M. (1970). *J. infect. Dis.*, **122**, 419
FUNKE, H. (1975). *Proc. IDF Seminar on Mastitis Control, Doc.*, **85**, 311
GREEN, E., ROBINSON, A.A.E., CHAMBERS, G. and MURRAY, J.G. (1967). *J. Soc. Dairy Tech.*, **20**, 3, 138
GREER, D.O. and PEARSON, J.K.L. (1973). *Br. vet. J.*, **129**, 544
HOWELL, D. (1972). *Vet. Rec.*, **90**, 654
JACKSON, G.G. (1974). *J. Amer. med. Assoc.*, **227**, 634
KAGAN, B.M., FANNIN, S.L. and BARDIE, F. (1973). *J. Amer. med. Assoc.*, **226**, 306
KEEFE, T.J. (1975). *Mastitis Symposium, Pennsylvania (Feb. 13th)*, p. 81
KELLY, W.R. and COLLINS, J.D. (1967). *J. Irish med. Assoc.*, **60**, 35
KUNIN, C.M., TUPASI, T. and CRAIG, W.A. (1973). *Annals of Int. Med.*, **79**, 555
LOVELL, R. (1962). In *Antibiotics in Agriculture*, p. 21. Ed. Woodbine, M. (Proc. Univ. of Nottingham. 9th Easter School in Agric. Sci.)
MADSEN, P.S., KLASTRUP, O., OLSEN, S.J. and PEDERSEN, P.S. (1975). *Nord. vet. Med.*, **27**, 305
MORSE, G.E. (1975). *Proc. IDF Seminar on Mastitis Control, Doc.*, **85**, 358
NEAVE, F.K., DODD, F.H. and HENRIQUES, E. (1950). *J. Dairy Res.*, **17**, 37
NEWBOULD, F.H.S. (1975). *Proc. IDF Seminar on Mastitis Control, Doc.*, **85**, 382
NYHAN, J.F. (1963) quoted by KELLY, W.R. and COLLINS, J.D. (1967)
O'REILLY, P.F. (1972). *Irish vet. J.*, **26**, 3, 41
OLSEN, S.J. (1975). *Proc. IDF Seminar on Mastitis Control, Doc.*, **85**, 410
OLSEN, S.J. (1976). Personal communication
PARKER, B.N.J. (1976). *Vet. Bull.*, **46**, 2, 83
PEARSON, J.K.L. (1950). *Vet. Rec.*, **62**, 166
PEARSON, J.K.L. (1951). *Vet. Rec.*, **63**, 215
PEARSON, J.K.L., GREER, D.O. and POLLOCK, D.A. (1976). *Br. vet. J.*, **132**, 588
PEARSON, J.K.L., GREER, D.O., SPENCE, B.K. and McPARLAND, P.J. (1972). *Vet. Rec.*, **91**, 615
PEARSON, J.K.L. and WRIGHT, C.L. (1969). *Vet. Rec.*, **84**, 294
PEDERSEN, P.S. (1975). *Proc. IDF Seminar on Mastitis Control, Doc.*, **85**, 352
PLOMMET, M. and LE LOUEDEC, C. (1975). *Proc. IDF Seminar on Mastitis Control, Doc.*, **85**, 265
SCHALM, O.W. (1968). *JAVMA*, **153**, 12, 1689
SCHULTZE, W.D. (1975). *14th Ann. Meet., Nat. Mastitis Council (U.S.A.)*, p. 41
SERIEYS, F. and ROGUINSKY, M. (1975). *Proc. IDF Seminar on Mastitis Control, Doc.*, **85**, 349
SIMMONS, H.E. and STOLLEY, P.D. (1974). *J. Amer. med. Assoc.*, **227**, 9, 1023
SMITH, A., WESTGARTH, D.R., JONES, M.R., NEAVE, F.K., DODD, F.H. and BRANDER, G.C. (1967). *Vet. Rec.*, **81**, 504
SMITH, H.W. (1962). In *Antibiotics in Agriculture*, p. 374. Ed. Woodbine, M. (Proc. Univ. of Nottingham, 9th Easter School in Agric. Sci.)

STEIGBIGEL, R.T., GREENMAN, R.L. and REMINGTON, J.S. (1975). *J. infect. Dis.*, **131**, 245

SWIDLER, G. (1971). *Handbook of Drug Interactions.* Wiley Interscience, New York

UVAROV, O. (1971). *Vet. Rec.*, **88**, 674

UVAROV, O., EVANS, J.M., MARSHALL, M. and SIZER, D. (1967). *Vet. Rec.*, **81**, 241

WILSON, C.D. (1961). *Vet. Rec.*, **73**, 1019

WILSON, C.D. (1976). Personal communication

WILSON, C.D. and BIRN, K.J. (1966). *Vet. Rec.*, **79**, 374

WILSON, C.D., LITTLE, T.W.A., ROBERTS, D.H. and HARDWICK, A.G. (1971). *Br. vet. J.*, **127**, 253

ZIV, G. (1975). *Proc. IDF Seminar on Mastitis Control, Doc.*, **85**, 314

16

TRIMETHOPRIM-SULPHONAMIDE SYNERGY IN SALMONELLA THERAPY

G. WHITE
Wellcome Research Laboratories, Berkhamsted

While it is comparatively easy to demonstrate a marked mutual potentiation of activity between trimethoprim and sulphonamides *in vitro* (Barnett and Bushby, 1970), the evaluation of a possible synergistic effect *in vivo* in bacterial diseases of animals presents great difficulties. *In vivo* activity depends not only on the activity of a drug against the pathogen, but also on the pharmacokinetic behaviour of the drug, which can vary markedly in the various species of domestic animals. One of the most important pharmacokinetic properties of a drug with regard to predictions of efficacy is its 'half-life', and whereas many sulphonamides have half-lives of several hours' duration in animals, that of trimethoprim is generally considerably shorter, and in cattle has the low value of about one hour (Davitiyananada and Rasmussen, 1974), which suggests that once daily administration in this species might be therapeutically inadequate. While field-trials in large numbers of cattle and pigs (Rehm and White, 1970) indicated that a combination of trimethoprim and sulphonamides gave superior results to the same sulphonamide when used alone at a higher dose rate, trimethoprim alone was not tested and the better results of the combination could have been due to the activity of trimethoprim. It was therefore decided to attempt to establish a disease model in cattle using an important pathogen, *Salmonella dublin*, to provide the opportunity to evaluate *in vivo* synergy under controlled experimental conditions.

Using a typical field strain of *S. dublin*, sensitive *in vitro* to about 0.25 μg ml^{-1} of trimethoprim and 25 μg ml^{-1} of sulphonamide, it was found that oral infection of young Friesian calves (2 to 4 weeks old) regularly produced a syndrome closely resembling field outbreaks of acute salmonellosis in calves, with peak mortality occurring at about 7 days after infection. The oral LD50 of this strain for calves under the experimental conditions was about 5×10^8 organisms, but in order consistently to produce the high mortality necessary to compare treatment regimes in comparatively small groups of animals (the maximum total number of calves was limited to 35), about 100 LD50s were given in the chemotherapy studies. A standard treatment schedule of five consecutive daily doses was used, the first dose being given 44 hours after infection, at which time nearly all calves had high pyrexia and severe enteritis.

The results of three experiments using various doses of trimethoprim and sulphadiazine are shown in *Tables 16.1, 16.2* and *16.3*. In experiment 1 (*Table 16.1*), the control mortality of 5/8 was unusually low, but it was conclusively demonstrated that sulphadiazine alone at daily doses of 40 mg kg^{-1} was therapeutically inadequate, whereas half this level in the presence of 4 mg kg^{-1} of trimethoprim gave a good therapeutic effect. In experiment 2 (*Table 16.2*), complete prevention of mortality (accompanied by rapid remission of symptoms) was produced by the two drugs in combination, but twice the level of trimethoprim (i.e. 8 mg kg^{-1}) when used alone was unable to prevent the death of 6 out of the 7 calves in this group, although some delay in mortality was apparent. In this experiment, it was shown that intravenous (i/v) administration was as effective as intramuscular (i/m), a surprising result since while i/m injection of the formulation used (an aqueous suspension of trimethoprim) produced low but prolonged serum levels of the drug, i/v administration resulted in a rapid decline of serum concentrations, the drug being usually undetectable (i.e. below 0.02 μg ml^{-1}) within 6 hours of injection. A possible explanation for the greater *in vivo* efficacy of trimethoprim than is suggested by the somewhat transient persistence in serum following i/v injection of cattle is provided by the fact that the drug is always found in higher concentrations in tissues than in serum (Bushby and Hitchings, 1968; Hansen *et al.*, 1973). It has also been shown (Chisholm *et al.*, 1973) by the subcutaneous implantation of plastic cages in dogs to collect samples of extracellular fluid, that trimethoprim not only reaches higher levels in extravascular fluid compartments than in serum, but also persists for much longer, and this property has also been confirmed in cattle in these laboratories by using a similar technique.

Table 16.1 Experiment 1. Calves infected with *Salmonella dublin* on day 0 and treated as indicated on days 2 to 6

SDZ (mg kg^{-1})	*TMP*	*Route*	*Cumulative mortality on day* 2	3	4	5	6	7	8	9	10	11	12	17+	*Total mortality*
20	4	i/m	0	0	0	0	0	0	0	0	0	0	1	1	1/8
–	8	i/m	0	0	1	1	1	1	1	1	1	1	1	2	2/8
40	–	i/m	0	3	4	4	4	4	4	4	4	5	5	5	5/8
–	–		0	0	0	2	3	3	3	4	5	5	5	5	5/8

Table 16.2 Experiment 2. Calves infected with *Salmonella dublin* on day 0 and treated as indicated on days 2 to 6

SDZ (mg kg^{-1})	*TMP*	*Route*	*Cumulative mortality on day* 3	4	5	6	7	8	9	11	12	14+	*Total mortality*
20	4	i/v	0	0	0	0	0	0	0	0	0	0	0/7
20	4	i/m	0	0	0	0	0	0	0	0	0	0	0/7
–	8	i/m	0	0	1	1	2	2	3	3	4	6	6/7
–	4	i/m	1	1	3	3	4	5	5	6	6	6	6/7
–	–		0	1	2	4	5	6	7	7	7	7	7/7

In experiment 3 (*Table 16.3*), graded doses of trimethoprim and sulphadiazine in 1:5 ratio were compared in order to assess the minimum effective daily dose. While 6 mg kg^{-1} of the combination was ineffective, a good result was produced by 12 mg kg^{-1}. At 24 mg kg^{-1} two calves died, but these calves were already moribund at the time of the first treatment and the pathological

Table 16.3 Experiment 3. Calves infected with *Salmonella dublin* on day 0 and treated (all i/v) as indicated on days 2 to 6

SDZ (mg kg^{-1})	*TMP*	*Cumulative mortality on day* 2	3	4	5	6	7	8	9	10	11	13	17+	*Total mortality*
20	4	1	1	2	2	2	2	2	2	2	2	2	2	2/7
10	2	0	0	0	0	0	0	1	1	1	1	1	1	1/7
5	1	0	1	1	1	2	3	5	5	5	6	6	6	6/7
–	8	0	0	0	0	1	1	3	4	4	5	6	7	7/7
–	–	0	1	3	5	6	6	6	6	7	7	7	7	7/7

changes were probably irreversible. The lack of efficacy of trimethoprim alone was confirmed in this experiment, although a delay in mortality was again apparent. *In vitro*, trimethoprim and sulphonamides are bacteriostatic when used alone, but a combination is often bactericidal. The delay in mortality, with death resulting from relapse after the end of treatment with trimethoprim alone, suggests that this may be due to the drug also having only a bacteriostatic effect *in vivo* when used alone, but this possible explanation needs further investigation.

The results of the three experiments described above demonstrate that while high doses of sulphonamide or trimethoprim when used alone are ineffective in the treatment of experimental salmonellosis in calves, effective therapy can be obtained by using lower doses of both drugs simultaneously. The marked *in vivo* potentiation results not only in a far better therapeutic effect, but also in a marked increase of the safety margin, particularly in comparison with the use of sulphonamides alone (often administered at dose levels of 100–200 mg kg^{-1} day), and in a reduction of the problems associated with the persistence of drug residues in treated food animals.

References

BARNETT, M. and BUSHBY, S.R.M. (1970). *Vet. Rec.*, **87**, 43

BUSHBY, S.R.M. and HITCHINGS, G.H. (1968). *Br. J. Pharmac. Chemother.*, **33**, 72

CHISHOLM, G.D., WATERWORTH, P.M., CALNAN, J.S. and GARROD, L.P. (1973). *Br. Med. J.*, **1**, 569

DAVITIYANANADA, D. and RASMUSSEN, F. (1974). *Acta vet. scand.*, **15**, 356

HANSEN, I., NIELSEN, M.L., HERRFORDT, L., HENRIKSEN, B. and BERTELSEN, S. (1973). *Chemotherapy*, **19**, 221

REHM, W.F. and WHITE, G. (1970). *Vet. Rec.*, **87**, 39

17

THE DEVELOPMENT OF β-LACTAM ANTIBIOTICS FOR THE TREATMENT OF BOVINE MASTITIS

ANNE M. HARRIS
P. W. MUGGLETON
Glaxo Research Ltd., Greenford

Antibiotics have been used for the treatment of mastitis for the last 30 years but the disease is still of economic importance in this country. Mastitis is a complex disease process in which environmental factors play a very important part. It is, therefore, recognized that control schemes must incorporate a series of techniques to reduce infection.

Intrammary preparations containing antibiotics have been widely used in the treatment and prevention of mastitis. These cerates, so called because they usually contain waxes, have been developed in response to changing patterns of infection and general approaches to the control of mastitis. In this communication we wish to outline the rationale behind cerate development, particularly for those containing β-lactam antibiotics and to show how theoretical approaches apply in the control of mastitis.

Mastitis

The disease was described by Dr. S. J. Edwards 14 years ago at the 9th Easter School as 'an inflammatory disease caused by bacterial invasion, chiefly streptococci and staphylococci. Other organisms may be implicated but less frequently.' This situation is not greatly changed today. Recently, more emphasis has been placed on infections caused by Gram-negative bacteria; these organisms often originate from the environment and probably take advantage of situations created by herd management, hygiene procedures and antibiotic preferences.

Mastitis is not static but is a disease process which requires evaluation and review at intervals. Each farm may be regarded as an ecological entity which has its own flora with attendant problems; these are profoundly influenced by environmental factors. Herd hygiene and management are therefore a major part of mastitis control and cannot be divorced from antibiotic treatment.

Cows are constantly exposed to bacteria from external sources and sub-clinical levels of infection are commonly found in 50–70% of most herds. Sub-clinically infected animals may develop clinical signs of mastitis and if antibiotic treatment is not given, the level of infection in the herd may rise further. At the end of lactation existing infections remain in the udder, and after calving the sub-clinical mastitis level may be significantly higher than during the previous lactation. The cycle continues, and the useful life of the animals may be ended sooner than necessary (*Figure 17.1*).

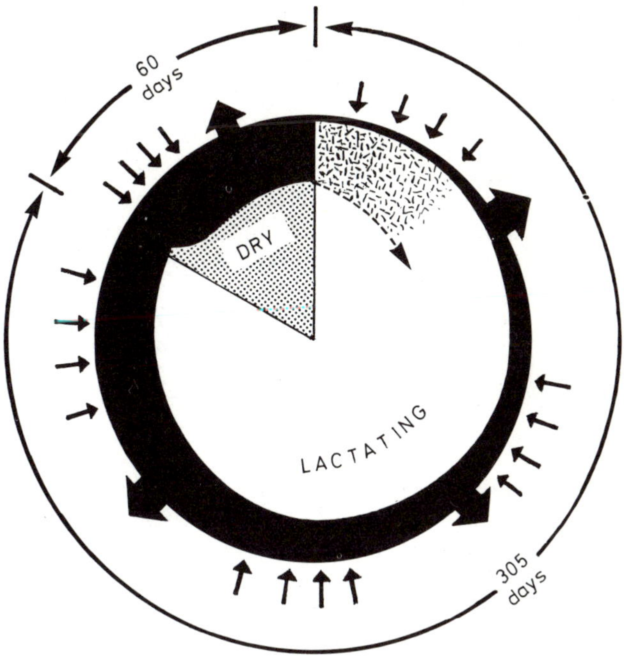

Figure 17.1 The build-up of sub-clinical infection in cows which receive no antibiotic treatment (by courtesy of J.M. Evans, unpublished data). ➡ *Outbreaks of clinical mastitis.* → *Infection from the environment.* ▒ *Sub-clinical infection in the second lactation.* ■ *Sub-clinical infection in the first lactation*

This cycle of infection has two points where antibiotics can be used: (*a*) to treat outbreaks of mastitis in milking cows as soon as they occur, and (*b*) to reduce sub-clinical infection during the dry period and hence increase the productive life of cows. Today, two types of cerate are available: those which are designed for milking cows and are excreted rapidly, and preparations for dry cows which provide prophylactic antibiotic cover for several weeks.

Cerate Development

The primary aims in cerate development are to produce safe and effective preparations. The safety of a cerate is usually assessed by monitoring the white cell count in milk; this may be used, in normal animals, as an index of the irritancy of a preparation. If an irritant cerate is infused, the cell count may rise dramatically and blood clots may be seen in the milk. Cerates for both milking cows and dry cows are tested to ensure that no significant cell count rise occurs after infusion. In mastitic cows, cell counts of 10 millions ml^{-1} are often recorded; after treatment with a non-irritant cerate this count should be reduced to less than 1.0 million ml^{-1}.

Recently, considerable emphasis has been placed on the importance of cell counts as indicators of levels of herd infection. Many farms now take part in schemes to monitor bulk tank cell counts and we are moving towards the point where cell counts may be used to assess the milk quality. Several E.E.C. countries already differentiate grades of milk using cell counts and impose penalties for high counts. It is, therefore, important to consider cell counts when new cerate preparations are developed.

Effective treatment of mastitis depends on two main points: (*a*) the antibiotic or antibiotics selected, and (*b*) the excretion characteristics of the drugs *in vivo*. The selection of antibiotics for formulation in cerate preparations must be based primarily on considerations of the aetiology of the disease and the spectrum of activity and mode of action of the antibiotics. Mastitis treatment is usually empirical and based on previous experience at a given farm. The aetiology of a case is rarely established before treatment is initiated. Other characteristics of the antibiotic are important, particularly physical properties such as solubility which may influence antibiotic excretion. In addition, drugs must be active in the presence of milk at concentrations which can be attained *in vivo*.

Antibiotic excretion in the udder is significantly influenced by the base in which the drug is formulated. It is the base which determines whether an antibiotic is released quickly (QR cerates) or slowly (long-acting, LA cerates) in the udder. QR bases often contain beeswax, oils and wetting agents to ensure that antibiotic diffuses quickly through the udder and is excreted within a stated time. Milk must be discarded throughout periods of antibiotic treatment and so formulations must be designed to strike a balance between economic loss of milk and effective therapy.

Long-acting cerates are formulated in geis without wetting agents. No milk waste occurs as these cerates are intended for dry cows; the aim is therefore to extend the antibiotic cover for as long as possible during the normal 8 to 10-week dry period.

The timing of antibiotic release from the base is important in attaining therapeutic levels in the udder, and when two or more antibiotics are used it is important that all the components of the cerate diffuse at appropriate rates. This is particularly relevant when additive or synergistic drugs are used. The antibiotics may act optimally when they are present in defined proportions, and so both the levels of antibiotic chosen and the type of base must be adjusted to ensure that optimal excretion occurs *in vivo*.

Additional factors in the development of cerates are the stability and presentation of the preparations. Cerates may be badly stored before use and so 'shelf-life' must be assessed over a range of temperatures. The presentation of the final product must be suitable for administration by untrained personnel because cerates are frequently infused by farmers or stockmen rather than veterinary surgeons. Tubes or syringes are usually used and these must be compatible with the cerate inside them; no toxic products should leach from the container into the preparation.

Cerates in Clinical Use

Penicillin was the first β-lactam antibiotic discovered and was used initially in the prevention of 'summer mastitis' caused chiefly by *Corynebacterium pyogenes* (Pearson, 1948, 1951). In the early experiments during the late 1940s the protective effect of aqueous penicillin was assessed, followed by trials using penicillin in oil and wax. The latter protected cows from 'summer mastitis' during the dry period. Penicillin in various bases was subsequently used to treat clinical mastitis, chiefly caused at that time by *Streptococcus agalactiae.*

By the mid 1950s mastitis caused by penicillin-resistant staphylococci became prevalent, probably as a result of increased use of penicillin, the only antibiotic then available for use in mastitis. Cerates were subsequently developed using more than one antibiotic; penicillin activity was complemented by novobiocin or streptomycin which acted against penicillin-resistant *Staph.aureus* strains. Streptomycin was also used in the relatively rare cases of *E.coli* mastitis.

Cloxacillin was the first semi-synthetic β-lactam antibiotic used in mastitis control during the 1960s. The compound is resistant to staphylococcal penicillinase and has been successfully used in the treatment of mastitis caused by *Staph.aureus.* Cloxacillin is, however, less active than penicillin against streptococci and corynebacteria.

During the late 1960s several facets of mastitis began to change. Farmers became more aware that the disease could be treated and controlled with the help of antibiotics. Dry cow therapy became popular as a control measure, and schemes were recommended incorporating hygiene procedures such as teat-dipping together with antibiotic therapy. More frequent cerate infusions were given and longer milk discard times following treatment became accepted in the attempt to balance effective therapy against economic milk production.

The aetiology of the disease appeared to change during this time; Gram-negative infections were reported more frequently. This could be the result of hygiene, management procedures or prolonged use of narrow-spectrum antibiotics which has resulted in opportunist growth of Gram-negative commensal organisms.

Cerates developed since 1970 have reflected these changes in aetiology and approach to mastitis control. Streptomycin/penicillin preparations containing 100 or 300 mg of each antibiotic have been used for many years. Newer preparations have been formulated with high potencies (up to 1 g) of each drug. These preparations ensure high antibiotic levels in the udder, following and between infusions. The overall treatment period is longer; antibiotic is usually present for six or seven days during the treatment and discard period. Both penicillin and streptomycin are bactericidal antibiotics which act additively or synergistically to provide broad-spectrum antibiotic cover. *In vivo* results show that these preparations are effective in the treatment of clinical mastitis.

High-potency streptomycin/penicillin cerates have also been successfully used in routine dry cow therapy; sub-clinical infections are significantly reduced during the dry period. Antibiotic levels have been demonstrated in secretion samples for 4 or 5 weeks in the dry udder (Pugh *et al.*, 1973).

The concept of complementing penicillin with streptomycin has been exploited for many years because the combination of drugs can be synergistic;

recent clinical evidence in comparison with *in vitro* sensitivity tests has demonstrated this phenomenon. Fifty-eight cases of mastitis caused by penicillin or streptomycin-resistant organisms were treated with preparations containing high potencies of both antibiotics. The causative organisms were resistant to one or other antibiotic when individual antibiotic discs were used but all the isolates were sensitive to penicillin/streptomycin combination sensitivity discs. Clinical results showed that 52/58 cases (90%) responded to therapy (Evans *et al*., 1975). These results demonstrate that when combinations of antibiotics are used, sensitivity testing may more accurately predict clinical response if appropriate combination discs are used.

During the same trials, 15/15 isolates which were resistant to both penicillin and streptomycin, responded to treatment with the drug combination; whereas 5/23 cases caused by organisms which were sensitive to both drugs, failed to respond to therapy. This finding serves as a reminder that antibiotic-resistant strains are not necessarily highly virulent or pathogenic; indeed, it is more likely that the reverse is true.

Recently new β-lactam antibiotic combinations have been introduced: ampicillin/cloxacillin mixtures and streptomycin/penicillin/nafcillin cerates. These preparations contain the penicillinase-resistant drugs cloxacillin and nafcillin and complement their narrow-spectrum with ampicillin and streptomycin to provide broad-spectrum activity.

Present-day interest in new preparations for mastitis focuses attention on broad-spectrum antibiotics or combinations of drugs; these are formulated to give higher levels of antibiotic for longer periods of time. For dry cow therapy, longer-acting preparations are being used and more than one infusion may be given to afford complete protection.

Cephalosporin Cerates

Semi-synthetic cephalosporins are a class of β-lactam antibiotics which have not been widely used in veterinary medicine in this country although they are well established for human use. We have examined a range of experimental cerates containing different cephalosporins and report our laboratory and clinical findings with two of these preparations. The two cephalosporins were initially selected because they had suitable *in vitro* activity against organisms which commonly cause mastitis. The compounds were subsequently formulated in suitable bases and studied *in vivo* in experimental animals and under field conditions.

Cephoxazole, 7-(3-*o*-chlorophenyl-5-methylisoxazole-4-carboxamido)-cephalosporanic acid, was formulated with procaine penicillin in a quick release base. This antibiotic combination was used because surveys of mastitis aetiology showed that streptococci are still an important cause of the disease and penicillin remains the most active antibiotic against these organisms. Cephoxazole has activity against penicillin-resistant strains of *Staph. aureus* and thus complements the activity of penicillin. In addition, cephoxazole is an efficient inhibitor of the β-lactamases produced by *Staph. aureus* and many Gram-negative bacteria. The cephalosporin therefore protects penicillin from degradation and the combination of drugs is active *in vitro* against both Gram-positive and Gram-negative bacteria which cause mastitis.

The additive antibacterial action of cephoxazole and penicillin is most effective when the drugs are combined in 1:1 mixtures. The experimental cerate therefore contained 250 mg of each antibiotic in a quick release base. This formulation was well tolerated in the udder after three infusions were given at 24-hour intervals. Both cephoxazole and penicillin were excreted at similar rates; concentrations of the antibiotics in milk were in the ratio of 1:1.

The efficacy of the preparation was evaluated against clinical cases of mastitis under field conditions. The cerate was effective in the treatment of mastitis caused by *Staph. aureus, Streptococcus* spp., *Corynebacterium* spp. and *E.coli*: 174 quarters showing clinical signs of mastitis were treated and 139 (80%) of these were clinically normal one week after the last infusion. The preparation was non-irritant in mastitic quarters and assisted in reducing the cell count during treatment. Initially, 89% of quarters had counts greater than 2.0×10^6 ml^{-1} of milk. After treatment 62% of these quarters had counts of less than 0.5×10^6 ml^{-1}. There was a reduction of 5.0×10^6 ml^{-1} or more in 92% of quarters following infusion.

A second cephalosporin was formulated as an experimental cerate in a long-acting base. Cephalonium, 3-(4-carbamoyl-1-pyridiniomethyl)-7-(2-thienylacetamido)-3-cephem-4-carboxylate, is relatively insoluble in water. It was considered that the physical properties of the antibiotic and the base should ensure prolonged antibiotic activity in the dry udder.

Cephalonium is active *in vitro* against most of the organisms which cause mastitis. The antibiotic has rapid antibacterial activity against Gram-positive and Gram-negative bacteria. An experimental cerate containing 250 mg cephalonium in LA base was infused into cows in an experimental herd. The preparation was well tolerated in milking cows, no rise in cell count having occurred in 21 days after a single infusion. Antibiotic levels were prolonged in milking cows and, in dry cows, cephalonium was detected for up to 10 weeks in most quarters.

The efficacy of cephalonium cerate was assessed in dry cows in seven commercial herds: 396 quarters were infused immediately after the last milking of the lactation. Milk samples were examined immediately before infusion and at 4 days after calving. The preparation was effective in eliminating infections in 120 out of 148 quarters (81%) which were infected at the beginning of the dry period. Of the 248 quarters which were uninfected initially 230 (93%) remained free from infection 4 days after calving. The incidence of new infections and mastitis at calving was low in quarters infused with the experimental preparation; 5% of quarters had new infections and 5 cases of mastitis occurred among treated quarters.

The results obtained with experimental cerates containing cephalosporins indicate that these antibiotics are of considerable value in the treatment of mastitis. The results further demonstrate that the cephalosporin cerates described fulfilled the criteria outlined previously for the design of intramammary preparations. Both preparations were active *in vitro* and *in vivo* against the organisms which cause mastitis; antibiotic excretion was designed to ensure that the compounds were present in the udder at optimum concentrations for appropriate periods of time; the cerates were well tolerated *in vivo* and contributed to a reduction in cell count in mastitic quarters.

General Comments

The International Dairy Federation in 1973 took the view that mastitis eradication is not attainable. The disease is a very complex process in which aetiology and environment cannot be separated. We now have available a wide selection of cerates containing antibiotics for use in the treatment and prevention of the disease. Perhaps our next objective should be to ensure that we use the preparations we have in the best possible way. Antibiotic policies may be of value in some circumstances, used together with scrupulous hygiene and sensible herd management. Antibiotics may then become even more valuable tools in the control of mastitis.

References

EDWARDS, S.J. (1962). *Antibiotics in Agriculture.* Ed. Woodbine, M. Butterworths, London

EVANS, J. M., WATSON, D. J., HARRIS, A. M. and LLEWELLYN, G. G. (1975). *Vet. Rec.*, **97**, 248

INTERNATIONAL DAIRY FEDERATION. (1973). *Annual Bulletin,* no. 76, Secretariat General, International Dairy Federation, Brussels

PEARSON, J. K. L. (1948). *Proc. Soc. appl. Bact.*, **11**, 27

PEARSON, J. K. L. (1951). *Vet. Rec.*, **63**, 215

PUGH, K. E., HARRIS, A. M., MARSHALL, M. J. and EVANS, J. M. (1973). *Vet. Rec.*, **93**, 212

18

DETECTION OF ANTIBIOTIC RESIDUES IN SLAUGHTERED ANIMALS

ANN McCRACKEN
Veterinary Research Laboratories, Stormont, Belfast, Northern Ireland

Over the past few years there has been increasing concern over the extensive use of antibiotics in animal husbandry and their addition to animal feedstuffs has heightened the problem. Public opinion has demanded that food of animal origin for human consumption be free from the residues of substances like DDT, organophosphates and antibiotics.

I will describe briefly the method we use in Northern Ireland to detect antibiotic residues in animal tissues and the efficiency and sensitivity of our method. The antibiotics we look for are those most commonly used in animal husbandry in Northern Ireland, namely penicillin, ampicillin, neomycin and oxytetracycline – these are detected by a microbiological assay. Chloramphenicol has also been included to ascertain the extent of its use. The method used for meat or organ samples is shown in *Table 18.1*. The sample is chopped up finely and macerated

Table 18.1 Method of detection of antibiotic residues

Meat + antibiotic ↘ ↙ Test meat sample

Maceration
|
Extraction
|
Concentration
|
Resuspension
|
Microbiological assay

in a Stomacher with a suitable extractant, spun and the fluid phase concentrated to dryness in a rotary evaporator. Two ml of an appropriate buffer is added and the sample placed in a cylinder cup on a seeded agar plate. Samples are allowed to diffuse for 3 h at room temperature and incubated overnight at 30°C.

Different extractants and different conditions are required for each antibiotic (*Table 18.2*); any variation of these conditions can affect the sensitivity of the assay quite dramatically. An antibiotic residue is detected by a clear zone around the cup and is measured using an overhead projector equipped with a photo-transparency of metric graph paper.

Table 18.2 Optimal conditions for detection of antibiotics in meat

Antibiotic	*Extractant*	*Test organism*	*Medium**	*Buffer for resuspension*
Ampicillin	Acetonitrile/buffer pH 7.9 (2/1)	*S. lutea*† ATCC 9341	XI (pH 7.9)	III (pH 7.9)
Chloramphenicol	Acetone	*S. lutea*† ATCC 9341	I (pH 6.5)	I (pH 6.0)
Penicillin	Acetone	*S. lutea*† ATCC 9341	I (pH 6.5)	I (pH 6.0)
Neomycin	Buffer pH 7.9	*S. epidermidis* ATCC 12228	XI (pH 7.9)	III (pH 7.9)
Oxytetracycline	Methanol/HCl (98/2)	*B. cereus* var *mycoides* ATCC 11778	VIII (pH 5.6)	IV (pH 4.5)

*Designations as quoted by Kirshbaum and Arret (1967).
†*Micrococcus luteus* (Baird-Parker, 1974).

Routinely large assay plates are used. The samples are placed in quadruplicate in a random manner according to a 10 × 8 Latin square design to counter any variations within the plate. The cylinder cup measures 8 mm and values >14 mm are considered significant.

Standard curves are prepared for each antibiotic. To ensure that results from different batches can be compared, standards are always included and if they fall within the standard deviation limits of the curve the experimental results can be used.

Having developed and standardized the method we then decided to compare the sensitivity of our test with standards set down by the F.A.O./W.H.O. Committee (1969) (*Table 18.3*). These standards state the maximum acceptable level of antibiotics allowed in 1 g of meat.

Table 18.3 Comparison of limits of detection of antibiotic residues

Antibiotic	*Lowest limit (μg g^{-1} muscle)*	*F.A.O./W.H.O. maximum acceptable level (μg g^{-1} muscle)**
Ampicillin	0.005	0.06
Penicillin	0.001	0.06
Oxytetracycline	0.05	0.25
Neomycin	3.5	0.5
Chloramphenicol	0.5	–

*F.A.O./W.H.O. (1969).

It can be seen that our method is capable of detecting levels of ampicillin, penicillin and oxytetracycline well below these standards; however, neomycin can only be detected at a level of 3.5 μg g^{-1} muscle and chloramphenicol at 0.5 μg g^{-1} muscle, which does not satisfy the suggested acceptable levels.

Having developed a satisfactory test to detect residues, experimental work was initiated to determine the extent of drug residues.

When animals are injected with an antibiotic the elimination rate is fairly rapid but the antibiotic also forms complexes with proteins in the tissues. Up to this point we had been looking at antibiotic solutions which were added to meat; now we had to investigate meat from animals previously injected with antibiotic since this is the type of sample which any legislation would require to be tested.

Calves were injected (i/m) with two consecutive therapeutic doses of either ampicillin, penicillin, oxytetracycline, neomycin or chloramphenicol. They were killed 24 h later and samples of muscle, kidney and urine were examined (*Table 18.4*). Ampicillin, penicillin and oxytetracycline were detected in all the

Table 18.4 Detection of antibiotic residues in calves slaughtered 24 h after therapeutic injections

Antibiotic	*Dose administered* (mg kg^{-1})	*Tissue tested*	*Amount of antibiotic* (μg g^{-1} *tissue) recovered*
Ampicillin	10	Muscle	>0.04
		Kidney	>0.04
		Urine	>0.04
Penicillin	3	Muscle	>0.04
		Kidney	>0.04
		Urine	>0.04
Oxytetracycline	3	Muscle	>0.20
		Kidney	>0.20
		Urine	>0.20
Neomycin	100	Muscle	0.0
		Kidney	>3.5
		Urine	>3.5
Chloramphenicol	5.5	Muscle	5.7
		Kidney	7.0
		Urine	0.0

tissues examined; neomycin, however, could only be detected in kidney and urine. We have previously shown that a solution of neomycin in muscle can only be detected in very high concentrations and it may be that such high concentrations are not achieved in muscle tissue of the live animal. Chloramphenicol was detected in muscle and kidney but not in urine. It may be that chloramphenicol is present in a degraded form in urine and was thus not detectable by the assay method used – the method only detecting biologically active residues. From these results it was concluded that kidney seemed to be the best tissue for detection of antibiotic residues.

It was decided to investigate this a little further and examine tissues from various sites of calves previously injected with a therapeutic dose of either penicillin, ampicillin or oxytetracycline. Thirteen sites were examined, ranging from rump steak and choice fillet to urine and serum (*Table 18.5*). The important points from this Table is that 6/6 diaphragm, kidney, heart, urine and serum samples were positive for each antibiotic. In other words, using this method, these sites will detect these antibiotics if present in calves. From the

Table 18.5 Number of samples showing a positive reaction when tested for antibiotic residues

	Number of samples showing positive reaction		
	(0.04 μg g⁻¹ tissue)	*(>0.15 μg g⁻¹ tissue)*	*(>1 μg g⁻¹ tissue)*
Sites	*Calves injected with penicillin*	*Calves injected with ampicillin*	*Calves injected with oxytetracycline*
Gluteus muscle (injection site)	6/6	6/6	6/6
Gluteus muscle (opposite injection site)	6/6	5/6	6/6
Psoas muscle	5/6	5/6	6/6
Pectoral muscle	6/6	4/6	6/6
Diaphragm	6/6	6/6	6/6
Oblique abdominal muscle	3/6	4/6	6/6
Longissimus dorsal muscle	6/6	4/6	6/6
Masseter muscle	6/6	5/6	6/6
Kidney	6/6	6/6	6/6
Heart	6/6	6/6	6/6
Liver	6/6	5/6	5/6
Urine	5/5*	6/6	4/4*
Serum	6/6	6/6	6/6

*Urine not available at slaughter from the other group members.

economic point of view, diaphragm, urine and serum have minimal commercial value and thus would be easily obtainable. However, a point worth bearing in mind is that some animals will urinate involuntarily after stunning and urine samples may not always be available.

Over the past five years kidney has been used in the Netherlands as the test sample from slaughtered animals. Our results and those of other workers (Takacs and Kovacs, 1969; Schothorst and Leusdem, 1972; Nouws and Smulders 1974) have shown that kidney is a perfectly suitable organ to detect the presence of antibiotic residues. We therefore decided to compare the official testing method of the Netherlands with our method using the calves previously injected with antibiotic.

The Netherland kidney test is extremely simple requiring only a paper assay disc and a piece of kidney. The disc is placed in an incision in the kidney and

Table 18.6 Number of samples showing a positive reaction when tested for antibiotic residues

	Calves injected with penicillin		*Calves injected with ampicillin*		*Calves injected with oxytetracycline*	
Site	*Method 1*	*Method 2*	*Method 1*	*Method 2*	*Method 1*	*Method 2*
Kidney	6/6	3/6	6/6	4/6	6/6	1/6

Method 1: McCracken, O'Brien and Campbell (1976).
Method 2: Schothorst and Peelen-Knol (1970).

removed after 2 h; it is then placed on a seeded agar plate, incubated overnight and any zones measured. The results of this comparison are shown in *Table 18.6.*

Method 1 detected residues in all kidneys whereas method 2 detected 3/6 of the kidneys from penicillin positive calves, 4/6 of the ampicillin positive kidneys and 1/6 of the oxytetracycline positive kidneys. The lack of detection of oxytetracycline is particularly outstanding, but it can probably be accounted for by the fact that *S. lutea* only is used as the test organism in method 2 and other workers have shown that tetracyclines are rarely detected using this organism. The general conclusion from comparison of the two methods using kidney samples is that method 1 is more efficient at detection of residues than method 2.

The kidney test method was extended to other organ and muscle samples. *Table 18.7* shows the number of samples showing a positive reaction when tested

Table 18.7 Number of samples showing a positive reaction when tested for antibiotic residues

	Calves injected with penicillin		*Calves injected with ampicillin*		*Calves injected with oxytetracycline*	
Sample	*Method 1*	*Method 2*	*Method 1*	*Method 2*	*Method 1*	*Method 2*
Kidney	6/6	3/6	6/6	4/6	6/6	1/6
Heart	6/6	4/6	6/6	2/6	6/6	0/6
Liver	6/6	4/6	5/6	3/6	5/6	0/6
Urine	5/5*	1/5*	4/4*	2/4*	4/4*	2/4*
Serum	6/6	0/6	6/6	1/6	6/6	0/6
Gluteus muscle (injection site)	6/6	4/6	6/6	6/6	6/6	0/6
Gluteus muscle (opposite injection site)	6/6	3/6	5/6	1/6	6/6	0/6
Psoas muscle	5/6	2/6	5/6	1/6	6/6	1/6
Pectoral muscle	6/6	2/6	4/6	1/6	6/6	0/6
Diaphragm	6/6	1/6	6/6	2/6	6/6	1/6
Oblique abdominal muscle	3/6	2/6	4/6	2/6	6/6	0/6
Longissimus dorsi muscle	6/6	2/6	4/6	0/6	6/6	0/6
Masseter muscle	6/6	2/6	5/6	0/6	6/6	0/6

*Urine not available at slaughter from other group members.
Method 1: McCracken, O'Brien and Campbell (1976).
Method 2: Schothorst and Peelen-Knol (1970).

for penicillin. Method 1 came out very well, oblique abdominal muscle being the poorest detector of the presence of penicillin residues; however, method 2 gave rather surprising results. Heart, liver and muscle injection site gave better results than kidney – the organ on which the test is based. Results from calves injected with ampicillin show once again that method 1 has better recovery of antibiotic residues than method 2 in all organs. The indication from the kidney test is further exemplified in the results from calves injected with oxytetracycline. Method 2 is virtually unable to detect oxytetracycline residues in slaughtered calves.

Table 18.8 Lowest limits of detection of antibiotic residues by methods 1 and 2

Antibiotic	*Lowest limit of detection* *Method 1** *(μg g⁻¹ tissue)*	*Method 2†* *(μg ml⁻¹ 'renal fluid')*	*F.A.O./W.H.O.†† maximum acceptable level* (μg g⁻¹)
Penicillin	0.001	0.04	0.06
Ampicillin	0.005	NT	0.06
Oxytetracycline	0.05	0.8	0.25

*McCracken, O'Brien and Campbell (1976).
†Schothorst and Peelen-Knol (1970).
††F.A.O./W.H.O. (1969).
NT = not tested.

Table 18.8 shows a comparison of the limits of detection of both methods. Assuming the units are comparable (the term renal fluid is not well defined in the original text), method 1 can detect much lower concentrations of antibiotic than method 2.

It is hoped this work will serve to point out the difference already existing between methods of detection of antibiotic residues and the need for a generally accepted, sensitive method. I think we should also decide just how important antibiotic residues are in our Sunday joint.

References

BAIRD-PARKER, A.C. (1974). *Bergey's Manual of Determinative Bacteriology*, 8th edn, p. 479. Williams and Wilkins Co., Baltimore

KIRSHBAUM, A. and ARRET, B. (1967). *J. Pharm. Sci.*, **56**, 511

McCRACKEN, A., O'BRIEN, J.J. and CAMPBELL, J.N. (1976). *J. appl. Bacter.*, **40**, 61

NOUWS, J. F. M. and SMULDERS, A. H. J. W. (1974). *Tidschr. Diergen.* **99**, 1155

SCHOTHORST, VAN, M and PEELEN-KNOL, G. (1970). *Netherland J. Veter. Sci.* **3**, 85

SCHOTHORST, VAN M. and LEUSDEM, VAN F. M. (1972) *Tidschr. Diergen.* **97**, 1043

TAKACS, J. and KOVACS, S. (1969) *Acta Veter. Acad. Sci. (Hungary)*, **19**, 11

19

NON-SPECIFIC RESISTANCE TO INFECTION IN RELATION TO MASTITIS

K. G. HIBBITT
A. W. HILL
Institute for Research on Animal Diseases, Compton, Newbury

Non-Specific Resistance to Infection in Relation to Mastitis

Protection of the mammary gland of the cow against invading pathogens depends on many defence mechanisms, most of which are non-specific and together constitute the animals natural resistance to infection. Pathogens invading the mammary gland may be subjected to these natural defences at two levels, in the teat canal and in the mammary gland itself. A number of workers in the past have recognized the teat canal as a barrier to infection (Murphy and Stuart, 1953; Fincher *et al.*, 1956; Plastridge, 1958). It functions not only as a simple mechanical barrier, but as an antimicrobial barrier, since substances such as fatty acids (Adams and Rickard, 1963) and antimicrobial proteins (Hibbitt, Cole and Reiter, 1969) can be isolated from the sebum-like teat canal keratin.

Microorganisms escaping destruction in the teat canal may be destroyed, or their growth inhibited, by the milk. The inhibitory activity of milk may be attributed to the phagocytic activity of polymorphonuclear leucocytes which accumulate during the early stages of infection, and to the presence of antimicrobial factors in the non-cellular fraction of the milk which may be partly of serum origin. Investigations are still being made into the mode of action and the chemical nature of the intracellular substances responsible for killing phagocytosed microorganisms, the soluble factors in the milk and the teat canal antimicrobial factors. Evidence is accumulating which suggests that the non-specific antimicrobial systems involved are capable of being stimulated.

Teat Canal Defences

Murphy and Stuart (1955) found no relationship between the length of the teat canal and resistance to *Streptococcus agalactiae* infections, but McDonald (1970) in a histological study, showed a marked difference in the cross-sectional diameter between teat canals from susceptible and resistant glands. The teat canals from the susceptible quarters had a larger diameter and a thinner keratinous lining than the canals from resistant quarters. This study was repeated recently using a radiographic technique (McDonald, 1975) when it was confirmed that teat canal diameter was a most important factor in controlling resistance to new intramammary infection.

Substantial evidence exists for the protective barrier afforded by the teat canal. This was shown in a study involving six lactating goats, when 6×10^{-4} ml of a culture of *Str. agalactiae* (containing 1.5×10^2 to 1.5×10^4 CFU) were deposited in the teat canals. Two of the 12 injected glands developed clinical signs of mastitis whereas 6 of the 12 glands became infected when 12 CFU were deposited directly into the teat cistern. Two more glands developed mastitis when the six resistant glands were reinfected directly into the teat cistern with 9×10^3 CFU (Hibbitt and Jones, 1967).

The environment within the teat canal does not encourage bacterial growth. The commensal organisms which colonize the teat canal of the healthy cow consist mainly of coagulase negative staphylococci (Cullen and Herbert, 1967); they grow very feebly *in vivo* and in experiments involving eight cows, were shown to have a mean percentage viability of 0.15% (Hibbitt, Benians and Rowlands, 1972).

The keratinous lining of the teat canal is important in the defence of the mammary gland. Murphy (1959) showed that a partial removal of the keratin by a reaming process produced a temporary decrease in resistance of the canal to invading pathogens. The investigation of the antimicrobial factors in the keratin has attracted considerable attention. Adams and Rickard (1963) isolated lipids from fresh teat canal keratin which were lethal to *Str. agalactiae*. They showed that certain non-esterified fatty acids were very antimicrobial and that larger amounts of these fatty acids were present in mastitis-resistant compared with mastitis-susceptible cows. This role of the lipids in the defence of the

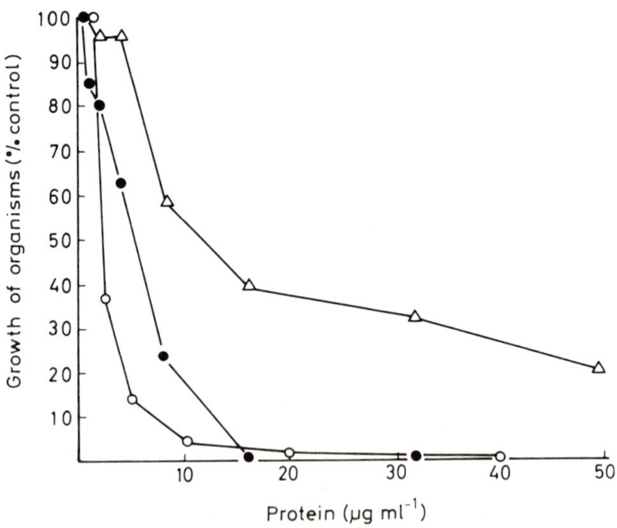

Figure 19.1 The inhibitory effect of proteins isolated from teat canal keratin on the growth of microorganisms. ○–○ = Staphylococcus aureus *42D;* ●–● = Staphylococcus aureus *52B;* △–△ = Streptococcus agalactiae *S13. (Hibbitt, Cole and Reiter, 1969)*

mammary gland nevertheless remains in some doubt, since these findings were not confirmed by Treece, Morse and Levy (1966).

Antimicrobial basic proteins have been isolated from the teat canal keratin of the cow (Hibbitt and Cole, 1968; Hibbitt, Cole and Reiter, 1969). These antimicrobial proteins were obtained by an acidic extraction followed by chromatography on a carboxymethyl cellulose column.

The proteins were soluble in water and dilute acids and were resolved by polyacrylamide gel electrophoresis into six bands at pH 3.0. They were poorly resolved at pH 7.0 but still positively charged and moved towards the cathode, whereas at pH 9.0 all but a trace were anionic. The antimicrobial activity of these proteins was investigated using two strains of *Staphylococcus aureus* (42 D and 52 B phage type) and one strain of *Str. agalactiae*. The effect of various concentrations of the isolated proteins on the growth of these organisms is shown in *Figure 19.1*. The growth of the two strains of *Staph. aureus* was inhibited by 50% at a concentration of 2–5 μg protein ml^{-1} while the *Str. agalactiae* was inhibited at 11.5 μg ml^{-1}.

This antimicrobial activity was lost in the presence of anionic proteins isolated from the teat canal. Similarly, if the cationic fractions were pre-incubated at pH 7.0 for 15 min at 37°C with anionic polymers such as DNA or heparin, complexes were formed which were devoid of biological activity (*Table 19.1*).

Table 19.1 The effect of DNA and heparin on the antibacterial activity of the teat canal proteins (Hibbitt and Benians, 1971)

Organism	*Treatment*	*Growth (%)*
*Staphylococcus aureus**	Nil	100.0
	Incubated† with cationic proteins	0.0
	Incubated with cationic proteins complexed with:	
	0.4 μg DNA	0.0
	0.8 μg DNA	0.7
	1.6 μg DNA	49.2
	3.2 μg DNA	100.0
	0.2 μg heparin	0.0
	0.4 μg heparin	2.1
	0.8 μg heparin	5.0
	1.6 μg heparin	69.2
	3.2 μg heparin	100.0

*Approximately 70 colony-forming units of *Staph. aureus* were incubated for 30 min in 1 ml 0.01 M citric acid + Na_2HPO_4 buffer (pH 7.0), then grown in Oxoid nutrient broth containing 1% Davis agar.
†*Staph. aureus* was incubated for 30 min in 1 ml of the buffer described above containing 8 μg of the cationic proteins.
‡The protein complex was prepared by incubating 8 μg of the cationic proteins with DNA or heparin in 1 ml of the buffer described above at 37°C for 15 min.

This loss of biological activity was not surprising since at physiological pHs it was necessary for the positively charged groups on the cationic proteins to bind electrovalently to the negatively charged microorganisms before inhibiting their growth.

The changes produced in the fine structure of staphylococci were studied after incubation with the teat canal antimicrobial proteins, using electron microscopy. Organisms incubated with these proteins showed damage to the cell wall and the underlying membrane. Many organisms showed a shrinkage of the protoplasm from these damaged regions, and all the organisms appeared to

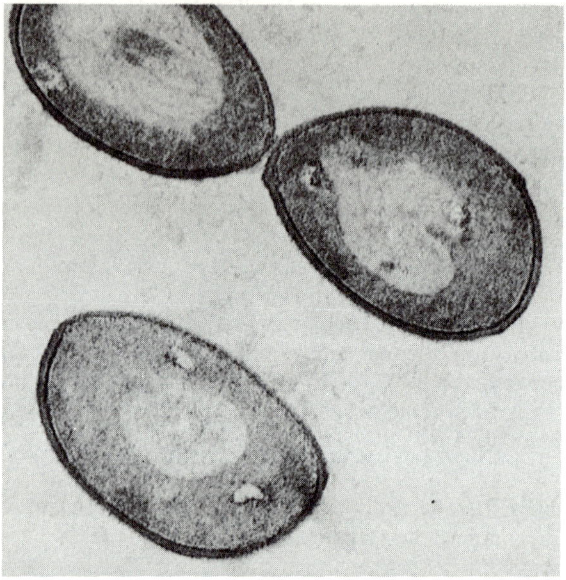

Figure 19.2 Normal staphylococci (× 80 000)

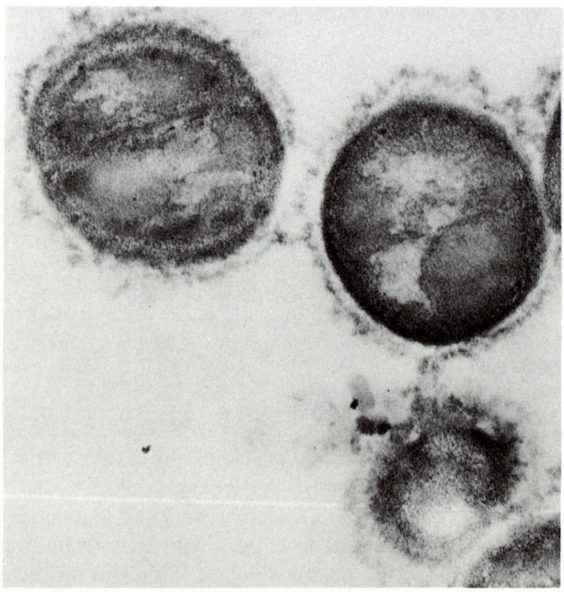

Figure 19.3 Staphylococci treated with antimicrobial proteins isolated from teat canal keratin (250 μg ml^{-1}) (× 80 000)

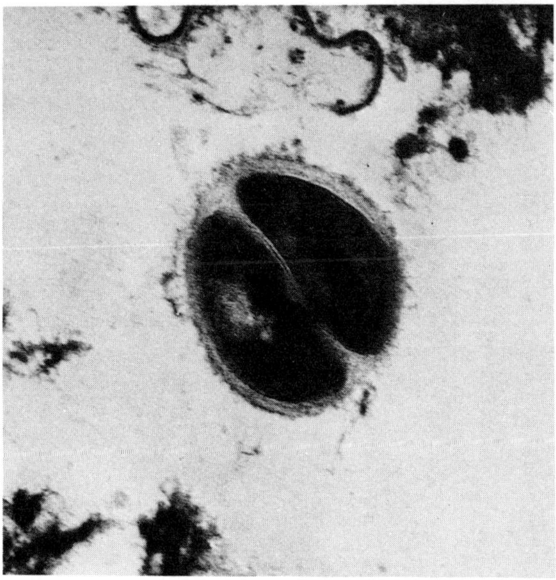

Figure 19.4 Staphylococcus aureus *recovered after 24 h in the teat canal of the cow (× 80 000)*

be surrounded by a layer of fibrillar material. *Figure 19.2* shows a group of staphylococci incubated at 37°C in isotonic saline for 1 h, and *Figure 19.3* shows organisms incubated under the same conditions but in isotonic saline containing teat canal antimicrobial proteins (250 $\mu g\ ml^{-1}$). Similar changes in morphology were observed in *in vivo* experiments when staphylococci were deposited in the teat canals of healthy cows and recovered after 24 h (*Figure 19.4*).

Damage to the cell wall and plasma membrane was expected to lead to a leakage of the cell contents to the exterior; this was studied in a series of experiments in which staphylococci were grown in a nutrient broth containing [1-^{14}C] valine. The organisms which incorporated the labelled amino acid into their protoplasmic proteins, were thoroughly washed in isotonic saline to remove free labelled amino acid, and incubated for 5 h at 37°C with cationic proteins dissolved in isotonic saline. Samples of the incubation mixture were removed at regular intervals and the staphylococci sedimented by centrifugation. Any labelled protein leaking from the organisms was precipitated in the particle-free supernatant with trichloracetic acid, solubilized and counted in a liquid scintillation counter. *Figure 19.5* shows that labelled protein leaked from the staphylococci treated with cationic proteins, whereas there was no significant leakage from organisms treated with isotonic saline or bovine serum albumin (Hibbitt and Benians, 1971).

The results of *in vitro* experiments on the teat canal defences require careful interpretation since the environment in these artificial conditions cannot be compared with the living teat canal, where protein synthesis is actively proceeding and where invading pathogens are being subjected to newly synthesized antimicrobial factors. Teat canal keratin was not antimicrobial under *in vitro*

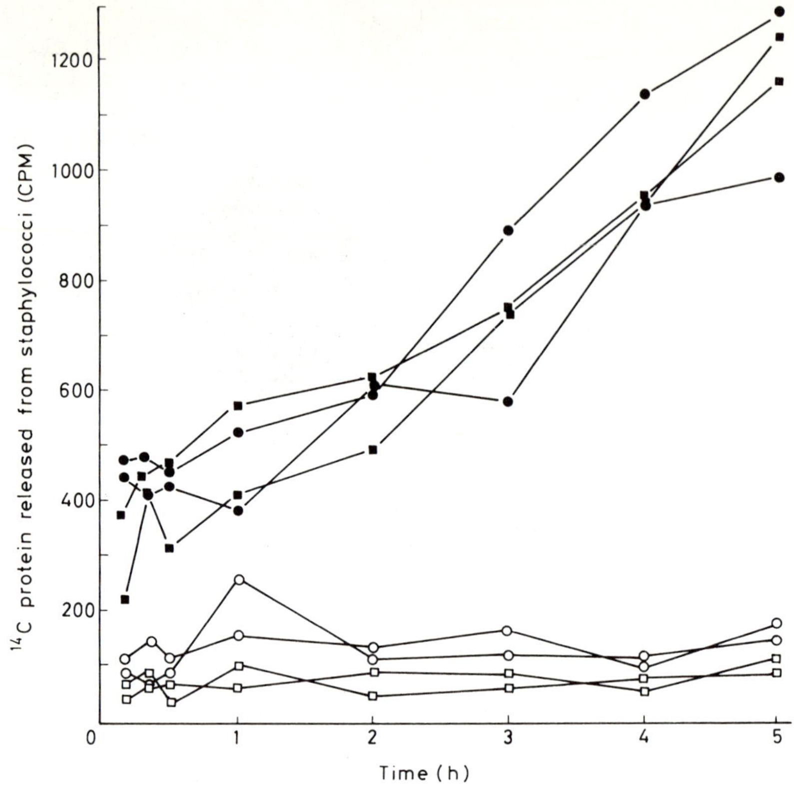

Figure 19.5 The release of ^{14}C-labelled protoplasmic proteins from staphylococci incubated with with teat canal cationic proteins, calf thymus histone F2A, bovine serum albumin and isotonic saline. ●–● = Calf thymus histone F2A; ■–■ = teat canal cationic proteins; ○–○ = bovine serum albumin; □–□ = untreated control. (Hibbitt and Benians, 1971)

conditions. The *in vitro* experiments of Russell, Brooker and Reiter (1975), while showing a definite loss of antimicrobial activity of calf thymus histone F 11A (pI 10.0–11.5) in the presence of milk or casein, would not reflect the conditions existing within the living teat canal where proteins with lower pI values (7.0–9.0) are being synthesized continually. There is strong evidence to suggest that staphylococci deposited in the teat canals of normal cows are

Table 19.2 The binding of ^{131}I Bovine serum albumin to microorganisms recovered from the teat canals of the cows (Hibbitt and Benians, 1971)

Cow number	^{131}*I Bovine serum albumin* (ng 10^{-8} organisms) *binding to* *Control organisms*	*Recovered organisms*
1	7.9	423.0
2	7.7	202.0
3	0.0	272.0
4	75.0	1694.0
5	0.0	802.0

coated with these basic proteins. The studies shown in *Table 19.2* involving five cows, demonstrated that staphylococci deposited and then recovered from the teat canal after 24 h were more positively charged than untreated control organisms (Hibbitt and Benians, 1971).

Mammary Gland Defences

Pathogenic organisms escaping the defences afforded by the teat canal are subjected to the defences of the mammary gland. These mammary gland defences consist of a wide range of antimicrobial proteins in the cell-free milk and the phagocytic activity of some of the milk cells. The humoral and cellular factors may be considered together since efficient phagocytosis depends largely on the presence of opsonins and other humoral substances.

Cell-free milk contains a number of non-specific antimicrobial substances which can play an important role in the defences of the mammary gland in the early stages of infection. These substances are not antibodies and have been described in the past as 'lactenins'.

Lactoferrin is a lactenin, an iron-binding protein which, in the presence of bicarbonate, inhibits the growth of microorganisms which have a high requirement for iron. Lactoferrins compete for the iron and inhibit the bacterial growth (Oram and Reiter, 1966; Oram and Reiter, 1968). This antimicrobial system is inhibited by the presence of citrate which competes with the lactoferrin for the available iron and makes the iron available to the invading bacteria. Lactoferrin may be of limited value as a defence system in colostrum and milk, but could be of greater importance in the dry cow when the mammary secretion has a lower citrate and higher bicarbonate concentration (Reiter and Bramley, 1975).

The lactoperoxidase/thiocyanate/hydrogen peroxide system is also antimicrobial and inhibits the growth of some strains of streptococci which produce lactic acid (Reiter *et al*., 1963; Mickelson, 1966). More recently the system has been shown to inhibit the growth of *Escherichia coli, Pseudomonas aeruginosa, Salmonella typhimurium* and *Staphylococcus aureus* (Reiter and Bramley, 1975). Lactoperoxidase is present in milk, but the levels of the SCN^- can be variable and will depend on the feeding regime. Some bacteria produce their own hydrogen peroxide which leads to their 'self-destruction' while other organisms such as *E. coli* and *Staph. aureus* are killed only in the presence of an exogenous supply of peroxide (Reiter and Bramley, 1975). This antimicrobial system has obvious limitations, but should receive further attention.

In the early stages of infection of the mammary gland there is a considerable increase in the number of somatic cells in the milk and is associated with an increased resistance of the mammary gland to infection (Schalm, 1970). This resistance may be partly due to an enhanced antimicrobial activity of the cell-free milk, since Brownlie (1972) showed that cationic proteins isolated from the whey of cows injected with *E. coli* lipopolysaccharide (LPS) were antimicrobial to staphylococci, streptococci and *E. coli* whereas the whey from normal cows had no antimicrobial activity. The constituents of the mammary secretion during a mild inflammation of the mammary gland are of local and systemic origin. Shah and Morse (1964) demonstrated a movement of proteins from the systemic circulation into the mammary gland during the early stages of infection. An influx of immunoglobulins, complement units and other antimicrobial systems would contribute to the defences of the gland. This passage of serum factors to the mammary gland in some animals may be too slow to be of use in the protection against invading pathogens.

The proteins released from milk leucocytes during inflammation had an antimicrobial activity and possessed antigenic and chromatographic properties similar to the cationic proteins isolated from the milk leucocytes (Brownlie, 1971). Goldstein *et al.* (1973) also observed a release of proteins from polymorphonuclear leucocytes in association with an activation of the alternate complement pathway. This pathway may be activated by *E. coli* endotoxins (Kane, May and Frank, 1973).

Most of the immunoglobulin in the colostrum and milk of cattle is derived from the blood, the levels of all classes are low in normal milk but are elevated considerably in colostrum. Inflammation of the glandular epithelium changes its permeability to the serum proteins (Lascelles and McDowell, 1974) so the immunoglobulin levels increase rapidly during infection or if the gland is stimulated by endotoxins. The precise role of the immunoglobulins in mammary secretions is not clear since there is evidence to suggest that complement activity is very low or even absent (Reiter, Sharpe and Higgs, 1970). The passage of immunoglobulins from the systemic circulation to the inflamed mammary gland is accompanied nevertheless by a movement of complement units and the provision of opsonins for phagocytosis.

The importance of the cell response in infection of the mammary gland remains in some doubt. A pre-existing leucocytosis induced by endotoxin will protect the udder against infection by low numbers of staphylococci and other pathogens (Blobel and Katsube, 1964; Newbould and Neave, 1965; Reiter, Sharpe and Higgs, 1970). More recent *in vitro* studies however, have suggested that phagocytic killing is less efficient in the mammary gland than in blood due to the inhibitory effect of casein (Russell and Reiter, 1975). Some inhibition may be attributed to the casein, but endotoxin can also affect the efficiency of the neutrophil so the behaviour of endotoxin-stimulated cells in the *in vitro* studies may not reflect truthfully the conditions in the infected mammary gland. Nies *et al.* (1971) were one of many groups who have reported a release of lysosomal enzymes from neutrophils in the presence of endotoxin, and in another laboratory the release of these enzymes was accompanied by a reduced ability to kill injected *Staph. aureus* (Koch, 1975). It is possible that the protection afforded by a pre-existing leucocytosis induced by endotoxin is due partly to the diminished killing ability of the neutrophils together with an increased antimicrobial activity of the cell-free milk, since antimicrobial cationic proteins in milk leucocytes (Hibbitt, Brownlie and Cole, 1971) are released into the milk whey after endotoxin stimulation of the mammary gland (Brownlie, 1971, 1972).

Stimulation of Resistance to Infection

Non-specific resistance to infection was studied further in experiments investigating the changes which occur in tissues and body fluids when resistance is stimulated after injections of endotoxin. Earlier studies by many workers have shown that endotoxin will stimulate the resistance of laboratory animals against pathogenic organisms. More recently these endotoxin studies in the mouse have been extended to the protection of the mouse mammary gland against staphylococcal infection. Anderson (1976) showed that intramammary inoculation of endotoxin in mice three days before intramammary challenge with staphylococci induced resistance to staphylococci. A similar resistance was induced if the endotoxin was injected into the peritoneal cavity three days before challenge. The enhanced resistance was not due to the presence of neutrophils in the mammary alveoli at the time of challenge, but was associated with the stage of lactation. Endotoxin injected intraperitoneally or into the mammary gland produced an accelerated mammary gland involution. The mechanism leading to this involution remains in doubt and the reason for the enhanced resistance of the involuted gland requires further investigation.

Experiments demonstrating an enhanced resistance to infection in laboratory animals following parenteral endotoxin injections have been repeated in studies on the dairy cow. The antimicrobial activity of the serum of the cow against *E. coli* increases after endotoxin is injected intramuscularly (Hill, Shears and Hibbitt, 1976). This antimicrobial activity is complement-dependent and can be removed by heat treatment at 56°C for 30 min (*Figure 19.6*). The enhanced antimicrobial activity is accompanied by various changes in the levels of serum

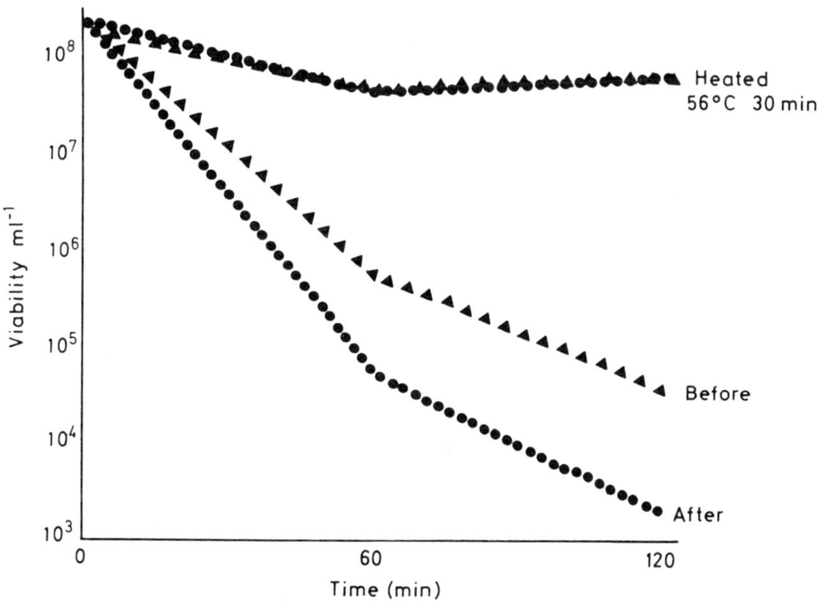

Figure 19.6 The antimicrobial activity against E. coli *of serum from cows before and after endotoxin treatment*

components (Hibbitt *et al.*, 1977). The level of total serum protein increased by 9% and this increase was attributed largely to the increases in the levels of transferrin (74%), IgG (22%) and IgM (30%). The immunoglobulin levels were increased partly by the formation of endotoxin-specific antibody which could be precipitated by absorption with endotoxin. In addition, non-specific immunoglobulins were formed and were found to be mainly of the IgG class in the endotoxin absorbed sera. This immunostimulant activity of endotoxin is not understood fully, but it may be due to a stimulation of protein synthesis (Koj and McFarlane, 1968) and/or a release of preformed immunoglobulin as reported by Hill and Rowley (1967) in experiments involving guinea pigs. Endotoxin has been reported in the literature to stimulate the classical and alternate complement pathway (Kane, May and Frank, 1973) in laboratory animals. Polyacrylamide gel electrophoresis studies, in the investigations on dairy cows, revealed consistent changes in the levels of certain α and β globulins after endotoxin injections. These proteins have not been identified, but the changes in their levels may be consistent with a complement activation and the associated increase in the complement-dependent antimicrobial activity.

The advantage to the mammary gland of being able to stimulate antimicrobial activity in the serum may lie in the possibility of achieving an enhanced antimicrobial activity in the serum components of the inflammatory response. The rate at which serum components pass from the systemic circulation to the mammary secretion during early infection requires further study since it may be associated with the animal's susceptibility or resistance to mastitis.

References

ADAMS, E. W. and RICKARD, C. G. (1963). *Am. J. vet. Res.* **24**, 122

ANDERSON, J.C. (1976). *Res. vet. Sci.,* **21**, 64

BLOBEL, H. and KATSUBE, Y. (1964). *Am. J. vet. Res.,* **25**, 1085

BROWNLIE, J. (1971). *Biochem. J.*, **125**, 81P

BROWNLIE, J. (1972). *Ph.D. thesis.* University of Reading

CULLEN, G. A. and HERBERT, C. N. (1967). *Br. vet. J.,* **123**, 14

FINCHER, M. G., HODGES, H. G., MURPHY, J. M. and MORSE, G. E. (1956). *Mastitis Research and Control Programme*. Report N.Y. State vet. College

GOLDSTEIN, I. M., MELCHIORRE, B., OSLER, A. G. and WEISSMANN, G. (1973). *J. Immunology,* **111**, 33

HIBBITT, K. G. and BENIANS, M. (1971). *J. gen. Microbiol.,* **68**, 123

HIBBITT, K. G., BENIANS, M. and ROWLANDS, G. J. (1972). *Br. vet. J.*, **128**, 270

HIBBITT, K. G., BROWNLIE, J. and COLE, C. B. (1971). *J. Hyg. Camb.,* **69**, 61

HIBBITT, K.G. and COLE, C.B. (1968). *Biochem. J.,* **106**, 39P

HIBBITT, K. G., COLE, C. B. and REITER, B. (1969). *J. gen. Microbiol.*, **56**, 365

HIBBITT, K.G., HILL, A.W., YOUNG, J.L. and SHEARS, A.L. (1977). *J. comp. Path. Ther.,* **87**, 195

HIBBITT, K. G. and JONES, G. W. (1967). *Vet. Rec.*, **80**, 270

HILL, A.W., SHEARS, A.L. and HIBBITT, K.G. (1976). *Infec. Immun.,* **14**, 257

HILL, W. C. and ROWLEY, D. (1967). *Aust. J. exp. Biol. med. Sci.,* **45**, 693

KANE, M.A., MAY, J. E. and FRANK, M. M. (1973). *J. clin. Invest.,* **52**, 370

KOCH, C. (1975). *Acta path. microbiol. scand.,* Sect. C, **83**, 195

KOJ, A. and McFARLANE, A. S. (1968). *Biochem. J.,* **108**, 137

LASCELLES, A. K. and McDOWELL, G. H. (1974). *Transplant. Rev.* **19**, 170

McDONALD, J.S. (1970). *Proc. 3rd Int. Conf. Cattle Diseases,* Phildelphia, pp. 97–103

McDONALD, J.S. (1975). *Cornell Vet.,* **65**, 492

MICKELSON, M. N. (1966). *J. gen. Microbiology,* **43**, 31

MURPHY, J.M. (1959). *Cornell Vet.,* **49**, 411

MURPHY, J. M. and STUART, O. M. (1953). *Cornell Vet.,* **43**, 465

MURPHY, J.M. and STUART, O.M. (1955). *Cornell Vet.,* **45**, 112

NEWBOULD, F. H. S. and NEAVE, F. K. (1965). *J. Dairy Res.,* **32**, 163

NIES, A. S., GREINEDER, D. K., CLINE, M. J. and MELMON, K. L. (1971). *Biochem Pharm.,* **20**, 39

ORAM, J. D. and REITER, B. (1966). *Report National Institute for Research in Dairying,* p.93

ORAM, J. D. and REITER, B. (1968). *Biochem. Biophys. Acta,* **170**, 351

PLASTRIDGE, W. N. (1958). *J. Dairy Sci.,* **41**, 1141

REITER, B. and BRAMLEY, A. J. (1975). *Proc. Seminar on Mastitis Control.* International Dairy Federation

REITER, B., PICKERING, A., ORAM, J.D. and PAPE, G.S. (1963). *J. gen. Microb.,* **33**, XII

REITER, B., SHARPE, M.E. and HIGGS, T.M. (1970). *Res. vet. Sci.,* **11**, 18

RUSSELL, M. W., BROOKER, B. E. and REITER, B. (1975). *Res. vet. Sci.,* **20**, 30

RUSSELL, M. W. and REITER, B. (1975). *J. Reticuloendothelial Soc.,* **18**, 1

SCHALM, O. W. (1970). *VIth Int. Conf. on Cattle Diseases,* Philadelphia, p.25

SHAH, P. C. and MORSE, G. E. (1964). *Am. J. vet. Res.,* **25**, 714

TREECE, J.M., MORSE, G.E. and LEVY, C. (1966). *J. Dairy Sci.,* **49**, 1240

V

ANTIBIOTICS, ANTIBIOSIS AND FEED

20

A MECHANISM OF GROWTH PROMOTION: NON-LETHAL FEED ANTIBIOTIC INDUCED, CELL WALL LESIONS IN ENTERIC BACTERIA

J. R. WALTON
Department of Veterinary Preventive Medicine, University of Liverpool, Wirral

The mechanism of growth promotion in young actively growing animals or birds will inevitably involve a complex interaction of many factors. The fact that known growth-promoting agents (GPA) fail to stimulate growth in germ-free animals is in itself an indication that serious attention should be paid to the direct effect of GPAs on enteric bacteria. With this in mind I shall discuss in detail the effect of one well established GPA, namely zinc bacitracin on *Escherichia coli* isolated from pigs and poultry (Walton and Bird, 1975).

In order to understand fully the mechanism of action of bacitracin the structure of the bacterial cell envelope, which is composed of cell wall and cytoplasmic membrane, needs to be described in some detail.

Gram-Positive Bacterial Cells

These bacteria have a relatively simple cell envelope composed basically of three layers (*Figure 20.1*).

(1) *Cytoplasmic membrane*. This is the innermost layer and while not strictly a component of the cell wall it is immediately underlying and adherent to it.

(2) *The peptidoglycan or murein layer*. This second layer is interspersed with teichoic acid and this usually extends over the peptidoglycan layer as an outer coat.

(3) Various other structures may be present around the cell such as *protein* or *carbohydrate capsules*. In general the whole framework of the Gram-positive cell wall has an open fibrous structure which will allow the passage of many types of molecules.

Gram-Negative Bacterial Cells

These bacteria have a very complex cell envelope composed of about five layers. The innermost layer is the cytoplasmic membrane which lies directly underneath

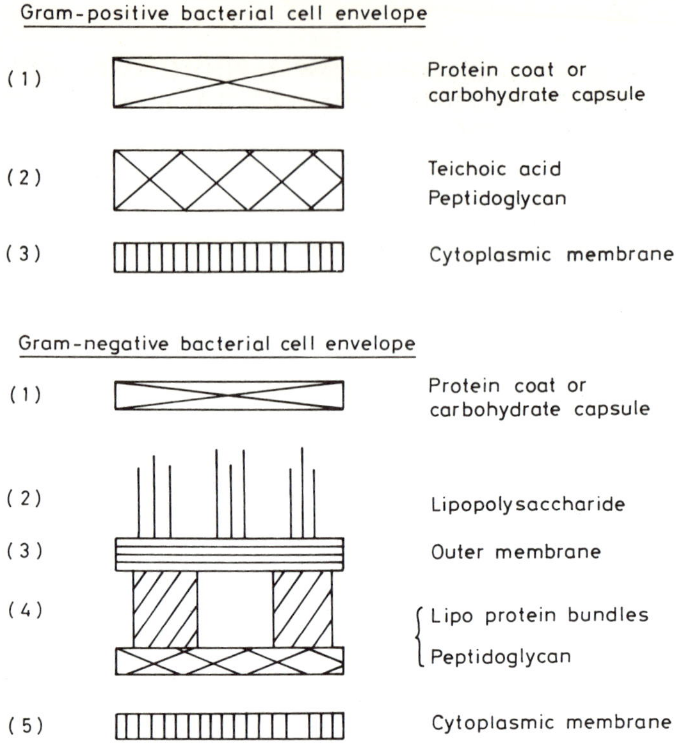

Figure 20.1 Diagramatic representation of the basic structures comprising the bacterial cell envelope

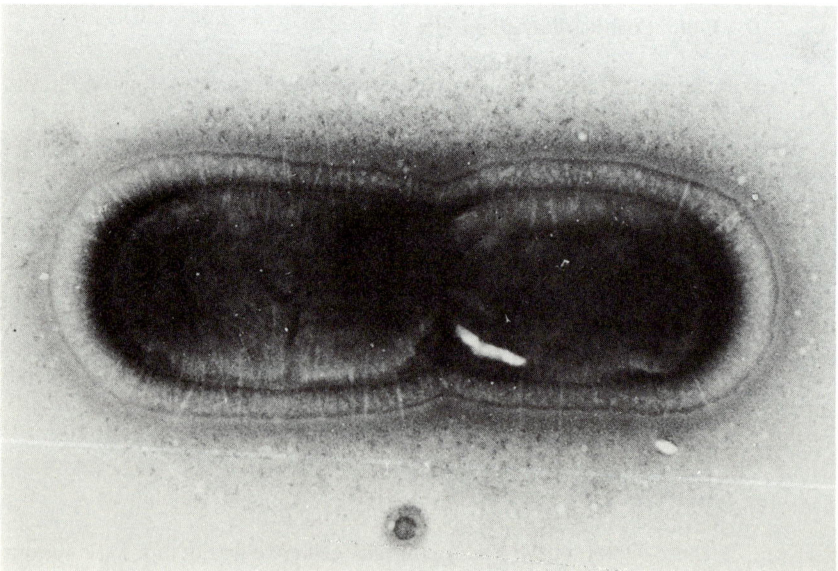

Figure 20.2 Strain of Escherichia coli *showing a well demarcated capsule*

a layer of peptidoglycan. Distinct from the Gram-positive cells, teichoic acids are not present at this level; instead, there is a combination of peptidoglycan with lipoprotein molecules which extend outwards in bundles. The outer membrane provides a permeability barrier limiting the outward and inward movements of various molecules and in particular prevents the penetration of many antibiotics. Permeability is dependent to a large extent on the content of lipopolysaccharide (LPS) and any alteration in LPS content, as in the conversion from the smooth to the rough phase, will automatically result in an alteration in cell permeability. Certain types of R factor-mediated resistance result from the formation of a specific protein which is intercalated into the outer membrane and this decreases its permeability.

The final layer of the cell envelope may either be a protein or a carbohydrate capsule, depending on the nutritional status of the organism and the condition of its environment. If this layer becomes very dense, as in mucoid strains of bacteria (*Figure 20.2*), certain antibiotics may be absorbed to it but generally this capsular layer provides no barrier to the passage of antibiotics (Costerton and Cheng, 1975).

Bacitracin is a polypeptide antibiotic which remains almost entirely unabsorbed after oral administration. Following the Swann Committee report, zinc bacitracin was accepted as a feed antibiotic and could therefore be added, without veterinary prescription, to animal feed.

Bacitracin is generally considered to have activity only against Gram-positive bacteria, and the main effect on these bacteria is the inhibition of peptidoglycan synthesis with the accumulation of peptidoglycan precursors. There is also a secondary effect on the cell membranes but the mechanism of the latter is not entirely clear. The effect of bacitracin on Gram-negative enteric bacteria has received little attention as it is generally considered to be active only against Gram-positive organisms.

Most of the data available on growth promotion indicates that the increase in metabolic performance is most likely due to some interference with the viability of one or more groups of enteric bacteria. In the U.K. numerous growth-promoting agents are widely used in pig and poultry nutrition and, contrary to common belief, all these agents exhibit some form of antibacterial effect which may be much more subtle than simple destruction of bacterial cells. The recognition of this antibacterial effect depends in part upon such indirect methods as increased sensitivity to certain chemotherapeutic agents or replacement of a certain species of bacteria by another of the same genus but with a different biochemical profile. This replacement phenomenon is especially seen with members of the Group D streptococci in pigs and poultry. Many types of bacteria have been examined for the effects of GPAs and a reduction in toxin production has been recognized in *Cl. perfringens (welchi)*, but despite previous experiments to detect changes in enteric Gram-negative bacteria none have been found.

In an attempt to determine if Gram-negative bacteria like *E. coli* are involved in growth promotion a series of experiments were made both in animals and in the laboratory in order to detect any alterations in bacterial numbers and other more subtle changes in cell structure.

Examination of faeces from cattle receiving zinc bacitracin in the diet revealed no difference in viable *E. coli* count compared with faeces from cattle receiving unsupplemented food. Strains of *E. coli* were then cultured on agar medium containing zinc bacitracin and incubated aerobically overnight at 37°C. After incubation the organisms were examined in the electron-microscope using a negative staining technique. *Escherichia coli* cultured on agar medium without added zinc bacitracin possessed the structural appearance of typical undamaged cells (*Figure 20.3*). Examination of *E. coli* grown on agar containing zinc bacitracin revealed the presence of structural lesions in the bacterial cell wall. Defined areas of cell wall damage were recognized along the long axis of the bacterial cell (*Figures 20.4* and *20.5*).

The lesions described were not present on all the cells examined. Almost all the damaged cells are in the early stages of growth while cells in the stationary phase appear to be undamaged. This observation may indicate that cells may be susceptible to damage only during the early growing phase.

When zinc bacitracin-treated cells were examined for susceptibility to therapeutic antibiotics it was shown that the minimal inhibiting concentrations (MIC) of these drugs were reduced when compared with data obtained prior to zinc bacitracin treatment. This was not totally unexpected because if zinc bacitracin is interfering with membrane integrity and inhibiting the synthesis of peptidoglycan then the permeability of the cell wall will increase and the damaged cells will thus become more susceptible to penetration by other antibiotics. One could postulate that cell wall-damaged bacteria would also be more susceptible to the variable environment present in the intestinal tract and also to the normal defence mechanisms of the host. Either of these could result in a local reduction of bacterial numbers resulting in an increased availability of essential nutrients to the host animal, and hence growth promotion.

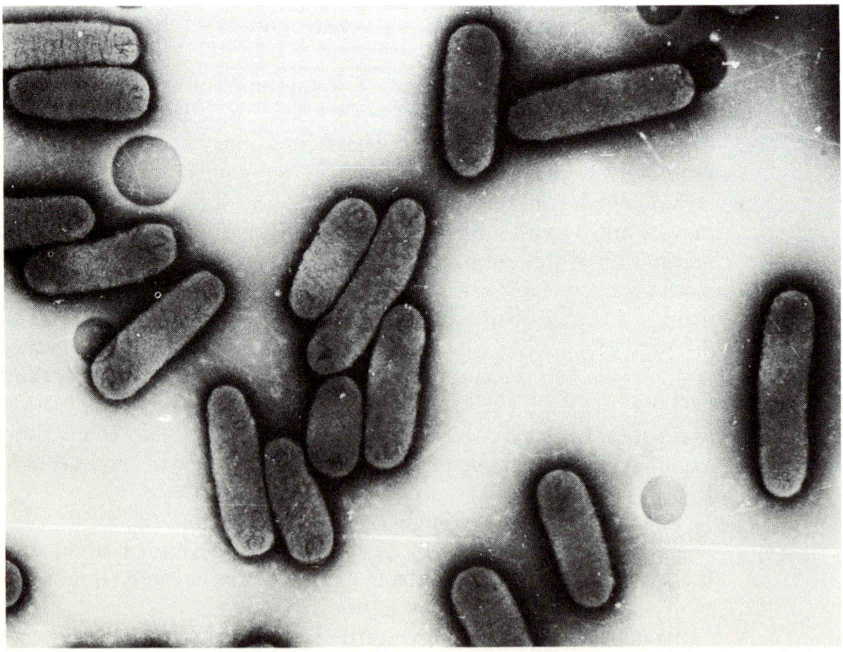

Figure 20.3 Escherichia coli *from agar medium without added zinc bacitracin (× 15 600)*

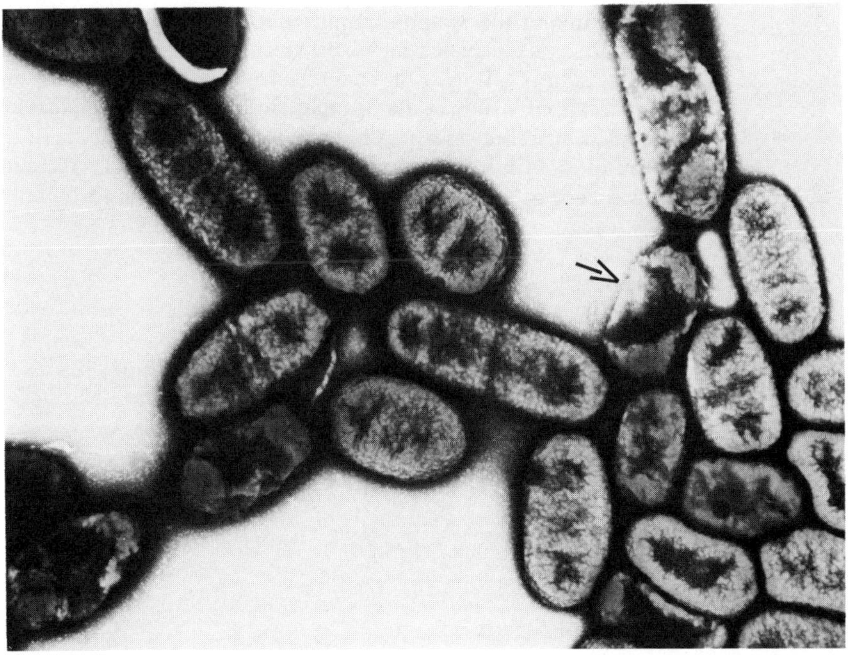

Figure 20.4 Escherichia coli, *grown in the presence of 100 μg ml^{-1} zinc bacitracin, showing discreet cell wall lesions (× 25 600)*

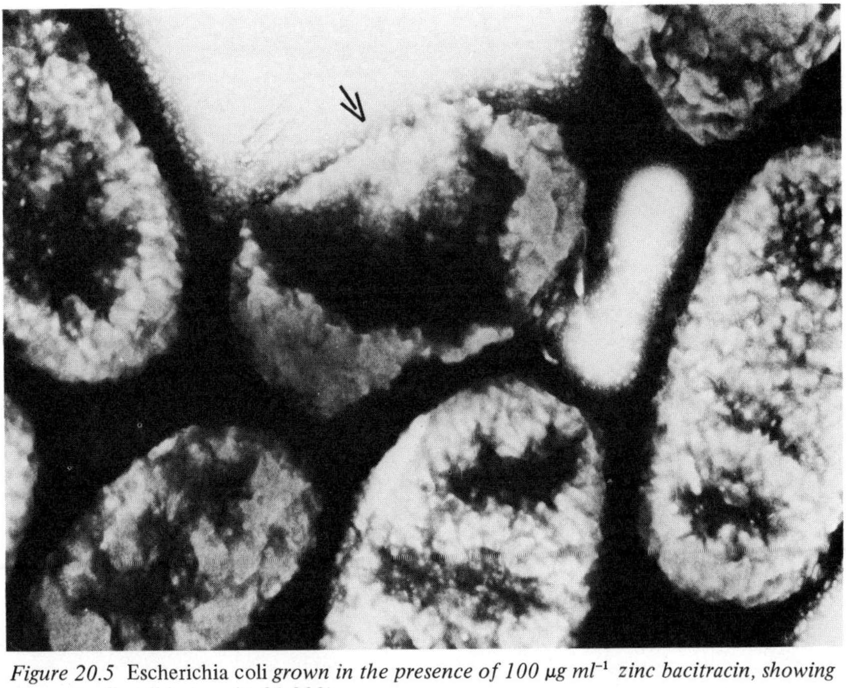

Figure 20.5 Escherichia coli *grown in the presence of 100 μg ml^{-1} zinc bacitracin, showing discreet cell wall lesions (× 81 900)*

The adoption of the Swann Committee recommendations that a special group of feed antibiotics be created may have given rise to an unexpected bonus to the agricultural industry. If by using these feed antibiotics to promote growth, the overall susceptibility of bacteria to other antibiotics can be increased, this will provide major benefits in respect of prolonging the effective life of the therapeutic antibiotics for intestinal use and also may lead to a decrease in antibiotic resistance of enteric bacteria in the general environment.

References

COSTERTON, J. W. and CHENG, K. J. (1975). *J. Antimicrob. Chem.*, **1**, 363
WALTON, J. R. and BIRD, R. G. (1975). *Zbl. Vet. Med. B*, **22**, 318

21

CHEMICAL CONTROL OF CROP CONSERVATION

A. D. DRYSDALE
B.P. Nutrition (U.K.) Ltd, Witham, Essex

Introduction

Although the word 'antibiotic' has developed a specific meaning in the area of human and animal health as 'a substance produced by a microorganism and able in dilute solution to inhibit or kill another microorganism', the original dictionary definition of 'tending to prevent, inhibit or destroy life' can be applied to the action of chemicals used in the protection against spoilage of stored agricultural crops.

The use of propionic acid for the treatment and storage of moist grain, developed within The British Petroleum Company, is one example of this second definition, and the use of this method of crop storage is widespread in many countries and is still growing. The biocidal and biostatic effects of some of the aliphatic acids, particularly acetic acid, have been known for centuries but it is only since the 1930s, when relatively small quantities of propionic acid were introduced to protect some foods against surface spoilage, that more attention has been paid to individual acids and the differences between them.

Huitson (1968) reported some of the early work using propionic acid in the treatment and storage of moist grain destined for animal feed. This showed that moist grain could be stored aerobically for long periods at any moisture level, by spraying it with propionic acid to ensure good coverage of the grain. The biocidal properties of undiluted propionic acid resulted in virtual sterilization of the grain, and through retention and absorption into the grain prevented subsequent deterioration by microbial contamination. More recently a review of the practical applications of this work using the product Propcorn*, essentially propionic acid, has been made (Drysdale, 1973). This reported on the growth of the moist grain storage system in the United Kingdom and some of the important factors involved in its practical use.

Before further discussing the treatment and use of acid-treated grain the alternatives available should be considered. Ripe grain consists of a living embryo, the endosperm as a store of food and various protective coatings. In a normal life process the grain gives off water, heat and carbon dioxide as its store of food is consumed. The rate at which these processes continue depends on its moisture

*Propcorn is a trade mark of The British Petroleum Company Limited

content, its temperature and the availability of oxygen. By adjusting these conditions the life-rate of the grain is altered as in the systems of drying (moisture content), ventilation and refrigeration (temperature) and ensiling in the absence of air (oxygen). All these systems are well known but differ from the acid system which preserves the characteristics of the grain harvested.

The Effect of Different Acids on Keeping Quality of Grain

Various chemical products have been shown to have a preservative effect but chiefly it is the group of volatile fatty acids that have been studied because of their lack of toxicity in feed. Most of these organic acids show some preservative properties but propionic acid has apparently a much greater and specific effect against moulds and yeasts as shown by a recent study of the preservative action of formic, acetic, propionic, butyric and some acid mixtures. This work by Sauer (1973), shown in *Table 21.1*, lists the number of weeks that maize of

Table 21.1 Mould-free storage time (weeks) of maize at 24% moisture content stored at 24°C

Acid applied	*Application rate (%)* 0.4	0.5
None	Less than 1 week	
Formic	1	2
Acetic	1	2
Iso-butyric	2	9
Propionic	22+	22+

24% moisture content stored at 23°C remained mould-free. These figures constitute the summary table of a series of experiments done under laboratory conditions. Over the 22-week period of the study, formic and acetic acid-treated grain remained mould-free for only two weeks when treated with 0.5% acid. At the same rate grain treated with iso-butyric acid stored for nine weeks, whilst with propionic acid it was still well preserved when the trial finished at 22 weeks.

In our laboratories a similar study with different rates of acid showed the same general pattern (*Table 21.2*). With barley at 20, 25 and 30% moisture content, stored at 23°C, propionic acid was always superior to acetic acid which was itself better than formic. Both *n*-butyric and iso-butyric acids have been

Table 21.2 Treatment rate (% acid) for 12 months mould-free storage under laboratory conditions at 23°C

Acid applied	*Grain moisture content (%)* 20	25	30
Formic	0.6	1.5	2.3
Acetic	0.8	1.0	1.6
Propionic	0.3	0.35	0.45

studied and although approaching propionic acid in effect, they suffer from the disadvantage of their characteristic smell. As a result, field trials have shown a strong reluctance to the acceptance of butyric acid.

Sogn (1973) has reported Norwegian experiments where formic and propionic acids were compared on grain at 28% moisture content. The 1% formic acid level failed to preserve the grain, the temperature rising to 65°C within four weeks. Propionic acid completely preserved the grain at the lowest level of application, 0.3%. Formic acid, however, is used to a limited extent in practice for winter storage in Scandinavia at between 1.8 and 2.0 times the rate of propionic acid. Temperatures of stored grain in winter are in the region of 0–5°C and it is logical that these low temperatures can significantly assist in maintaining the quality of stored grain.

In some cases binary and ternary mixtures of formic, acetic and propionic can be more effective than individual acids (British patent 1 155 485). There are many references to mixed acids in the literature but few products are available commercially. A mixture of 80% propionic and 20% acetic acids is marketed in the U.S.A. but application rates are recommended at 20% above the rate for propionic acid. Sauer and Burroughs (1973), using mixed acids, showed the dominant effect of propionic acid in binary mixtures. There have been reports of a high level of corrosion where mixed acids have been used and this has precluded the use of these potentially cheaper mixtures of the readily available organic acids.

In conclusion, work in Britain, the U. S. A., Scandinavia and elsewhere has indicated that propionic acid is a better mould inhibitor than any of the other readily available materials with application in farm conditions.

Control of Mycotoxin Production

In grain, heating followed by mould growth is visually dramatic and has sufficient economic repercussions to demand that precautions be taken to prevent spoilage. Sporadic outbreaks of mycotic disease and mycotoxicosis arise in livestock and in humans where storage conditions deteriorate. These can arise under any grain storage system although moist grain, because of its higher water content, may predispose some stored feeds to microbial attack. Even where propionic acid has been applied this may not prevent harmful mycotoxin effects in livestock where the mould growth has developed *in the field* before treatment (Miller *et al*., 1973).

Aflaxtoxicoses and other mycotoxin problems appear of greater significance in maize crops where moisture levels in the field are maintained at a higher level, and for longer periods, than with the small grains, barley, oats, wheat and sorghum. With more stringent control of feedstuffs it is less likely that these will cause an acute problem at a national level as has happened previously. However, with more emphasis on home-grown and home-mixed feeds a more sporadic but incipient type of sub-clinical mycotoxicosis is likely in certain farming systems, particularly in maize-growing areas.

In hay there has not been the same ability to provide an economic system of protection against mould growth as in grain and much of the mycotic disease in Britain originates from badly preserved hay. Lacey (1975) has suggested that of the 80% of conserved grass stored as hay, on average one third of this is spoiled by moulds. Of mouldy samples examined at Rothamsted, over half contained moulds noted for their disease-producing characteristics. Farmer's Lung organisms were found in 40% of the samples and in 15% of the samples at a level above 2×10^5 colonies g^{-1} dry wt.

The use of propionic acid on hay has been studied by our group for some years but it is only recently that control of fungal heating in hay has been achieved under field conditions, although this effect was shown quite conclusively in the laboratory many years ago. Factors contributing to the difficulties in translating from the successful field treatment of grain to hay include: the greater surface area of hay, the inability to determine the moisture content of hay in the field, the variability in moisture within a field and the very large problem of distribution of the correct level of preservative acid over the crop.

The system being introduced now for hay utilizes the fungicidal effect of propionic acid but produces a much smaller droplet size by means of a spinning disc applicator, than that produced in the treatment of grain. Applied at the baler or perhaps by a special applicator in a separate pass before baling, this technique should permit a significant improvement in hay quality. The *British Medical Journal*, discussing Farmer's Lung disease from hay in a recent editorial (Anon., 1975), stated that 'What is needed is a substance which, while harmless to cattle would inhibit one or more of the steps in this process and could be added to hay baled in wet conditions; such a development would constitute an important contribution to the health of farmers'. It is believed that with hay, as with grain, chemical control of this conserved crop is now attainable.

The Effect of Different Acids on Mould and Yeast Growth

Concern was expressed in the early days of acid preservation that some species of mould might continue to grow at marginal levels of acid application and as a result develop a resistance to the acid applied. Laboratory studies in the early stages of acid storage used various application rates and from these it was apparent that at the lower levels there were species differences in the tolerance of added acids. Pelhate (1973) reported on the differential growth of moulds where treatment was made by propionic, sorbic, acetic and formic acids at different rates. *Paecilomyces* spp and *Monascus* spp continued to grow at the maximum rate used in the study, 0.5% by weight of propionic and acetic acids. In contrast, formic acid showed good control of these species but had little effect on *Aspergillus flavus* which is a known hazard in feeds. Acetic and formic acids showed better control of yeasts than did propionic acid. Kozakiewicz and Clarke (1973) also suggest that grain residues from feed grains treated over successive seasons could harbour such fungi as *Paecilomyces varioti* and provide inoculum for the next batch of freshly treated grain.

Application rates in practice have been placed well above the levels found to control microbial growth in the laboratory (up to five times higher). An abbreviated list of recommended application rates for various lengths of storage are shown in *Table 21.3*. Now, with widespread use of propionic acid on farms, one can only report that there are no indications of an increasing mould problem nor of any detectable signs of resistant strains developing.

Table 21.3 Recommended Propcorn application rate for treatment of moist grain

Grain moisture content (%)	*Application rate* (litre per tonne) *for different lengths of storage*			
	Months			
	12	*6*	*3*	*1*
15	5	4.5	4.0	4.0
20	7.5	6.5	5.5	4.5
25	10.0	9.0	7.5	6.0
30	13.0	11.5	10.0	8.0
35	17.0	14.0	12.5	10.5
40	20.5	18.0	16.0	14.0

Applications made on farms now are better than those in the early days of the system. This appears to be almost entirely due to the improvement in applicators themselves as well as to the improved technique of application.

Among the practical items causing problems were:

(1) Incorrect measurement of the moisture in grain, either because a moisture meter was not used or it was not used correctly, or it did not have a scale appropriate to the high moisture often treated.

(2) Incorrect measurement of grain flow through applicators on farm augers particularly in the drying phase where a drop of five percentage units in moisture is known to double the rate of grain movement through the application system. Without adjustment under these drying-out conditions, under-treatment could easily result and it has been observed that it is in these conditions farmers assume they may be over-applying rather than the true situation of under-applying.

(3) Grain which has been allowed to sit untreated for some hours, and where respiration followed by bacterial growth leads to a rise in temperature, requires an application rate of 25% higher than that recommended. However, in extreme conditions this 'crop' provides one of the most difficult to preserve.

Feeding Value of Treated Grain

There is a clear case on management considerations, and in many situations on economic considerations also, for the storage of acid-preserved high-moisture grain. To be fully integrated the grain has also to be acceptable to the consumer. The use and palatability of treated grain for human food is beyond the scope of this paper but it should be recorded that work is already in progress on the acceptance of treated rice in some countries and that treated wheat has been successfully used in bread making.

Much work has been published on the use of treated grain in livestock feeds. Wilson (1973) has summarized eight trials with beef cattle in which treated high-moisture maize was fed and compared with dry maize. In six of these trials an improvement in daily weight gain was recorded and over the eight trials this averaged 3.3%. The efficiency with which the treated grain was converted into liveweight averaged 6.5% higher than the dry grain. Various reasons have been put forward for this improvement: an increase in acceptability of treated grain, the energy value of the added acid and the improved texture of the processed grain have all been implicated.

Since propionic acid is itself a significant source of energy for ruminants, the amount added to grain will be metabolized and utilized for production. In normal use at say 30% moisture, an application of 1.3% acid would be required for complete storage. A high intake of 10 kg treated grain would provide 125 g propionic acid which is less than 10% of the propionic acid produced naturally in the rumen daily. In the work of Jones, Donefer and Elliot (1970) it was estimated that treatment added 68 g propionic acid to the daily intake of cows and Jorgensen, Larsen and Barrington (1973) estimated 123 g per 10 kg grain consumed. Livingstone *et al*., estimated that pigs gained 21 g per day more as a direct result of the energy value of the acid. The energy value of propionic acid, therefore, can be expected to contribute to the production of the animal although in a practical situation this is likely to be too small to be recorded. Dairy cows have been fed Propcorn-treated maize with good results. Eight investigations reported by Jorgensen, Larsen and Barrington (1973) concluded that both dry matter intake and the resultant milk yield were similar with acid-treated grain and dry or ensiled grain. Milk constituents were not altered by treatment, although it was expected that the fat level might fall since this is known to be reduced by feeds that result in a high proportion of propionic acid in total rumen acids. It was concluded that the fineness of grinding of other feeds in the diet could influence the fat content of milk more than the direct addition of relatively low levels of propionic acid.

The physical form of the moist grain is different from dry grain, particularly after processing. Dry grain is broken into smaller particles and becomes more dusty than moist grain when processed by rolling or by hammer milling. Livingstone *et al*., (1971) compared moist acid-treated rolled barley with the normal system of dry, milled grain. Liveweight gains of 732 and 729 g per day were found with the dry and Propcorn-treated barley, respectively. Here the apparent digestibility of dry matter and nitrogen was reduced by 2–4 percentage units although this was compensated for by the acid, which was estimated to have contributed directly about 21 g weight gain per day. Lawrence (1976), using one-year old maize at 37% moisture, treated with 2.6% Propcorn and fed to pigs from weaning until slaughter, found identical weight gains of 700 g per day between the dry and the moist treated grain. The apparent digestibilities of dry matter and protein were virtually the same with the dried and the moist treated grain. These comparable results with dry and treated grain show that rolled grain can be quite satisfactory for pigs if it is well rolled. Other benefits can result from the coarser texture of the moist feed since finely milled grain is known to cause stomach ulceration and intestinal upsets.

In conclusion, nutritional benefits in cattle and pigs can be traced to the coarser texture of the feed. Acid-treated grain has also improved digestibility of the feed and there are indications that protein might be better utilized. Treated grain is generally more acceptable than dry grain for livestock and suffers less from dustiness which can be a hazard.

References

ANON. (1975). *Br. med. J.*, **3**, 189

DRYSDALE, A. D. (1973). *Ann. Technol. Agric.*, **22**, 615

HUITSON, J. J. (1968). *Process Biochem.*, **3**., 31

JONES, G. F., DONEFER, E. and ELLIOT, J. I. (1970). *Can. J. Anim. Sci.*, **50**, 483

JORGENSEN, N. A. LARSEN, H. J. and BARRINGTON, G. P. (1973). *34th Minnesota Nutrition Conference*, pp. 129–138

KOZAKIEWICZ, Z. and CLARKE, J. H. (1973). *Trans. Br. mycol. Soc.*, **61**., 355

LACEY, J. (1975) *Trans. Br. mycol. Soc.*, **65**., 171

LAWRENCE, T. L. J. (1976). *J. agric. Sci.*, (*Camb*.), **86**, 315

LIVINGSTONE, R. M., DENERLEY, H., STEWART, C. S. and ELSLEY, F. W. H. (1971) *Anim. Prod.*, **13**., 547

MILLER, J. K., HACKING, A., HARRISON, J. and GROSS, V. J. (1973). *Vet. Rec.*, **93**, 555

PELHATE, J. (1973). *Ann. Technol. Agric.*, **22**, 647

SAUER, D. B. (1973). *Report U.S. Grain Marketing Research Center,* Manhattan, Kansas

SAUER, D. B. and BURROUGHS, R. (1973). Paper 73–307 presented at 1973 Meeting Amer. Soc. Agric. Eng.

SOGN, L. (1973). *Ann. Technol. Agric.*, **22**, 675

WILSON, L. L. (1973). *Proc. Grain Conditioning Conf.*, Univ. Illinois, pp. 68–84

VI

PRACTICAL CONSIDERATIONS

22

CHEMICALS AND HEAT AS ASCOSPORE ACTIVATORS

V.M. PALMER
I.J. McEVOY
Department of Industrial Microbiology, University College, Dublin, Eire

It has been known since 1933 that *Byssochlamys fulva* can cause spoilage of thermally processed fruit (Oliver and Smith, 1933). Later, Put and Kruiswijk (1964) showed that *Byssochlamys nivea* frequently caused this problem also. McEvoy and Stuart (1970) reported *Aspergillus fischeri* var. *glaber* as a contaminant of canned strawberries and that like *B. nivea* and *B. fulva*, its ascospores were extremely heat-resistant and constitutively dormant.

Emerson (1948) activated ascospores of *Neurospora crassa* using furfural. Since then many other chemicals including derivatives of furfural and organic solvents were shown to be activators of dormant spores (Sussman, 1953; Sussman, Lowry and Tyrrell, 1959).

Yates, Seaman and Woodbine (1968), investigating dormancy of *B. nivea* ascospores, found acetate to stimulate germination, but only when used in conjunction with a heat treatment. Recently, chemical activation of ascospores of *B. nivea, B. fulva* and *A. fischeri* var. *glaber*, using acetaldehyde, was reported (Palmer and McEvoy, 1974).

Materials and Methods

B. nivea, CMI 146520 and *B. fulva*, CMI 140021 were grown in one-ounce universal bottles at 25°C on Potato Dextrose Agar (Difco). *A. fischeri* var. *glaber*, CMI 144207 was grown in a similar manner on a medium consisting of: 1.41 g NH_4NO_3, 1.0 g K_2HPO_4, 0.5 g $MgSO_4.7H_2O$, 0.5 g KCl, 0.01 g $FeSO_4.7H_2O$, 30 g sucrose, 15 g agar (Oxoid No. 3), 1000 ml distilled water.

Ascospore suspensions were obtained by macerating the surface growth of slope cultures in sterile distilled water. Cultures were at least six months old when used. Asci of *B. fulva*, which remained intact after maceration, were broken by vigorous agitation with 2.0 mm glass beads on a wrist action shaker.

A constant-temperature water bath was used to heat test tubes containing spore suspensions of approximately 10^6 spores ml^{-1}. After the desired period of time, tubes were withdrawn and cooled in water. Spores were then spread, using a sterile Pasteur pipette, onto 1.0% plain water agar (PWA) and incubated at 30°C in darkness. After 24 h, percentage germination was assessed microscopically. Three lots of at least 100 spores were counted per treatment.

Chemical treatment of ascospores was done by immersing the spores in 15 ml of chemical solution of chosen concentration. After treatment, usually for 1 h, spores were centrifuged free of chemical and resuspended in sterile distilled water.

All chemicals were of Analar grade unless otherwise stated. Acetaldehyde was of Laboratory Reagent Grade (Hopkin and Williams).

Results

Ascospores of the three fungi were found to respond to high concentrations of acetaldehyde. Using one-hour treatments, optimal activation occurred with 2.0 to 4.0 M solutions (*Figures 22.1* and *22.2*). Inhibition of germination occurred when higher concentrations were used or when duration of treatment was increased (*Figure 22.3*).

It should be noted, however, that while the response of particular spore suspensions was consistent and could be repeated, extreme variation was observed between suspensions from different cultures. Variation was virtually eliminated in the case of *A. fischeri* var. *glaber* by using suspensions from cultures of the same batch. Unfortunately, *B. nivea* and *B. fulva* showed great variation even within the same batch of cultures. Other authors have reported this problem (Yates, Seaman and Woodbine, 1968). This variation is illustrated in *Table 22.1*, where the response of three ascospore suspensions of *B. nivea* to acetic acid is given.

Acetic acid was initially tested as an ascospore activator because it was known that acetaldehyde contained a small quantity (0.4%) of contaminating

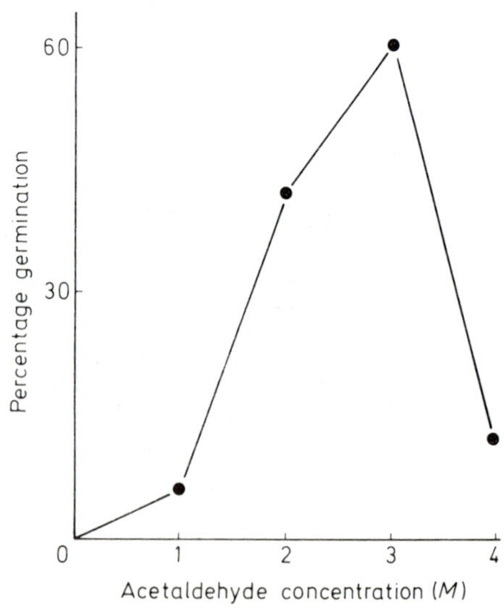

Figure 22.1 Percentage germination of ascospores of Aspergillus fischeri *var.* glaber *on PWA, 24 h after immersion in 1 to 4 M acetaldehyde for 1 h*

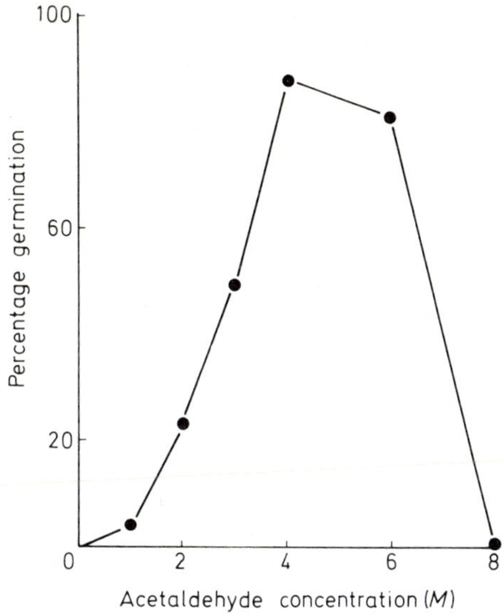

Figure 22.2 Percentage germination of ascospores of Byssochlamys fulva *on PWA, 24 h after immersion in 1 to 8 M acetaldehyde for 1 h*

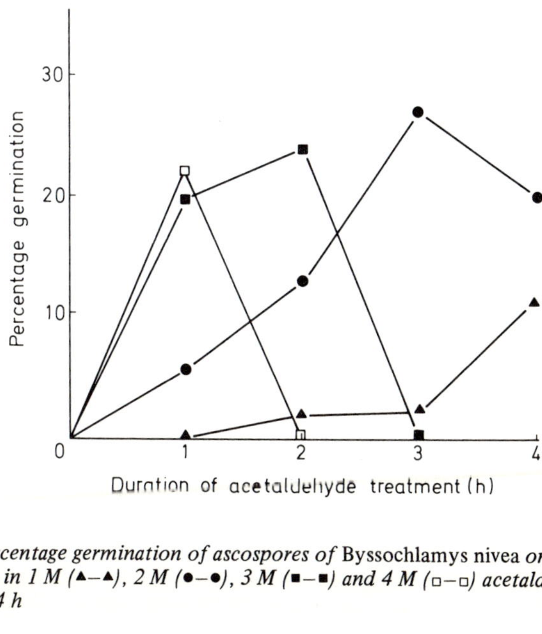

Figure 22.3 Percentage germination of ascospores of Byssochlamys nivea *on PWA, 24 h after immersion in 1 M (▲–▲), 2 M (●–●), 3 M (■–■) and 4 M (□–□) acetaldehyde for periods of 1 to 4 h*

Table 22.1 Percentage germination of ascospores of *Byssochlamys nivea* on PWA, 24 h after immersion in acetic acid for 1 h and 3 h. Ascospores were taken from three slope cultures of the same batch

Normality of acetic acid	*Culture 1*		*Culture 2*		*Culture 3*
	1 hour	*3 hours*	*1 hour*	*3 hours*	*1 hour*
0.0	0.0	0.0	0.0	0.0	0.0
0.01	–	–	–	–	0.0
0.05	–	–	54.2±2.8	76.5±5.6	–
0.1	–	–	59.1±0.6	80.9±2.2	11.0±1.8
0.5	–	–	53.1±2.0	78.8±1.9	22.4±1.1
1.0	–	–	46.9±5.9	72.2±4.9	18.4±3.1
2.0	0.0	18.4±2.0	34.6±2.6	51.0±3.4	20.7±4.2
3.0	0.0	20.8±1.5	20.7±4.1	40.2±5.3	–
4.0	0.0	14.2±0.8	34.3±1.5	32.2±3.6	–
5.0	0.0	8.5±3.3	21.3±6.2	30.6±1.6	–
8.0	–	–	18.7±3.5	21.7±2.2	–

acetic acid. Acetic acid was found to be an activator in its own right (*Figure 22.4, Table 22.2*) but at concentrations much higher than those which could possibly be present in solutions of acetaldehyde. Due to the presence of acetic acid, the pH of acetaldehyde solutions ranged from 2.84 for an 8.0 M solution to 3.49 for a 1 M solution. The pH of acetic acid solutions ranged from 1.2 for a 10 N solution to 3.6 for a 0.01 N solution. Immersion of ascospores in HCl solutions at these low pH values was not found to cause activation, so the effect obtained with acetic acid apparently was not due to a pH shock. The data presented in *Figure 22.4, Table 22.1* and *Table 22.2* served to establish which

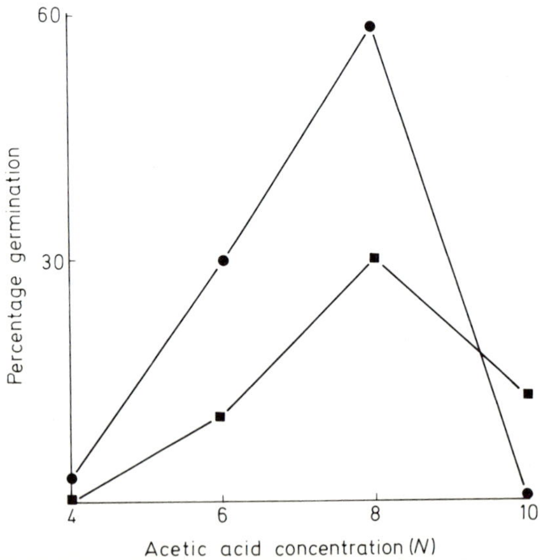

Figure 22.4 Percentage germination of ascospores of Aspergillus fischeri *var.* glaber *on PWA, 24 h after immersion in 4 to 10 N acetic acid for 1 h (■–■) and 3 h (●–●)*

Table 22.2 Percentage germination of ascospores of *Byssochlamys fulva* on PWA, 24 h after immersion in 1 to 10 N acetic acid for 1 h and 3 h

Normality of acetic acid	*1 hour*	*3 hours*
1	>1.0	7.2±2.4
3	14.0±4.2	18.2±3.4
5	17.1±3.2	24.7±3.4
6	35.2±3.1	81.2±3.4
8	43.2±2.9	76.5±3.5
10	30.8±4.4	77.9±4.4

concentrations of acetic acid were effective for ascospore activation and this information was used in later experiments.

The pH of the heating medium was found to influence ascospore activation (*Table 22.3*). Phthalate buffer was used to obtain pH 3.0, 4.0 and 5.0 and phosphate buffer to obtain pH 6.0, 7.0 and 8.0. Low pH was found to facilitate activation of ascospores of *A. fischeri* var. *glaber* at 70°C. However, at 80°C, pH 3.0 appeared to have a killing effect. It is interesting that activation can be obtained using 80°C with pH as high as 8.0. Both heat treatments gave almost complete activation at pH 4.0. Yates, Seaman and Woodbine (1968) found this pH most suitable for heat activation of ascosopores of *B. nivea.*

Table 22.3 Percentage germination of ascospores of *Aspergillus fischeri* var. *glaber* on PWA, 24 h after heat treatment (70°C and 80°C for 20 min) in buffers of pH 3.0 to 8.0

pH	*70°C*	*80°C*
6.8 (Control, distilled water)	4.8±0.7	84.0±1.8
3.0	81.9±6.0	<1.0
4.0	91.5±0.6	91.3±2.7
5.0	30.7±9.3	84.0±3.4
6.0	3.0±0.3	83.0±4.4
7.0	1.5±0.4	82.3±2.8
8.0	2.7±0.9	86.1±3.4

The strain of *B. nivea*, which was used in this work, produced ascospores which germinated after heat treatment only to the extent of about 0.1%. They were heat-resistant however, since ascospores which failed to germinate after heat treatment could subsequently be activated by chemicals.

The combined effect of heat and chemical treatment was studied using ascospores of *A. fischeri* var. *glaber* and *B. fulva*. When ascospores were heat treated, cooled and immersed in acetaldehyde or acetic acid and then incubated, synergic effects were observed using treatments which alone did not produce a high percentage germination (*Tables 22.4, 22.5, 22.8* and *22.9*). Synergism was not as obvious when chemical treatments were followed by heat treatments (*Tables 22.6, 22.7, 22.10* and *22.11*).

Table 22.4 Percentage germination of ascospores of *Aspergillus fischeri* var. *glaber* on PWA, 24 h after heat treatments of 60°C, 70°C and 80°C for 20 min followed by immediate immersion in 1M and 3 M acetaldehyde for 1 h

Acetaldehyde treatment	*Heat treatment*			
	None	*60°C*	*70°C*	*80°C*
None	0.0	0.9±0.1	5.4±2.5	91.1±2.4
1 M	1.9±0.1	90.9±2.0	90.1±3.2	92.5±2.6
3 M	49.0±2.2	86.3±2.5	84.6±2.2	73.7±2.5

Table 22.5 Percentage germination of ascospores of *Byssochlamys fulva* on PWA, 24 h after heat treatments of 60°C, 70°C and 80°C for 10 min followed by immediate immersion in 1 M and 4 M acetaldehyde for 1 h

Acetaldehyde treatment	*Heat treatment*			
	None	*60°C*	*70°C*	*80°C*
None	0.0	0.7±0.2	2.5±0.6	10.4±3.7
1 M	3.9±2.2	31.5±2.4	70.0±1.0	92.7±3.1
4 M	61.4±4.9	88.0±3.5	97.1±1.8	84.9±2.8

Table 22.6 Percentage germination of ascospores of *Aspergillus fischeri* var. *glaber* on PWA, 24 h after immersion in 1 M and 3 M acetaldehyde for 1 h followed by heat treatments of 70°C and 80°C for 20 min

Heat treatment	*Acetaldehyde treatment*		
	None	*1 M*	*3 M*
None	0.0	3.7±0.6	53.2±2.0
70°C	5.4±2.5	5.9±0.5	77.1±5.1
80°C	91.1±2.4	92.7±0.9	84.7±4.9

Table 22.7 Percentage germination of ascospores of *Byssochlamys fulva* on PWA 24 h after immersion in 1 M and 4 M acetaldehyde for 1 h followed by heat treatments of 70°C and 80°C for 10 min

Heat treatment	*Acetaldehyde treatment*		
	None	*1 M*	*4 M*
None	0.0	4.4±1.4	53.9±0.1
70°C	2.5±0.6	4.8±3.4	10.9±4.3
80°C	10.4±3.7	10.3±1.3	13.1±0.9

Table 22.8 Percentage germination of ascospores of *Aspergillus fischeri* var. *glaber* on PWA, 24 h after heat treatments of 70°C and 80°C for 20 min followed by immersion in 4 N and 8 N acetic acid for 1 h

Acetic acid treatment	*Heat treatment*		
	None	*70°C*	*80°C*
None	0.0	4.7±2.9	92.2±1.0
4 N	2.2±1.4	88.5±1.0	93.9±0.9
8 N	52.9±1.9	91.2±2.8	83.8±3.8

Table 22.9 Percentage germination of ascospores of *Byssochlamys fulva* on PWA, 24 h after heat treatments of 70°C and 80°C for 10 min followed by immersion in 3 N and 6 N acetic acid for 1 h

Acetic acid treatment	*Heat treatment*		
	None	*70°C*	*80°C*
None	0.0	2.5±0.6	10.4±3.7
3 N	15.2±1.3	36.1±3.7	25.4±6.2
6 N	35.0±6.3	67.4±2.6	20.3±1.7

Table 22.10 Percentage germination of ascospores of *Aspergillus fischeri* var. *glaber* on PWA, 24 h after immersion in 4 N and 8 N acetic acid for 1 h followed by heat treatments of 70°C and 80°C for 20 min

Heat treatment	*Acetic acid treatment*		
	None	*4 N*	*8 N*
None	0.0	2.2±1.4	52.9±1.9
70°C	4.7±2.9	6.2±2.0	89.5±2.1
80°C	92.2±1.0	91.4±0.7	88.7±2.6

Table 22.11 Percentage germination of ascospores of *Byssochlamys fulva* on PWA, 24 h after immersion in 3 N and 6 N acetic acid for 1 h followed by heat treatments of 70°C and 80°C for 10 min

Heat treatment	*Acetic acid treatment*		
	None	*3 N*	*6 N*
None	0.0	15.2±1.3	35.0±6.3
70°C	2.5±0.6	4.2±1.2	20.0±3.5
80°C	10.4±3.7	11.3±2.2	16.1±4.0

Dilution-plate techniques have been used for selective isolation of fungi from soil and other natural substrates. In this investigation, soil samples were taken from fields known to contain the fungi under discussion. Samples were heat treated or were suspended in dilutions of acetaldehyde or acetic acid. Chemicals were removed by centrifugation or diluted with culture medium prior to plating. Three media were used:

(1) Martin's Peptone Dextrose Agar, at pH 5.2, containing Rose Bengal at 33 mg l^{-1} and streptomycin at 30 mg l^{-1} (Martin, 1950);
(2) Potato Dextrose Agar, at pH 5.6, containing streptomycin at 50 mg l^{-1};
(3) Plain Water Agar (2% agar) adjusted to pH 4.0 with dilute HCl.

A. fischeri var. *glaber* was isolated from soil which had been:

(1) heated at 80°C for 20 min;
(2) treated with 2.0 M acetaldehyde for 1 h with subsequent removal;
(3) treated with 3.0 N acetic acid for 1 h with subsequent removal.

The fungus grew on all three culture media.

B. nivea was isolated from soil which had been:

(1) heated at 80°C for 20 min;
(2) treated with 0.1 M acetaldehyde for 30 min with subsequent dilution to 0.005 M;
(3) treated with 1.0 N acetic acid for 30 min with subsequent dilution to 0.05 N.

The final pH of the medium in this case was 4.0. The fungus grew on Potato Dextrose Agar and on Plain Water Agar. Streptomycin did not appear to be inhibitory.

Byssochlamys fulva was not isolated from any of the soils tested. However, Put (1964) noted that *B. fulva* was completely inhibited by streptomycin at one part per million, so that it would not have been expected to appear on any media containing this antibiotic.

Heat treatment is probably the most effective means of isolating *A. fischeri* var. *glaber* from soil. Acetic acid at 1.0 N is a suitable selective agent for *B. nivea* and possibly for *B. fulva* also. High initial concentrations are tolerated. Dilution, rather than removal, is sufficient to prevent toxicity. Residual acetic acid depresses the pH of the medium to approximately 4.0, thus further inhibiting bacterial growth.

Discussion

The high concentration of chemicals required for activation of these ascospores is remarkable. However, Sussman, Lowry and Tyrrell (1959) also used high concentrations of organic solvents to activate the *Neurospora* ascospore. This was in contrast to extremely low concentrations of furfural. It is interesting to note that furfural does not appear to activate ascospores of *A. fischeri* var. *glaber* (Palmer and McEvoy, unpublished) or of *B. nivea* (Yates, Seaman and Woodbine, 1968).

It seems unlikely that the activation effects of acetic acid are due simply to a pH shock since no activation was obtained with HCl at low pH levels and in view of the stimulatory role of acetate reported by Yates, Seaman and Woodbine

(1968). Furthermore Splittstoesser, Wilkison and Harrison (1972) reported that the response of ascospores of *B. fulva* to heating at low pH depended on the type of inorganic acid in the activation medium.

It is possible that acetaldehyde activation under the experimental conditions used here was facilitated by the presence of contaminating acetic acid. The high concentrations of acetic acid (8.0 N) required to activate *A. fischeri* var. *glaber* argues against this supposition. Also, activation by acetaldehyde can be obtained even at pH 8.0. However, this aspect is currently being investigated.

Synergic effects have been observed between heat and chemicals previously. Yates (1973) observed stimulation of respiration in ascospores of *B. nivea* using heat and acetate. Sussman (1954) reported heat-sensitization to furfural activation in ascospores of *Neurospora*.

It is hoped that further work will elucidate the basis of these synergic effects and perhaps even the mechanism of activation.

References

EMERSON, M.R. (1948). *J. Bacter.*, **55**, 327

MARTIN, J.P. (1950). *Soil Sci.*, **69**, 215

McEVOY, I.J. and STUART, M. (1970). *Ir. J. agric. Res.*, **9**, 59

OLIVER, M. and SMITH, G. (1933). *J. Botany, Lond.*, **71**, 196

PALMER, V.M. and McEVOY, I.J. (1974). *Proc. Soc. Gen. Microbiol.*, **2**, 6

PUT, H.M.C. (1964). *J. appl. Bacter.*, **27**, 59

PUT, H.M.C. and KRUISWIJK, J.T. (1964). *J. appl. Bacter.*, **27**, 53

SPLITTSTOESSER, D.F., WILKISON, M. and HARRISON, W. (1972). *J. Milk Food Technol.*, **35**, 399

SUSSMAN, A.S. (1953). *J. gen. Microbiol.*, **8**, 211

SUSSMAN, A.S. (1954). *Mycologia*, **46**, 143

SUSSMAN, A.S., LOWRY, R.J. and TYRRELL, E.(1959). *Mycologia*, **51**, 237

YATES, A.R. (1973). *Can. Inst. Food Sci. Technol. J.*, **4**, 244

YATES, A.R., SEAMAN, A. and WOODBINE, M. (1968). *Can. J. Microbiol.*, **14**, 319

23

SOME FUNDAMENTAL REFLECTIONS ON 'ANTIMICROBIAL POTENCY'

A.J. ZWART VOORSPUIJ
Municipal Hospital, Dordrecht, The Netherlands

Antimicrobial potency is not a simple concept. It is one in which three essential elements can be distinguished:

(1) *An effect* (E), for instance a number or percentage of microbes killed or prevented from growing.

(2) *A quantity* (Q). If the processes involved can be related to equal volumes, 'concentration' may be read instead of quantity, for instance the measurement of the minimal effective concentration (MEC) by means of the serial dilution method.

(3) *A time* (t).

This is clear if we realize that the higher the potency, the better will be the effect obtained with a smaller quantity in a shorter time.

All this implies that it is impossible to express the potency in one value representing all the factors at the same time. Comparison of potencies, therefore, means either a comparison of effects with constant Q and t, or of quantities with constant E and t, or of times with constant E and Q.

It is evident that measurement of the potency according to each of these three possibilities requires an experimental arrangement of its own. But the results can be incorporated in one diagram, namely an $E/Q/t$ diagram. This is a spatial figure – in general a curved plane – with E, Q and t as coordinates. Every point in the $E/Q/t$ space stands for a total potency representing, therefore, each of its three factors.

The antimicrobial potency of a mixture can be compared with that of its components in two essentially different ways, discussed below.

First Method of Comparison

We simply compare the antimicrobial potency (measured as effect, concentration or time) of the mixture with that of the component substances A and B; we could also compare it with that of any other substance, whether it be simple or complex. The results of such a comparison can be described in the following way:

> Substance A gives a higher antimicrobial potency – measured for example as antimicrobial effect – than substance B because, in the time

t, one weight unit of substance *A* kills a higher percentage of microbes (which have grown under identical conditions in an untreated culture) than one weight unit of substance *B* in the same time.

For every mixture, that is for every mixing proportion, an $E/Q/t$ diagram can be determined, so that the potency can be compared in three different ways with those of the individual components.

In general the two individual components will have a different potency so, in general, five possibilities may be distinguished:

(1) The potency of the mixture is higher than that of the component with the best potency.
(2) The potency of the mixture is equal to that of the component with the best potency; for this case the term 'indifference' is widely used, but for reasons which will become clear later it is better to avoid this term.
(3) The potency of the mixture is less than that of the component with the best potency, but higher than that of the component with the lowest.
(4) The potency of the mixture is equal to that of the component with the lowest potency.
(5) The potency of the mixture is lower than that of the component with the lowest potency.

As can easily be seen in the case of a three-component mixture, there are in general seven possibilities. In fact, it is possible to introduce separate terms for each of these possibilities. This would not, however, simplify matters, particularly when there is an increasing number of components in the mixture. The most simple denomination for each of these possibilities is to speak of a simultaneous action of the first, second, third, fourth and fifth categories in the sequence given above (*see Figures 23.1* and *23.2*).

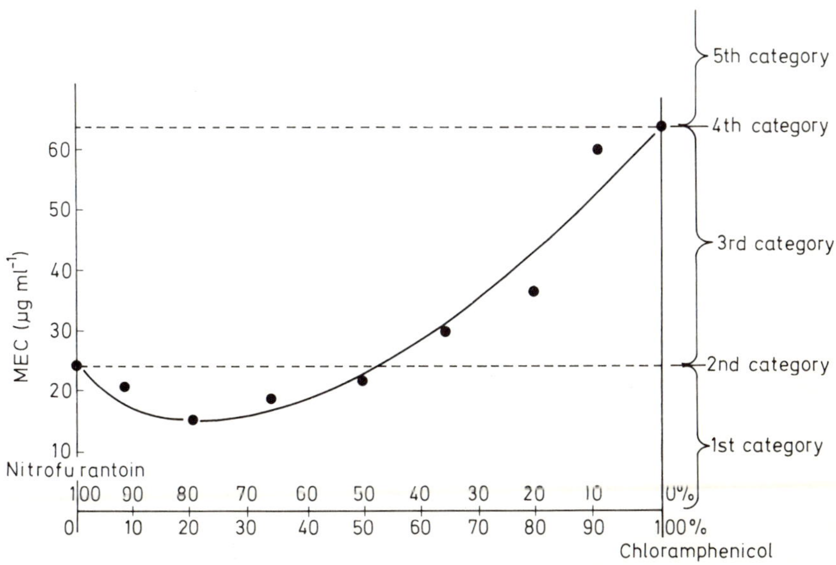

Figure 23.1 Combined action of nitrofurantoin and chloramphenicol on Proteus vulgaris in vitro, *expressed as MEC*

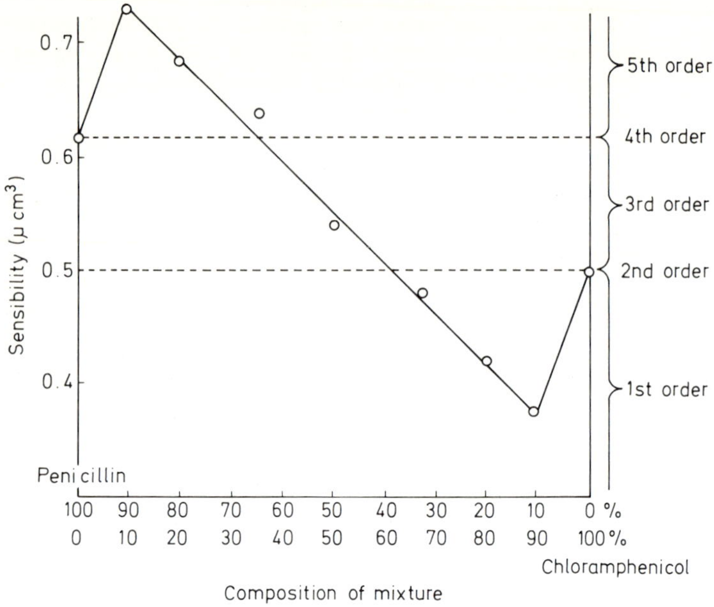

Figure 23.2 Combined action of penicillin and chloramphenicol on Haemophilus influenzae in vitro *expressed as MEC*

For reasons which will be understood later, it is undesirable in this method to use comparative terms like additivity, synergism and antagonism.

Second Method of Comparison

The potency of the mixture is compared with that of its components so that it can be determined whether the potency of the mixture is equal, higher or smaller than would be expected on the basis of its composition. In other words, the potency of the mixture is considered as a function of the potency of the component substances.

In this method of comparison there are three possibilities:

(1) Two substances *A* and *B*, mixed in a given proportion, yield a potency equal to the sum of the partial potencies of the components in the mixture. In such cases we use the term 'additivity', because this is associated with the addition, both as regards the original significance and its use in current language.

(2) Two substances *A* and *B*, mixed in a given proportion, yield a potency greater than the sum of the partial potencies of the components. In this case the mixture shows a surprisingly higher potency, and so we use the term 'synergism', which is generally used in the physical sciences for an unexpectedly high potency.

(3) Two substances *A* and *B*, mixed in a given proportion, yield a potency smaller than the sum of the partial potencies of the components. For analogous reasons, we speak of 'antagonism' in the case of such a surprisingly low potency.

It should be emphasized that these are the *only* three possibilities. In bacteriological literature and textbooks there is the almost universal misunderstanding that there should also be a fourth possibility, called 'indifference'. This should be considered as nonsense.

Indifference, as it is defined, is one of the five possibilities of our first method of comparison. While this is not a forbidden term, it should not be used alongside additivity, synergism and antagonism in the method of comparison of potencies under study. If desired, separate terms could be introduced for various degrees of synergism and antagonism, but this is not very useful.

We must be aware that the definitions given cannot be applied without being made more precise. It has been shown that the potency can be measured with three different criteria, and we must therefore investigate whether a sensible definition of additivity and thus also of antagonism and synergism can be based on each of them. In other words, we need to determine if and to what degree the addition of partial effects, of partial quantities or of partial times leads to useful definitions of such additivity.

Before proceeding to this, however, we wish to introduce the postulate that 'additivity' and 'replaceability' are identical. This seems clear enough, but we shall revert later on to the exact significance of this postulate.

Let us try out the following definition of additivity:

> Two substances A and B, in a previously chosen quantity and in a previously chosen time, show an additive activity if the antimicrobial effect

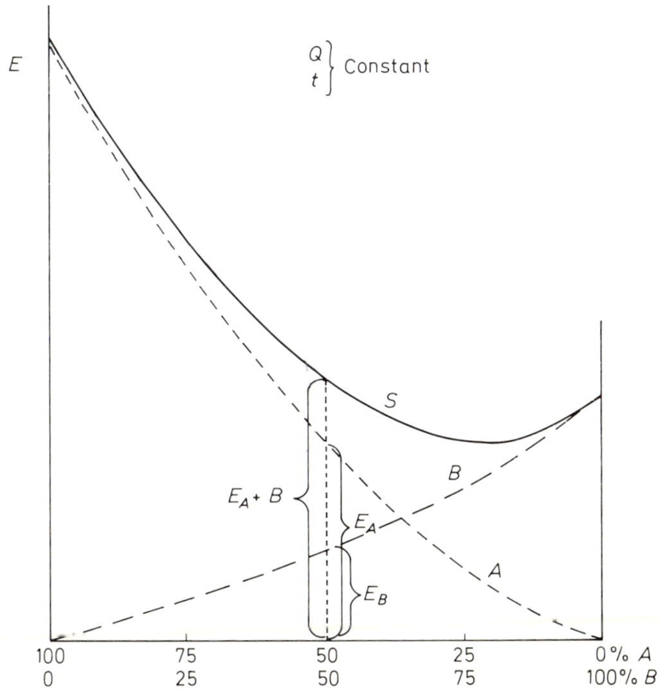

Figure 23.3 The proportion of the mixture is plotted on the horizontal axis and the effect on the vertical axis. The basic curves (A and B) are drawn for the separate substances; these curves indicate the change of the effect with the change of the quantities of these substances

of a mixture is equal to the sum of the partial effects of the separate components of the mixture.

In *Figure 23.3* the additivity curve is indicated by S. In agreement with the definition under investigation the points of this curve are obtained by accepting, for every proportion:

$$E_{A+B} = E_A + E_B$$

It is also possible to obtain a curve by experimental determination of the antimicrobial effect for the various mixing proportions, always with constant Q and t. If, for a given proportion, this curve runs above the additivity line, it would indicate a synergistic activity for that proportion; in the opposite case an antagonistic activity would be indicated.

We have also to investigate whether the definition under study is consistent with the postulate that additivity and replaceability are synonymous. In order to investigate this, we make use of a certain scientific trick. We choose for B a substance of which we know for certainty that it can be replaced by A, namely substance A itself. Let us therefore assume that substance B consists of a mixture of, for example, 50% A and 50% of an inactive substance C. If the basic curve for A is supposed to be known, the basic curve for B can be deduced from it, as the quantity of B is always half the corresponding amount of A. *Figure 23.4* will make clear the procedure.

The basic curve for substance A is drawn. From this has been derived the basic curve for B. From these curves, in accordance with the definition under

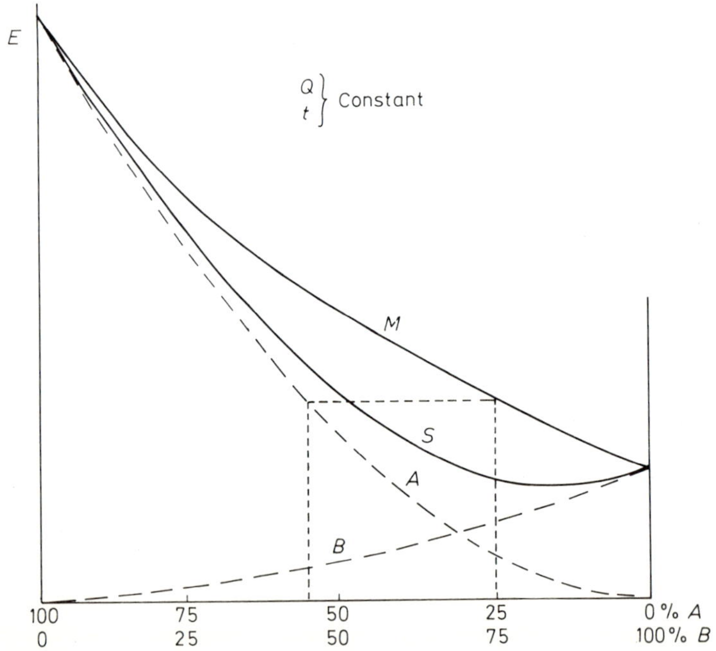

Figure 23.4 Try-out of a definition of additivity based on the adding up of partial effects

investigation, the additivity line S is constructed. The real activity of the mixture, for instance consisting of 25% A + 75% B can, however, also easily be predicted from the basic curve of A, as this mixture consists of 25 + 37.5 = 62.5% of A. A similar calculation can be made for every proportion; in *Figure 23.4* the experimental results that can be predicted with certainty, are represented by curve M.

According to the definition under study, the course of the curves would show that substances A and B act synergistically, while our postulate requires additivity. It means also that substance A acts synergistically with itself. It will be clear that if the basic curve for A has another form, the conclusion that substance A acts antagonistically with itself might likewise have been arrived at. The conclusion led to by the definition of additivity under study, proves to be inconsistent with our postulate and thus this definition must be rejected.

It should be pointed out that, in principle, one is completely free to accept the above definition of additivity, but this leads to the consequence that a substance must be called synergistic or antagonistic with itself. This is not forbidden in a formal reasoning, but then the terms synergism and antagonism refer to the course of the basic curves and no longer have the significance so far attributed to them, this significance being that in synergism the activity of the mixture is surprisingly high and in antagonism surprisingly small. If we wish to maintain this significance, we are forced to pose the postulate that 'additive' and 'replaceable' are synonymous. The postulate can also be formulated as follows: a substance is always additive with itself, never synergistic or antagonistic.

It will be clear that the untenability of the definition of additivity we have investigated is caused by the fact that the basic curves are not rectilinear. Conversely, we may say that a sensible definition of additivity can only be given if the basic curves are straight lines. One of the two variables of the basic curves – the one plotted at the horizontal axis – represents a quantity, i.e. the weight of the component involved. Straight lines will only be found fortuitously, whether the basic curve be considered in a relationship between E and Q, as we have just studied, or between t and Q.

This leads to the conclusion that all definitions of additivity, based on the addition of antimicrobial effects and of times, can be regarded as conflicting with our postulate and that they must be rejected. The only definitions of additivity left are therefore those based on the addition of quantities.

In this case the basic curve is not the result of an experiment, but by definition a straight line. The basic curve for substance A represents the incontestable truth that the quantity of substance A, for example in the mixing proportion 75% A/25% B, is three-quarters of that for 100% A. Thus we arrive at the conclusion that sensible definitions of additivity, and therefore also of synergism and antagonism, can only be based on the addition of quantities (*Figure 23.5*).

An example of an experiment *in vivo* may serve as an illustration of what is meant by all this. The experiment is carried out as follows. The antibacterial substance A is administered to a number of experimental animals, previously infected with a particular microorganism from which they would die in the time chosen if they were left untreated. The substance A is administered at regular intervals over the time and is given, for example, in the form of tablets. The number of tablets necessary to obtain for instance 50% survivors in the time t, is determined. Let us assume that this number is 60 for substance A.

The same experiment is carried out with substance B, and let us suppose that in this case 20 tablets of the same weight are required to obtain the same antibacterial effect in the same time. We may now say that 60 tablets of A may substitute 20 tablets of B, or 1 tablet of A may replace 1/3 tablet of B. If it is found in the experiment that this is indeed so for a given mixing proportion, we speak of additivity. Should the activity of the mixing proportion 50% A + 50% B be additive, 40 tablets of the same weight must therefore be required to obtain 50% survivors in the time t, because 30 tablets of A must be replaceable by 10 tablets of B. In an analogous manner we find 30 tablets for the proportion 25% A + 75% B. This case is represented in *Figure 23.5*.

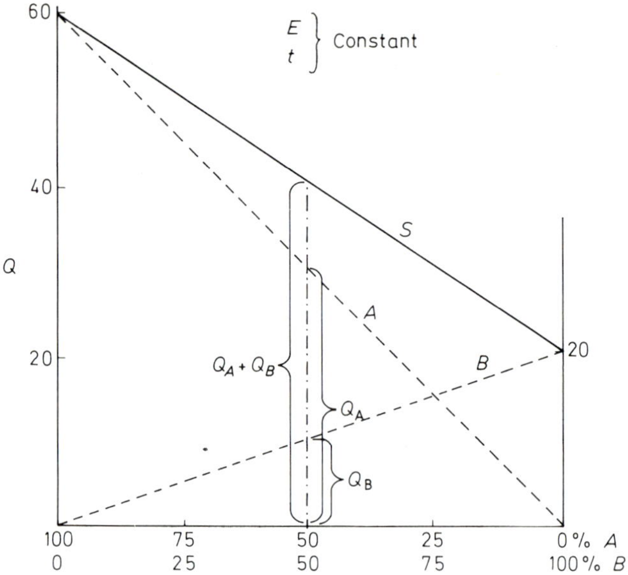

Figure 23.5 Additivity curve with rectilinear basic curves

The additivity curve now also becomes straight as is easily understood geometrically. For all the proportions it represents the sum of the numbers of tablets A and B:

$$Q_{A+B} = Q_A + Q_B$$

It should be emphasized, however, that we are dealing here with the sum of a number of tablets and not with the sum of the effects exerted by these tablets.

The picture given can be considerably simplified by taking the same number of tablets for both substances; this can be effected by making the weight of the B tablets one-third that of the A tablets. In this case the additivity curve takes a horizontal course, which means, that in additivity, it no longer matters which tablets (A or B) are taken, provided that the total number is 60. Thus, the replaceability comes even more to the fore.

If it appears experimentally that, in a given mixing proportion, our end can be attained with less than 60 tablets, we speak of synergism, if more are required, of antagonism.

The above *in vivo* experiment was chosen as an example because it offered the possibility of associating the reasoning with a dosage in tablets, but it is clear that the same argument can also be applied to the bacteriological investigation *in vitro*. In such an investigation one can even take a step further and, in an analogous way, one tablet of substance *A* can be supposed to be as heavy as 60 original tablets of this substance and one tablet of *B* equal to 20 of the first-mentioned tablets. In this way the total doses are obtained. We have introduced the term 'stop' for this quantity. A stop is therefore defined as that quantity of the simple substance which is just able to produce a given antibacterial effect in a given time.

The definition of additivity now becomes as follows:

> Two substances *A* and *B*, mixed in a given proportion, act additively if a previously chosen antimicrobial effect in a previously chosen time is obtained with a quantity of the mixture equal to 1, this being the sum of the partial quantities of the components in the mixture expressed in stops. If this sum is less than 1, we speak of synergism, if it is more, of antagonism.

A striking disadvantage of this method of representation is that for synergism only the range between 0 and 1 is available, while for antagonism the whole region between 1 and plus to infinity can be used. A symmetrical treatment of antagonism and synergism can, however, easily be restored by measuring the quantity on the vertical axis, not in stops but in the logarithms of the stops. The simultaneous activity of two substances is then expressed in an activity index, which is 0 for additivity, positive in the case of antagonism and negative in the event of synergism (*Figure 23.6*).

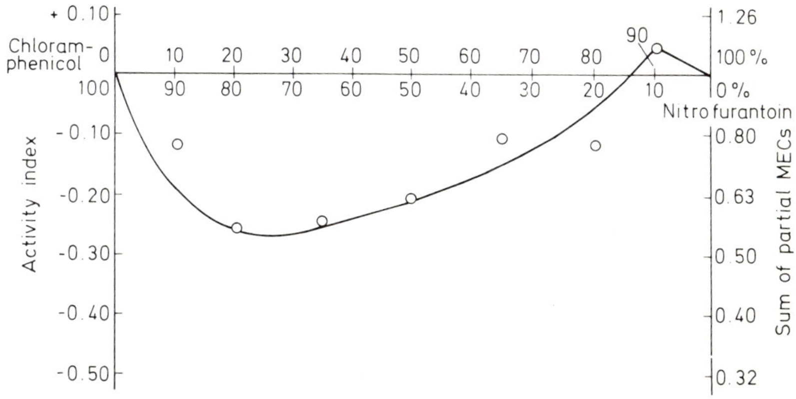

Figure 23.6 Combined action of nitrofurantoin and chloramphenicol on Proteus vulgaris in vitro, *showing mainly synergism*

An activity index of +2 means a quantity of 100 stops, i.e. an antagonism in which the quantity is 100 times as large as would be required if the mixture of the two substances in this proportion had acted additively.

The experimental arrangement can, for example, be set up as follows: by means of the serial dilution method the quantity of a substance is measured which is necessary to obtain a previously chosen antimicrobial effect – for example complete inhibition of growth – in a given time. The experiment must be carried out with the individual substances and with the mixing proportion under study, every mixture with a series of dilutions in which the proportion is constant and the quantity variable. *Table 23.1* shows how the calculation is done.

Table 23.1 Combined activity of isonicotinic acid hydrazide and *p*-amino salycylic acid on tubercule bacilli (strain $H_{37}R_V$)

Composition of mixture (%)		*Sensitivity* (μg ml⁻¹)			*Sensitivity (stops)*			*Activity index*
INH	*PAS*	*Total*	*INH*	*PAS*	*INH*	*PAS*	*Total*	
100	0	0.5	0.5	0	1	0	1	0
50	50	0.5	0.25	0.25	0.50	0.13	0.63	– 0.20
0	100	2	0	2	0	1	1	0

We have already dealt extensively with the addition of quantities in the comparison of potencies, measured according to the quantity. The addition of quantities can, however, also be used in the comparison of the potencies measured according to the antimicrobial effect and according to the time. This is done in the following way.

An antimicrobial effect and a time are chosen. The quantity necessary to realize this effect in the chosen time is looked up from $E/Q/t$ diagrams of the individual substances. These quantities are said to be one stop for each of the components. Then the quantity of the chosen mixing proportion, corresponding to one stop, is determined and from the $E/Q/t$ diagram of the mixture is read off the time which is necessary to obtain with one stop mixture the same antimicrobial effect. If this time is equal to the chosen time, we say that the potency of the mixture, measured according to the time, is additive.

In an analogous way one can use the addition of quantities in defining additivity, synergism and antagonism according to the antimicrobial effect.

Maximal Potencies

So far we have been dealing with cases where it was deemed possible to determine the quantity equivalent to one stop for the three competing agents. This is, however, not always possible, particularly when considering maximal potencies. Let us suppose that component A yields the maximal potency of killing (in time t) 90% of the microbes grown in an untreated blank culture, and that the corresponding maximum potency of B is 60%. If the maximal potency of A is chosen for the standard potency, measured according to the antimicrobial effect, the quantity equivalent to one stop cannot be determined for B.

For each of the five possibilities in our first method of comparison it can be shown that by accepting two conventions the current use of the terms additivity, synergism and antagonism is maintained. These two conventions are:

(1) For maximal potencies the greatest potency, achieved by the three competing agents – the two individual components and the mixture – is chosen as standard potency.

(2) For an agent, be it a simple component or the mixture, which never reaches the standard potency, the quantity equivalent to one stop is considered infinite.

Three Component Mixtures

In considering three component mixtures we first need to look for a method of presentation of such a system. In phase considerations in physical chemistry such a method is used.

Figure 23.7 shows an equilateral triangle, each side of which is divided into 100 equal parts. As can be shown geometrically, every point within the triangle

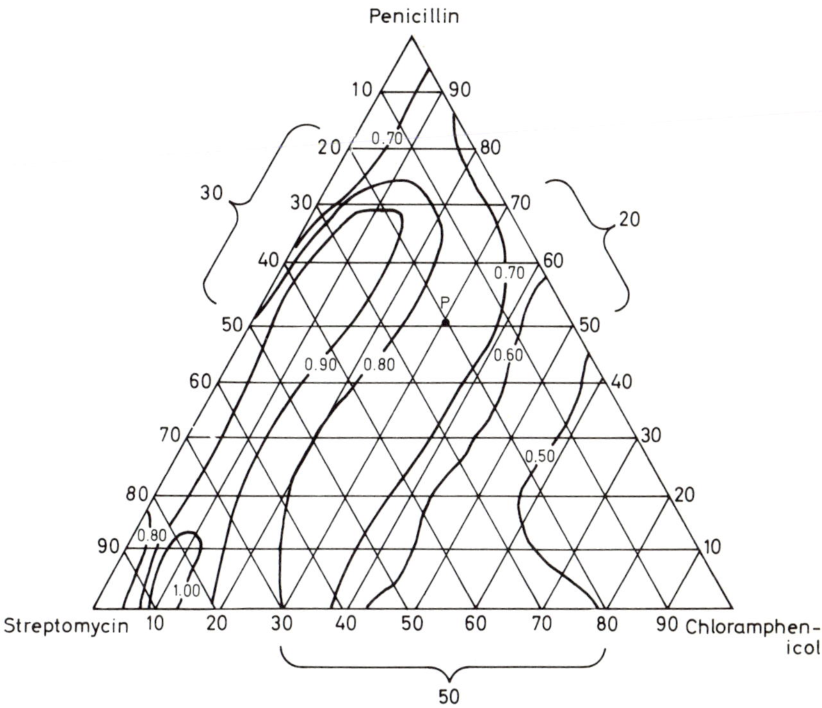

Figure 23.7 Antibacterial potency of mixtures composed of penicillin, streptomycin and chloramphenicol on Haemophilus influenzae *expressed as MEC*

represents the per cent composition of a mixture. Point *P* for example represents a mixture of 50% penicillin, 30% chloramphenicol and 20% streptomycin. The curves are drawn through points with equal MEC or equal activity indices.

Figure 23.8 is of the same kind. The MECs here are chosen in such a way that the regions or lines obtained represent the first, second, etc. categories.

The highest MECs are found for mixtures consisting of much streptomycin, little penicillin and little chloramphenicol (*Figure 23.7*).

In *Figure 23.9* the triangle is used to represent activity indices. In this three component mixture antagonism predominates. An example of a three component system in which synergism predominates is found in *Figure 23.10*.

It seems that the suggested terminological standards for the combined action of two or more antimicrobial agents offer very important advantages:

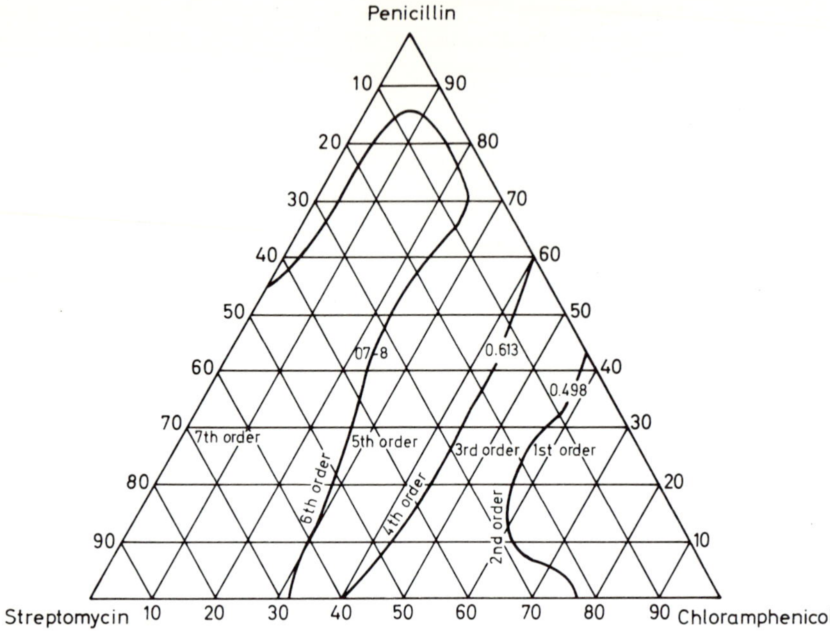

Figure 23.8 Mixtures of penicillin, streptomycin and chloramphenicol acting on Haemophilus influenzae *showing the regions of first, second etc. category*

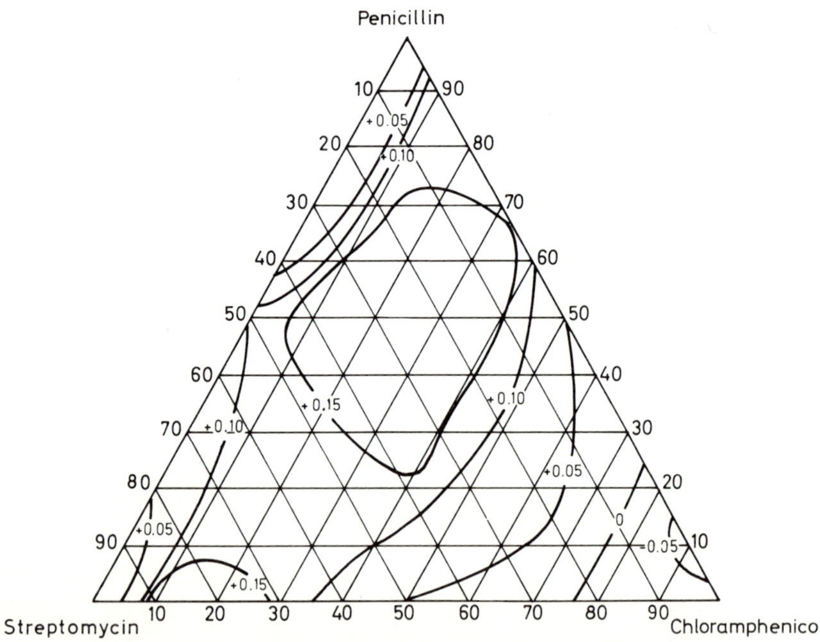

Figure 23.9 Mixtures of penicillin, streptomycin and chloramphenicol acting on Haemophilus influenzae *expressed as activity index*

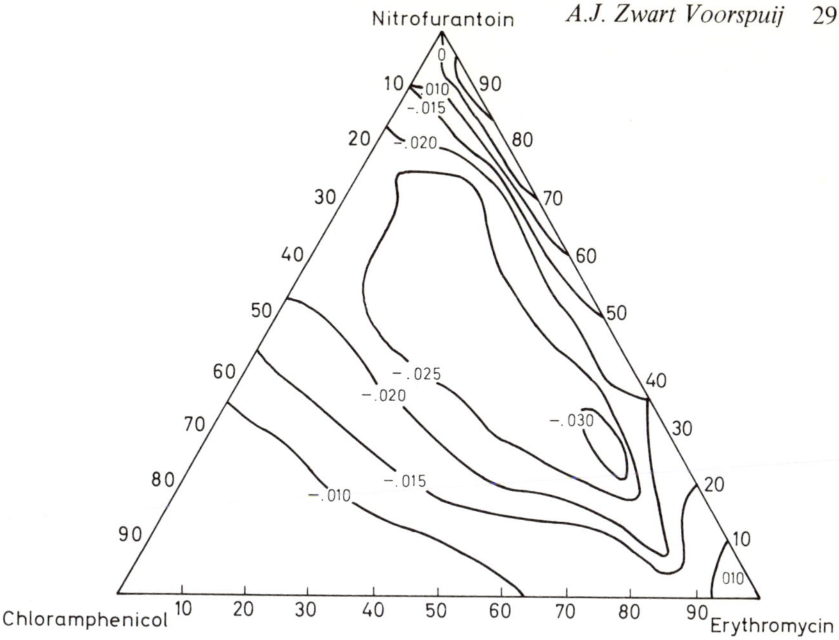

Figure 23.10 Mixtures of nitrofurantoin, chloramphenicol and erythromycin acting on Proteus vulgaris in vitro *expressed as activity index*

(1) All fundamental variables involved in the problem are related to each other in a logical way.
(2) With the help of the formulated concepts, the results of all methodologically correct experiments can be described in a simple and uniform manner.
(3) The defined results are simple and consistent with the terms currently in use as far as possible.
(4) The formulations chosen are also internally consistent.
(5) The degree of antagonism and synergism can be expressed numerically.
(6) The defined concepts remain constant regardless of the number of components of the mixture under study.
(7) Experimental results can be represented graphically in a simple and surveyable manner.
(8) Consistent use of the formulated results leads to an improved understanding of the problems of the subject.

These problems proved to be numerous but, nevertheless, soluble. We walk, however, in a field where one is easily lost.

References

ZWART VOORSPUIJ, A.J. and NASS, C.A.G. (1953). *Antonie van Leeuwenhoek,* **19**, 225

ZWART VOORSPUIJ, A.J., and NASS, C.A.G. (1957). *Arch. Intern. Pharmacodyn. et Ther.,* **109**, 211

ZWART VOORSPUIJ, A.J. and BOKMA, L.H. (1958). *Antibiot. Chemoth.,* **8**, 171

ZWART VOORSPUIJ, A.J. and BOKMA, L.H. (1958). *Ann. Inst. Pasteur,* **95**, 404

ZWART VOORSPUIJ, A.J. and BOKMA, L.H. (1958). *Antibiot. Chemoth.,* **9**, 27

24

SYNERGISM EXHIBITED: TOO SIMPLE A TECHNIQUE?

JANE C. FISHER
ANGELA C. LEAMAN
R.J.L. PAULTON
A. SEAMAN
M. WOODBINE

Microbiological Unit, Department of Applied Biochemistry and Nutrition, University of Nottingham, Sutton Bonington

A variety of approaches may be made in the search for the level of inhibition of an agent on a microorganism. This can operate through solid or liquid media; utilize optical density (Jouin Photometer); visible growth (Nephelometer); gas production (e.g. CO_2 evolution) or metabolite synthesis (lactic acid production).

However, if combined effects are the subject of interest, then the problems of the evaluation of two agents is not so simple and those of multiple agents difficult. For example, in solid media, having ascertained the minimum inhibitory concentration (MIC) the use of a gradient agar plate is possible (*see Figure 24.1 a, b*) with a more sophisticated approach to multiple interaction (*see Figure 24.1 c*).

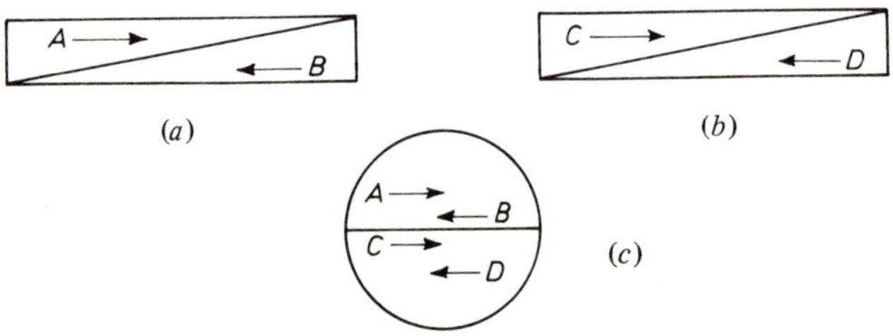

Figure 24.1 Use of gradient agar plates

The problems of diffusion may have to be faced – assuming the agents are diffusible from depots in the agar. It may be desirable to allow time for this and at a different temperature (refrigerator 4°C or room temperature).

If this sort of approach is not satisfactory then liquid media may have to be used. Steinberg (1939) introduced a concept of 'minimum salts:maximum growth' into the approaches of microbial (fungal) nutrition in which the overall nutritional need was found to be less than the sum of the individually assessed amounts – a 'sparing effect'. Here the converse is sought in maximum inhibition for minimum antibiotic(s). The sort of approach with liquid media may be of the form of a 10 × 10 tube layout (*see Figure 24.2*) in which a double dilution

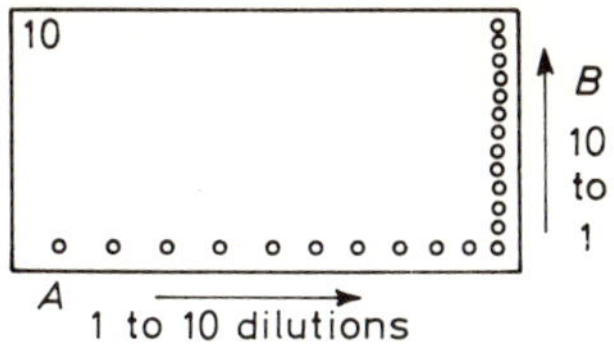

Figure 24.2 Double dilution approach for liquid media

approach may be used – a very time-consuming exercise with a relative high use of media, tubes and incubator space.

The approach used here is based on *Escherichia coli* type I, of different sero-types, with combined inhibition and may be assessed by antibiotic discs (both 'multodisks' and single) and a well technique. Some 30 strains of *E. coli*, largely associated with calf scours were obtained (courtesy of W.J. Sojka and R. Lovell). They included sero-types of 08, 09, 015, 026, 078, 086, 0128 and 0137 and two were β-haemolytic. They were all positive in relation to Eosin-Methylene Blue or MacConkey's agars; indole, methyl red and Eijkman reactions; negative for Voges-Proskauer and growth in citrate media (*see Table 24.1* based on the results of Leaman, Fisher and Paulton).

Table 24.1 Reactions of the *E. coli* type I strains

Strain	*Sero-type*	*Gram*	*Indole*	*MR*	*VP*	*E*	*Citrate*
* 1	08	–	+	+	–	+	–
5	09	–	+	+	–	+	–
7	015	–	+	+	–	+	–
10	026	–	+	+	–	+	–
*13	026	–	+	+	–	+	–
14	035	–	+	+	–	+	–
*15	055	–	+	+	–	+	–
16	078	–	+	+	–	+	–
19	086	–	+	+	–	+	–
21	0101	–	+	+	–	+	–
22	0103	–	+	+	–	+	–
23	0114	–	+	+	–	+	–
24	0115	–	+	+	–	+	–
25	0117	–	+	+	–	+	–
26	0119	–	+	+	–	+	–
28	0128	–	+	+	–	+	–
29	0137	–	+	+	–	+	–

The initial experiments (Leaman, 1963) used 'multodisks' which were placed on inoculated (1 ml of a 6 h broth culture to 9 ml agar) agar refrigerated for 1 h and allowed to diffuse for a further hour in the refrigerator. This was followed by incubation at 37°C. Any inhibition zone was enhanced by 0.01% of 2, 3, 5-triphenyltetrazolium chloride in the agar (Greaves, 1962). For the combinations, one 'disc' was superimposed on another. The results were difficult to assess as reciprocal combinations did not concur nor was any synergic manifestation apparent, i.e. greater than the three most effective – chloramphenicol, streptomycin, tetracycline.

Table 24.2 The antibiotics; concentrations used and zones (mm) of inhibition of individual discs

Agent	*Code*	*Concentration* (mcg or units*)	*24 h incubation* *Strain 1*	*Strain 13*	*Strain 15*
Ampicillin	PN	2	0	0	9
	PN+	25	15	21	26
Chloramphenicol	C	10	30	11	11
	C+	50	35	16	24
Cloxacillin	OB	5	0	0	0
Colistin	CS	50	17	23	18
	CS+	200	19	23	21
Compd. sulphas	S3+	300	30	32	31
Erythromycin	E	10	12	8	12
	E+	50	17	12	13
Fusidic acid	FD	10	6	0	11
Kanamycin	K+	30	19	18	21
Methicillin	CB	10	0	0	10
Neomycin	N+	30	18	12	20
Nitrofurantoin	F++	200	24	21	23
Novobiocin	NV	5	0	8	10
Penicillin G	P	1.5*	0	0	0
Phenethicillin	BX+	5*	0	0	0
Streptomycin	S	10	15	0	17
	S+	25	18	14	21
Tetracycline	TE	10	20	23	18
	TE+	50	26	27	25

A somewhat more sophisticated approach (Fisher, 1964) was then adopted in which 17 strains were used, pour plates in which 1 ml of culture (6 h at 37°C) was added to 9 ml Oxoid diagnostic sensitivity test agar (DST CM261) which were refrigerated and the antibiotic allowed to diffuse for 1 h at *c.* 4°C before incubation at 37°C (*see Table 24.2* which gives results after 24 h; the 48 and 72 h results were marginally greater).

Technique for Combinations

Arising out of the difficulties experienced with contiguous multodiscs, separation with individual discs was introduced. First, the agar (*c.* 6 ml) was poured into petri dishes which were refrigerated. The individual antibiotic discs – all of the same antibiotic and concentration – were then placed, labelled side *down*, on the agar (*Figure 24.3*). This allowed for smooth diffusion into the overlapping agar and for visibility through the base. A maximum of four combinations avoided overlap.

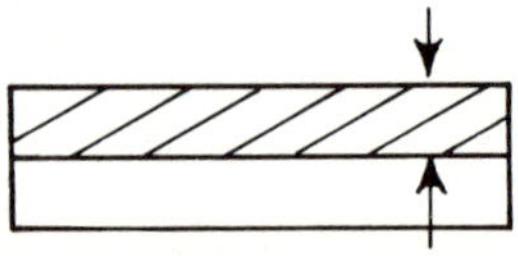

Figure 24.3

Next, 9 ml amounts of the DST agar were melted and maintained at 48°C while 1 ml of the *E. coli* was added and *well* mixed (for homogeneity). This was then placed on the plates which were then refrigerated. When the inoculated and diffused agar was set, a second disc was placed, labelled side *up*, upon the previous one (the 2 discs now being separated by the agar plus bacteria). The plates were then held for 1 h at 4°C and incubated for 18 h at 37°C. Each antibiotic was tested in combination with each of the range of 'antibiotics' against the three selected strains of *E. coli*.

It was found that there was a difference between the same combination when the position of the discs was reversed. The combined effect of two inhibitors was, therefore, obtained by taking the average of the two results. When *Penicillin G* (P), for example, was combined with *Ampicillin* (PN), *one* result was obtained when P was combined with other agents and was the *lower* disc of the pair (*Table 24.3*, column (*a*)) and the second result when PN was combined with other agents and in turn was the disc below P (*Table 24.3*, column (*b*)). The

Table 24.3 The effect of combining penicillin G with other inhibitory agents

	Strain 1				*Strain 13*				*Strain 15*			
Penicillin	*a*	*b*	*c*	*d*	*a*	*b*	*c*	*d*	*a*	*b*	*c*	*d*
PN	0	0	0	0	11	0	5.5	0	14	0	7.0	5.5
PN+	13	15	14.0	8.0	25	24	24.5	14.5	28	24	26.0	15.0
C	22	24	23.0	14.5	22	20	21.0	11.0	25	23	24.0	13.0
C+	29	33	31.0	17.0	29	28	28.5	15.0	30	32	31.0	17.5
OB	0	9	4.5	0	0	0	0	0	0	0	0	0
CS	14	19	16.5	9.0	13	19	16.0	9.5	13	16	14.5	9.0
CS+	19	24	21.5	12.5	17	23	20.0	11.5	17	21	19.0	12.0
S3+	32	35	33.5	17.0	30	35	32.5	20.0	30	35	32.5	17.5
E	12	35	23.5	17.0	9	10	9.5	6.0	12	18	15.0	7.0
E+	17	23	20.0	10.0	13	18	15.5	10.0	20	23	21.5	11.0
FD	0	0	0	0	0	0	0	0	0	0	0	0
K+	24	25	24.5	13.0	21	28	24.5	12.5	20	24	22.0	13.0
CB	0	0	0	0	0	0	0	0	0	0	0	0
N+	18	22	20.0	12.5	16	23	19.5	11.5	18	22	20.0	12.0
F++	23	29	26.0	14.5	23	30	26.5	15.5	22	27	24.5	14.5
NV	0	0	0	0	0	0	0	0	8	9	8.5	5.5
BX+	0	0	0	10.0	0	0	0	0	0	0	0	10.0
S	17	25	21.0	11.0	21	21	21.0	11.0	19	24	21.5	12.5
S+	19	24	21.5	15.0	20	23	21.5	14.0	22	25	23.5	13.0
TE	20	24	22.0	12.5	22	27	24.5	14.0	22	28	25.0	14.0
TE+	25	31	28.0	15.5	27	31	29.0	17.5	26	33	29.5	16.0

average is in column (*c*). Similarly, to find the effect of each agent alone, two discs of the same agent were superimposed and the results halved (*Table 24.4*).

Column (*d*) (*Table 24.3*) is obtained by adding the effect of the appropriate antibiotic to the effect of the other agent, e.g. for P, by adding the effect of ½(P + PN) (from *Table 24.4*) to the results, in the same column, for all the others. This gives the additive result, but the actual one is in column (*c*) (*Table 24.3*). If $c = d$, the combination is additive, if c is greater, it is synergic, if c is smaller, antagonism has occurred (and also if less than the more effective agent alone, i.e. for P and PN, also less than the larger of ½(P + PN) or ½(PN + RN). Differences of 2.0 or less have been assumed to arise merely from chance or variations in experimental technique.

Table 24.4 The effect of each antibiotic or agent alone

	Strain 1		*Strain 13*		*Strain 15*	
Agent	*i* (mm)*	*i*/2	*i*	*i*/2	*i*	*i*/2
PN	0	0	0	0	11	5.5
PN+	16	8	29	14.5	30	15
C	29	14.5	22	11	26	13
C+	34	17	30	15	35	17.5
OB	0	0	0	0	0	0
CS	18	9	19	9.5	18	9
CS+	25	12.5	23	11.5	24	12.0
S3+	34	17	40	20	35	17.5
E	34	17	12	6	14	7
E+	20	10	20	10	22	11
FD	0	0	0	0	0	0
K+	26	13	25	12.5	26	13
CB	0	0	0	0	0	0
N+	25	12.5	23	11.5	24	12
F++	29	14.5	31	15.5	29	14.5
NV	0	0	0	0	11	5.5
P	0	0	0	0	0	0
BX+	20	10	0	0	20	10
S	22	11	22	11	25	12.5
S+	30	15	28	14	26	13
TE	25	12.5	28	14	28	14
TE+	31	15.5	35	17.5	32	16

*The effect of two identical discs superimposed.

Each of the tables (21 or so Fisher, 1964) was followed by a histogram, showing the difference between columns *c* and *d* – as this shows more clearly the amount of synergism (or antagonism) for each strain and combination. With $c > d$ (synergism), the difference is to the right, antagonistic to the left (each mm = 1 mm difference) (*see Figure 24.4*).

Using this technique in a similar way to the illustration for penicillin G a sequence of results could be built up of potential (*in vitro*) combinations (*Table 24.5*).

Bearing in mind that these results were *in vitro* only and only apply to particular strains of *E. coli* I, to indicated concentrations of the inhibitors and the particular experimental conditions (all of which were as near the same as was possible), any differences should be due to either the inhibitor or the strain. The three strains differed only slightly, so any conclusion should be applicable to all coliforms.

What of anaerobiosis? The layer of inoculated agar was very thin, the differences between top and bottom discs was offset by the two positions per combination. So it is suggested that it could be a quick, easy, inexpensive method of assessing a potential combination; useful to indicate combinations worth further work, or those to avoid (antagonism), possibly by a tube dilution technique, in which diffusion rate problems would not necessarily apply.

Multiple combinations were then tried (Paulton, 1965). The idea of using a triple layer plate was considered but abandoned with enhanced anaerobiosis and the non-interaction of the top and third inhibition areas. The idea of using two

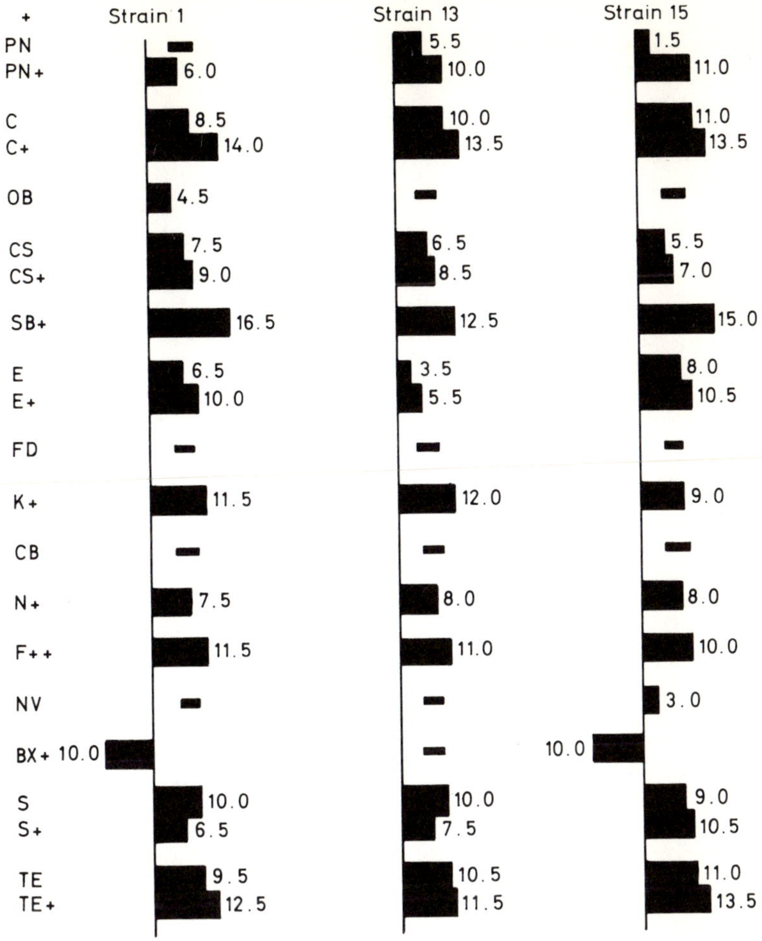

Figure 24.4 Penicillin G, 1.5 units

agents per disc with the third on a single disc was also possible (it could now be tried, e.g. with the trimethoprim-sulphonamide (Oxoid) discs). An approach, therefore, was adopted based on (*a*) the antagonism concept of Manten and Meyerman-Wisse (1962); (*b*) the criticism of 'the comparison of single drugs with combinations on the basis of their weights' (Jawetz and Gunnison, 1953) and the 'temptation . . . to claim synergism for a combination containing a fraction of the weight of one such minimal effective dose of each of two drugs and possessing greater activity than would be expected on the basis of algebraic summation, and (*c*) the theoretical desiderata of Zwart Voorspuij and Nass (1957) (*see also* Zwart Voorspuij, Ch. 23 this volume) who compared the efficacy of combinations with their constituents as *functions* of their respective weights. They defined:

> *addivity* as two substances, mixed in a given proportion, yield a performance equal to the sum of the partial performances of the components present in the mixture,

Table 24.5 The potential combinations

	PN	*PN+*	*C*	*C+*	*OB*	*CS*	*CS+*	*S3+*	*E*	*E+*	*FD*	*K+*	*CB*	*N+*	*F++*	*NV*	*P*	*BX+*	*S*	*S+*	*TE*	*TE+*
Ampicillin					+						+		+			+	+					
Chloramphenicol	+				+						+		+			+	+					
Cloxacillin		+	+	+		+	+	+	+	+		+		+	+				+	+	+	+
Compd. sulphas					+				+	+	+		+			+	+	+				
Erythromycin					+			+			+		+				+					
Fusidic acid		+	+	+		+	+	+	+	+		+		+	+	+			+	+	+	+
Kanamycin	+				+						+		+			+	+					
Methicillin		+	+	+		+	+	+	+	+		+		+	+				+	+	+	+
Neomycin	+				+						+		+				+					
Nitrofurantoin	+				+						+		+				+					
Novobiocin		+	+	+		+	+	+				+							+	+	+	+
Penicillin		+	+	+		+	+	+				+		+	+				+	+	+	+
Phenethicillin				+				+														+
Streptomycin	+				+						+		+			+	+					
Tetracycline	+				+				+		+		+				+					

synergism as two substances giving a greater performance, and
antagonism as two substances giving a lesser performance.

So, for each agent, solutions were made so that the same quantity of any pipetted (0.01 to 0.20 Emil micro-pipettes) into a seeded agar 'punch' plate, produced a specified zone of inhibition. If one, *A*, needed *a* mg, and similarly *B* needed *b* mg then in combination ½(*a* + *b*) was used. If this produced the same zone size, it was additive; if larger, it was synergic; if smaller, it was antagonistic. Volumes of 0.02 ml (0.01 ml of each of two agents were used) but the plates were not refrigerated before incubation (but higher concentrations offset this), and a constant inoculum was used (5 ml 6 h, then 5 ml 3 h and 1 ml of a 1:100 dilution) in DST agar. Combinations were also compared with their components (6 zones: 2 for combination, 2 for each component).

Using strain *B* in the first place (and then a further 7 to confirm), a 16 h incubation at 37°C the zone radius (½ zone diameter – 'ditch' diameter) was found to give good calibration curves against the log concentration (μg 0.02 ml^{-1}) for ampicillin, penicillin G, methicillin, phenethicillin, cloxacillin, kanamycin, neomycin, nitrofurantoin, polymyxin B, tetracycline, and reasonably adequate with streptomycin, erythromycin, novobiocin, chloramphenicol.

Using this technique, synergism (>5.5 mm) was found for ampicillin with penicillin G, methicillin; penicillin G with methicillin, phenethicillin, streptomycin, erythromycin and tetracycline; methicillin with streptomycin; phenethicillin with cloxacillin; cloxacillin with novobiocin; kanamycin with tetracycline; neomycin with novobiocin, polymyxin B and tetracycline; streptomycin with nitrofurantoin; erythromycin with chloramphenicol and tetracycline; novobiocin with chloramphenicol and polymyxin B. Such results would not be out of line with those of other workers (*see* Sutherland and Batchelor, 1964).

Using Three Agents

The method here was basically similar to that for two agents and the efficacy of such combinations was compared with the third agent and with the combination of all three. Now, if agents *A* and *B* are synergic, they will not produce a zone of 5 mm. So, the combination could be (*a*) diluted to produce such a concentration, or (*b*) a zone comparison could be compared of *A* + *B* with *A* + *B* + *C* and *C* alone. Method (*a*) was used as it was quicker and the results are based on 50% of the mixture; the synergic combinations were:

(1) ampicillin + penicillin with chloromycetin, erythromycin, streptomycin
ampicillin + neomycin with polymyxin B
ampicillin + streptomycin with novobiocin, erythromycin

(2) penicillin G + kanamycin with tetracycline
penicillin G + neomycin with tetracycline, polymyxin B, nitrofurantoin, novobiocin, erythromycin, streptomycin
penicillin G + erythromycin with tetracycline, polymyxin B, chloromycetin, nitrofurantoin
penicillin G + novobiocin with tetracycline
penicillin G + chloromycetin with tetracycline
penicillin G + polymyxin B with tetracycline

(3) kanamycin + neomycin with nitrofurantoin, erythromycin, streptomycin
kanamycin + streptomycin with polymyxin B
kanamycin + erythromycin with tetracycline
kanamycin + novobiocin with polymyxin B, chloromycetin
(4) neomycin + streptomycin with chloromycetin, novobiocin
neomycin + novobiocin with chloromycetin
neomycin + chloromycetin with tetracycline, polymyxin B
neomycin + polymyxin B with tetracycline
(5) erythromycin + nitrofurantoin with chloromycetin
(6) novobiocin + nitrofurantoin with polymyxin B
(7) polymyxin B + chloromycetin with tetracycline

Antagonistic combinations were also indicated, e.g.
(1) ampicillin, penicillin, tetracycline
ampicillin, neomycin, tetracycline
erythromycin, chloramphenicol, ampicillin
(2) ampicillin, penicillin, nitrofurantoin
ampicillin, novobiocin, nitrofurantoin
penicillin, novobiocin, nitrofurantoin
(3) nitrofurantoin, tetracycline, chloramphenicol
nitrofurantoin, novobiocin, chloramphenicol

Summary

An approach exists for a quick appraisal of a potential dual combination; this in turn, can be assessed in comparison with a third agent. But it must be emphasized that this is for one particular combination of the constituents (25 : 25 : 50%). It remains to be seen, now, whether others also find the approach justifiable.

References

FISHER, JANE C. (1964). Hons. Dissert., Nottingham
GREAVES, M.G. (1962). Hons. Dissert., Nottingham
JAWETZ, E. and GUNNISON, J.B. (1953). *Pharmacol. Rev.*, **5**, 175
LEAMAN, ANGELA C. (1963). Hons. Dissert., Nottingham
MANTEN, A. and MEYERMAN-WISSE, J. (1962). *Antonie van Leeuwenhoek*, **28**, 321
PAULTON, R.J.L. (1965). Hons. Dissert., Nottingham
STEINBERG, R.A. (1939). *Bot. Rev.*, **5**, 327
STEINBERG, R.A. (1950). *Bot. Rev.*, **16**, 208
SUTHERLAND, R. and BATCHELOR, F.R. (1964). *Nature, Lond.*, **201**, 868
ZWART-VOORSPUIJ, A.J. and NASS, C.A.G. (1957). *Arch. int. Pharmocodyn.*, **109**, 211

VII

PUBLIC HEALTH ASPECTS

25

STUDIES ON THE BIOAVAILABILITY, PHARMACOKINETICS AND RESIDUES OF SEMI-SYNTHETIC PENICILLINS IN RELATION TO THEIR VETERINARY APPLICATION

J.F. BUSWELL
G.H. PALMER
Beecham Pharmaceuticals, Tadworth

Introduction

A potential antibacterial chemotherapeutic agent must have certain basic properties. Firstly, it must exert an antibacterial action whether lethal or inhibitory at low concentrations against bacterial pathogens, and because it is frequently necessary to treat infections before or in the absence of an accurate laboratory diagnosis, or where the aetiology of the disease is complex, a broad spectrum of activity is desirable. Secondly, the antibacterial should be more or less without harmful effects on the tissues, organs and cells of the mammalian host with which, during chemotherapy, it will come into intimate contact.

Subsequent *in vivo* evaluation either in experimental infections in laboratory animals or in natural infections due to sensitive bacteria, will indicate its potential therapeutic usefulness. It follows, however, that any successful chemotherapeutic agent must reach the site of infection both at effective concentrations and for sufficient time to exert its antibacterial effect. The distribution of an antibacterial may therefore be as important as its spectrum of activity and lack of toxicity in the eventual outcome of a therapeutic regimen.

The following is an account of some of the studies which have been carried out in the determination of antibiotic distribution, in particular the semi-synthetic penicillins such as ampicillin, amoxycillin and cloxacillin with reference to their veterinary potential.

Methods of Analysis

Microbiological agar diffusion techniques are ideally suited for the analysis of antibiotics in body fluids and tissues over a wide range of concentrations. Relatively small quantities of biological material are required and extraction of antibiotic can usually be achieved by homogenization of tissue samples in an appropriate extractant such as phosphate buffer. For body fluids such as serum and milk, antibiotic standards are diluted in the appropriate control body fluid. Where it is known that tissue extracts interfere in the validity of an assay, standards are prepared in the appropriate tissue extract so that like is compared with like.

Occasionally, the presence of natural inhibitors such as lysozyme, antibody or lactoferrin may cause non-specific inhibition of some assay organisms. Fortunately, the majority of such inhibitors are relatively heat-labile compared to the penicillins and can be selectively inactivated. Treatment of samples with a specific enzyme, penicillinase, provides a simple confirmatory test for the presence of penicillins.

Table 25.1 shows the more usual assay organisms and their corresponding range of sensitivities for some semi-synthetic penicillins. It is therefore possible

Table 25.1 Assay organisms and their range of sensitivities for some semi-synthetic penicillins

	*Assay range (*mcg per ml *or* g *of tissue)*		
Antibiotic	*Bacillus subtilis*	*Sarcina lutea*	*Bacillus stearothermophilus (*var. *calidolactis)*
Ampicillin	10–0.5	0.8–0.2	0.1–0.01
Amoxycillin	10–0.5	0.8–0.2	0.1–0.01
Penicillin G	4–0.2	2.0–0.2	0.1–0.01
Cloxacillin	40–2.5	8.0–0.5	0.4–0.05 (Milk 0.01)

to carry out analyses of most semi-synthetic penicillins down to 0.01 mcg ml^{-1} or g of tissue or body fluid with a view to assessing their veterinary potential. Investigations of this type may supplement clinical experience but also have an important function in the selection of pharmaceutical preparations of antibiotics. In addition, knowledge of antibiotic distribution may act as a guide to the possible therapeutic applications of new antibiotics prior to field use.

A Distribution Studies

Table 25.2 shows a summary of the types of studies which may be involved in the overall assessment of antibiotics and their forms for veterinary use.

Table 25.2 Classification of distribution studies

A *Bioavailability*	(Basic)
	Blood levels
	Tissue and gut distribution
	Milk out
B *Supplementary*	(Specific points)
	Pharmacokinetics
	Tissue cages
	Thiry-Vella loops
C *Tissue residues*	(To establish withholding periods)

For a broad spectrum antibiotic with good oral and parenteral absorption and no toxicity, the range of veterinary applications is wide. Because the veterinary surgeon is concerned with a broad spectrum of bacterial infections in a number of animal species in both large and small animal practice, the possible range of distribution studies is correspondingly wide.

To illustrate the use of some of these techniques, some examples are shown of recent studies carried out in the assessment of amoxycillin* for veterinary use.

Amoxycillin is the hydroxy analogue of ampicillin and like ampicillin has broad spectrum activity for both Gram-negative and Gram-positive bacteria. It differs from ampicillin in some important respects. Firstly, it is better absorbed orally than ampicillin (Acred *et al.*, 1970). It has also been shown to exert a more rapid bactericidal action against certain strains of bacteria both *in vivo* and *in vitro* in small animal models (Hunter, Rolinson and Witting, 1973; Comber, Osborne and Sutherland, 1975).

For a wide range of infections involving bacterial invasion of organs and tissue, it is essential that antibiotic reaches therapeutic levels in the serum and that it is able to diffuse readily from the serum into the tissue at the site of infection.

Knowledge of the blood levels of antibiotic resulting from oral or parenteral administration provides basic information about drug distribution. The blood level is therefore a basic technique that provides information on bioavailability on an antibiotic and its various dosage forms. Furthermore, it is a dynamic procedure, and multiple sampling of blood or serum is a fairly simple operation in the majority of animal species used in our studies. For a multiple-species preparation such as a simple aqueous injectable, preliminary blood levels would be assessed in either dogs or calves. If the results are satisfactory then the preparation would be further evaluated in other species of veterinary interest such as horses, cows, pigs, sheep and perhaps poultry.

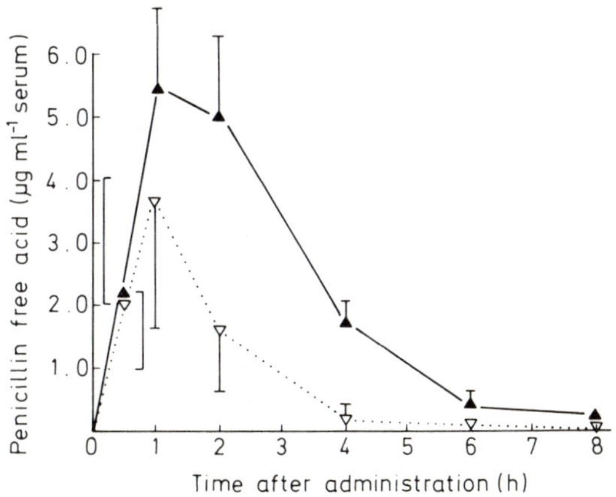

Figure 25.1 Serum levels following oral administration of ampicillin (△–△) and amoxycillin (▲–▲) trihydrate at the rate of 11 mg kg^{-1} in dogs. Vertical bars show the 95% confidence limits

For comparative blood levels to compare the relative serum bioavailability of two or more formulations of an antibiotic, cross-over studies in groups of 5–12 animals are satisfactory from the point of view of subsequent statistical analysis. *Figure 25.1* shows the results of such a study where amoxycillin and ampicillin

*Clamoxyl, Beecham Animal Health, Brentford.

were compared in Beagle dogs following oral dosing. It can be seen that the observed serum levels of amoxycillin exceeded those of ampicillin by a factor of 2–3 at 1–2 h after dosing and that this advantage was maintained over subsequent samplings.

TISSUE AND GUT DISTRIBUTION

Similar studies were carried out in other species and it was observed that amoxycillin was generally better absorbed than ampicillin. However for some infections, such as *Escherichia coli*, occurring either as the cause or as a complication of calf diarrhoea, concentrations of antibiotic in the tissues or contents of the alimentary tract are required for effective therapy. Groups of pre-ruminant calves were therefore killed at intervals following oral dosing with amoxycillin, and selected tissues and contents from the alimentary tract were removed for analysis. *Figure 25.2* shows the results of this study and it can be seen that considerable concentrations of amoxycillin were present in the various regions of the alimentary tract over the experimental period. The delay in the appearance of amoxycillin in the colon is a reflection of transit time along the gut. Peak

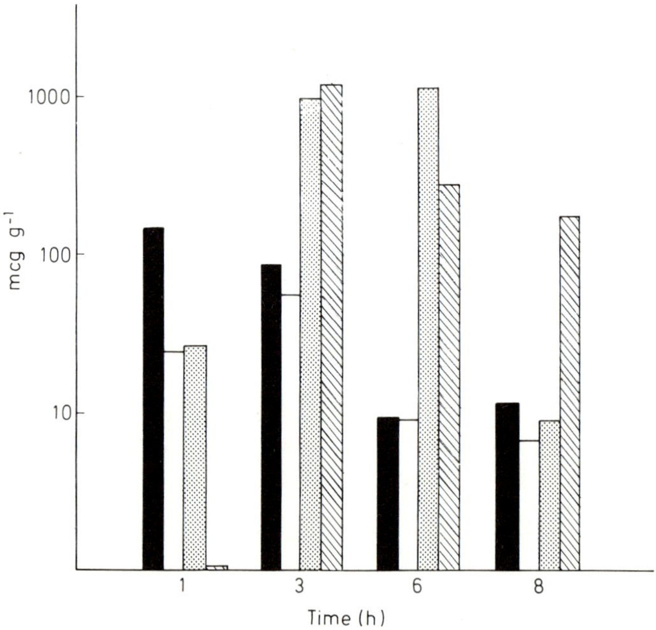

Figure 25.2 Concentration of amoxycillin in contents of the alimentary tract following oral administration at 7 mg kg^{-1} to pre-ruminant calves. ■ = Abomasum; □ = US (upper small intestine); ▨ = LS (lower small intestine); ▧ = colon

serum concentrations of amoxycillin were observed at 2–4 h which coincide with the high concentrations observed in the small intestine 3 h after dosing.

It is of interest to note that although a major portion of the dose was absorbed to give circulating concentrations of amoxycillin, sufficient of the dose remained in the alimentary tract to give amoxycillin concentrations well in excess of those bactericidal to most common pathogens.

MILK DISTRIBUTION

For intramammary preparations for the treatment of clinical mastitis, interest is focused on the distribution of antibiotic within the udder. For practical purposes, milk sampling at intervals after infusion serves as an indication of distribution throughout the udder. An example of such a study will be described under Synergic Considerations.

B Supplementary Studies

In this category are placed all those studies which provide basic information on the pharmacology of an antibiotic. For instance, pharmacokinetics is the study of mathematical models of drug distribution which enables antibiotics to be characterized and compared with each other. The representation of the body as a two-compartment open model has been described by Riggs (1972) and latterly by Ziv (1973) in the veterinary field. Essentially, it consists of a central compartment equivalent to plasma and a tissue compartment which is in fact a simplification of a heterogeneous collection of tissues. All drug is assumed to be removed irreversibly from the central compartment, i.e. into the urine. A drug administered intravenously will undergo simultaneous distribution and elimination processes and the shape of the subsequent serum curve will be dependent on both these processes. In essence, studies of serum concentration following intravenous infusion of a solution of an antibiotic is one of the simpler methods for studying its intrinsic character. The parameters derived from such models, for instance the apparent volume of distribution, are mathematical entities and complement studies of tissue distribution.

TISSUE CAGES

These are silicone rubber capsules which are surgically implanted under the skin or muscles. After a suitable time, they become lined with cells and capillaries and their lumen filled with interstitial fluid. Sufficient quantity of interstitial fluid is thus made available for assay. Such cages can be used to investigate movement of antibiotics from serum into intestinal fluid.

THIRY-VELLA LOOPS

Isolated loops of small intestine, opening onto the flank of an animal or Thiry-Vella Loops (Bywater, 1970), have a use in measuring the relative rates of absorption of antibiotics without the complication of stomach emptying or biliary secretion of antibiotic.

C Tissue Residues

The third major category of distribution study is the investigation of antibiotic residues following veterinary usage in order to establish a suitable withholding time, that is an interval at which no detectable antibiotic is present in edible tissues or body fluids.

Figure 25.3 illustrate a scheme for a typical study. In essence, groups of animals are checked in a pre-dose study to ensure that they are free of detectable antibiotic/antibacterials. The animals are then dosed at the maximum recommended level by the appropriate route of administration, and the urine and serum are monitored in the period following. Since for most penicillins the majority of the dose is excreted via the urine, it follows that when no detectable antibiotic is found in the urine, the tissues should also be free of antibiotic. At this point, the animals are slaughtered and at post mortem, representative tissues are removed and examined for the presence of antibiotic using the most sensitve assay techniques available. In the event of penicillin being detected, a further group of animals is slaughtered at a later interval following dosing and this procedure is repeated until negative residues are obtained.

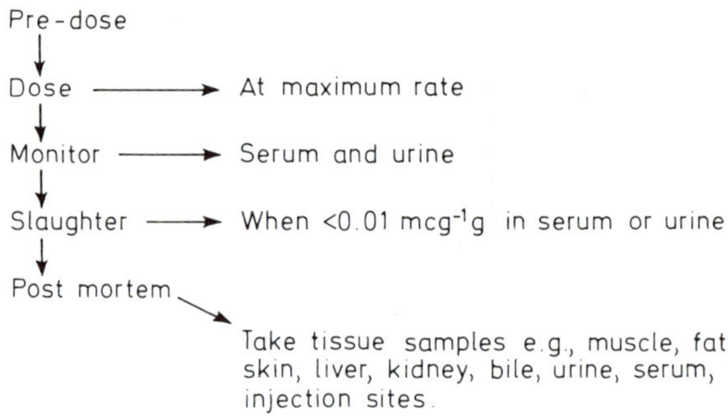

Figure 25.3 Tissue residue study

Synergic Considerations

In the use of semi-synthetic penicillins in the intramammary field for the treatment of bovine clinical mastitis, the persistence of antibiotic residues in milk subsequent to treatment of an infected quarter is of considerable interest to both the farmer and the pharmaceutical industry. The farmer is made well aware of economic loss due to depression of milk production from the infected animal during and subsequent to treatment, while the latter is subjected to legislation with regard to the withholding time – the period of several days in which milk from a treated cow must be discarded to protect the public from consuming antibiotic – and the dairy industries' ideal need for a cure allied to minimal milk revenue loss.

Within this field over recent years, trends have indicated an increasing incidence of coliform infections during lactation (Howell, 1972) brought about by overcrowding and poor hygiene. With this in mind and associated with the progressively more intensive methods used in dairy husbandry, it was decided to develop a lactation therapy with broad spectrum activity which would incorporate two semi-synthetic penicillins that had previously demonstrated synergistic activity in the context of human medicine.

The introduction of this combination, namely ampicillin and cloxacillin* for use in the intramammary field presented considerable technical difficulties. For the purpose of product registration with the Veterinary Products Committee of the Medicines Commission, it was initially hoped that the microbiological assay of the total combined penicillin content might be acceptable. However, it was requested that the separate levels for each component of the combination should be determined. For this purpose a selective assay procedure was developed. Following the usual milk out procedure where five lactating cows yielding two gallons daily were infused with Ampiclox LC in all quarters of the udder on three successive days at twenty-four hour intervals, individual bulk quarter milk samples were taken at twelve-hourly intervals and assayed for the respective antibiotics as shown in *Figure 25.4*.

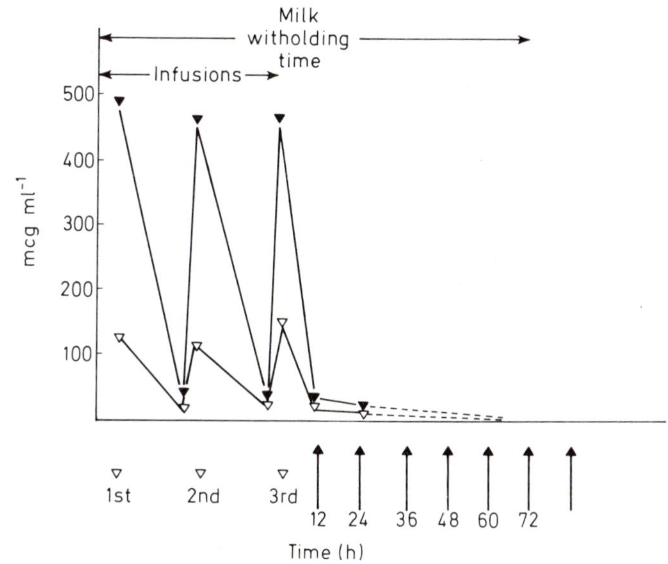

Figure 25.4 Concentrations of cloxacillin (▲–▲) and ampicillin (△–△) in milk following infusion with Ampiclox LC (– – –)

Cloxacillin and ampicillin content were estimated in the first instance by using specific organisms sensitive to one or other of the antibiotics to a detectable level of 1 mcg ml^{-1}. A staphylococcus was used for cloxacillin and a strain of *E. coli* for ampicillin. The staphylococcus used in this assay was selected for its sensitivity to cloxacillin and its ability to produce penicillinase, which conferred resistance to ampicillin. Conversely, the specific coliform was selected for its high degree of sensitivity to ampicillin yet displaying the innate characteristic of insensitivity to cloxacillin. Below the level of 1 mcg ml^{-1}, ampicillin

*Ampiclox LC, Beecham Animal Health, Brentford.

content was eliminated by using specific levels of penicillinase which ensured that residual cloxacillin remained intact and so available for bioassay against *Sarcina lutea* and *Bacillus stearothermophilus* var. *calidolactis*. For the inactivation of ampicillin, the following procedure was adopted. Twenty-five units of a suitable pure and preservative-free penicillinase were found to totally inactivate up to 4 mcg ml^{-1} ampicillin in the presence of 0.01 mcg ml^{-1} cloxacillin without affecting the latter. For the treatment of milk samples therefore, 0.1 ml of a sterile aqueous solution containing 1000 units of penicillinase per ml were added to each 4 ml sample and incubated at 37°C for 30 min. Having thus removed the ampicillin content, any residual penicillinase was inactivated by transferring the mixture to a water-bath at 80°C for 10 min followed by rapid cooling. Samples were then ready for assay against the appropriate organism for cloxacillin content.

Having determined the concentration of cloxacillin, the ampicillin content was estimated on the following day by diluting out the cloxacillin present with sterile milk known to be antibiotic- and inhibitor-free. This step reduced the cloxacillin content to less than the lowest detectable and assayable limit for either *S. lutea* or *B. calidolactis* and was carried out on duplicated milk samples that had been held deep frozen during the period of cloxacillin assay. Previous experience had shown that ampicillin in milk was stable when deep frozen for a considerable time.

By this method it was possible to meet the very stringent requirements of the Regulatory Authorities for 'lowest detectable limit' data on individual penicillins in milk. This limit is currently accepted to be less than 0.01 mcg ml^{-1} of milk.

Although fixed drug combinations do have their advantages for the user in terms of convenience, breadth of spectrum and possible synergism, they do pose special problems in their technical development. Not only are there the obvious formulatory and manufacturing difficulties, but there are special problems of detection and assay. The exercise quoted here demonstrates that such problems are not insurmountable.

References

ACRED, P., HUNTER, P.A., MIZEN, L. and ROLINSON, G.N. (1970). *Antimicrob. Agents and Chemother.*, **1**, 416

BYWATER, R.J. (1970). *J. comp. Path. Ther.*, **80**, 565

COMBER, K.R., OSBORNE, C.D. and SUTHERLAND, R. (1975). *Antimicrob. Agents and Chemother.*, **7**, 179

HOWELL, D. (1972). *Vet. Rec.*, **90**, 654

HUNTER, P.A., ROLINSON, G.N. and WITTING, D.A. (1973). *Antimicrob. Agents and Chemother.*, **4**, 285

RIGGS, D.G. (1972). *The Mathematical Approach to Physiological Problems.* MIT Press

ZIV, G. (1973). *Am. J. vet. Res.*, **34**, 1561

26

ANTIBIOTICS, ANIMALS AND MAN – AN APPRAISAL OF A CONTENTIOUS SUBJECT

A.H. LINTON
Department of Bacteriology, University of Bristol, Bristol

Introduction

After 30 years of antibiotic usage it is timely to appraise the situation as it exists today. Antibiotics have brought great benefits to man and animals in a variety of ways. Foremost would be the widespread relief of suffering and life-saving success of the therapeutic uses of antibiotics in the human and veterinary fields. Substantial amounts of antibiotics have also been used outside normal therapy for prophylaxis and growth promotion in animal husbandry and even in plant protection. There is no doubt that these wider uses have played a significant role economically in controlling losses due to infectious disease and in helping to meet the ever growing demands for animal protein foods.

The benefits have not been without certain disadvantages. The most important single factor, which in the last analysis decides the success or failure of an antibiotic in the treatment of microbial disease, is the sensitivity of the causal pathogen to the antibiotic being used. As antibiotics have been used more extensively so the number of strains typed and range of resistance in bacteria has increased and this has presented serious clinical problems. Consequently the treatment of choice, on the basis of the most favourable drug from both the pharmacological point of view and cost, have to be modified to meet the resistance properties of the infecting organisms.

Antibiotic resistant bacterial populations arise in man and animals by the use of antibiotics for therapy, prophylaxis or growth promotion (Siegal, Huber and Drysdale, 1974; Siegal, Huber and Enloe, 1974). The non-therapeutic uses therefore have come under heavy criticism by those concerned with the treatment of infectious disease. The immense value of antimicrobial agents as prophylactics, when raising animals under intensive husbandry practice, and the increased food conversion realized by the use of antibiotics in growth promotion, has to be balanced against these disadvantages. There is no simple answer to this problem since it is in essence a political one balancing one advantage for a community against another.

The most important question, on which more evidence is required, is whether the reservoir of resistant bacteria being built up by the continuing use of antibiotics in animals, constitutes a real threat to human health. The case for infections with salmonellae is well documented (Anderson, 1968a). In the outbreak of *Salmonella typhimurium* phage type 29 in calves, which lasted in Britain from 1963 to 1969, there was evidence that the emergence of resistant *S. typhimurium* correlated closely with the increasing range of antibiotics used and that resistant strains also caused infections in man.

The evidence for antibiotic resistant *Escherichia coli* of animal origin reaching man is less complete. It is not clear whether animal strains comprise a significant reservoir for man compared with cross-infection within the community of resistant *E. coli* arising from people who have recently received antibiotics. This paper is mainly concerned with assessing the risk to man of resistant *E. coli* of animal origin. It is concluded that antibiotic resistant *E. coli* in animals cannot, at present, be distinguished from those found in man and that the use of antibiotics in animals for whatever purpose contributes to the numbers of resistant *E. coli* potentially flowing to man. An attempt has been made to evaluate the relation of animal strains to human disease and it is concluded that only the prudent use of antibiotics, both in man and animals, will avoid an escalation of the problems of drug resistance in the therapy of infectious disease in the future.

THE IMPORTANCE OF TRANSFERABLE DRUG RESISTANCE *IN VIVO*

The mechanisms by which antibiotic resistance may arise in bacteria are common to animals and man, and since cross-infection of resistant strains between each is a strong probability, it is of first importance to investigate and to control the conditions under which antibiotic resistance arises and is spread.

R-plasmid infections constitute the most important mechanism by which antibiotic resistance can arise in a cell population. Under ideal *in vitro* conditions, transferable drug resistance (TDR) can spread like 'wildfire' throughout a susceptible bacterial population in a relatively short time (Richmond, 1972a). Without doubt TDR also occurs *in vivo*, both in animals and man, but the frequency with which it occurs is debated. A number of attempts to demonstrate TDR in animals and man have been made with varying success. *In vivo* transfer has been demonstrated in animals in which the gut flora was reduced in numbers or was non-existent. This was achieved by rearing mice in a germ-free environment (Salzmann and Klemm, 1968; Kasuya, 1964), by the use of chicks immediately after hatching (Walton, 1966a), by starving sheep and thereby replacing the rumen flora by a denser coliform flora (Smith, M.G., 1975) or by treating with antibiotics (Anderson, Gillespie and Richmond, 1973a; Anderson *et al.*, 1973b). Smith (1970a) was able to demonstrate TDR in chicken and calves but not in pigs, by feeding enormous numbers of donor strains to these animals, numbers which must be considered to be far in excess of those ingested naturally. In man, Smith (1969), fed a human subject with about 10^9 donor cells of human and animal origin to a volunteer and was able to demonstrate a small amount of transfer to resident flora but these did not persist for long in the alimentary canal. Anderson *et al.* (1973a, b) carried out similar experiments but were unable to demonstrate transfer unless a relevant antibiotic was administered whereupon transfer was detected at high frequency. Wiedemann (1972) concluded that the anaerobic conditions in the gut, the presence of bile salts, the metabolic activity of commensal organisms, variations in the growth kinetics of donor and recipient, and the cell wall characteristics of acceptor bacteria, all inhibit transfer. Anderson, J.D. (1974) has produced evidence that the *Bacteroides* sp. of the intestinal flora interfere with transfer presumably by liberating products inhibitory to conjugation. The different microbial gut flora in various animal species may therefore influence the chances of TDR occurring to varying degrees.

From these considerations it may be concluded that TDR occurs rarely in the normal gut but may be detected more regularly when certain conditions, such as the effects of antibiotics, are present (Lacey, 1975). The rare occasions when it does occur however may have far reaching effects, especially if drug resistance is transferred to a pathogen and opportunity for its spread to other hosts subsequently arises.

ANTIBIOTIC SELECTION PRESSURES

The *in vivo* transfer of drug resistance alone cannot be solely responsible for the prevalance of antibiotic resistance at the present time. The view has been expressed that environmental selection by antibiotics and colonization of patients with resistant organisms have far greater epidemiological significance than R-factor transfer in the gastrointestinal tract (Gardner and Smith, 1970). Two additional factors are therefore of major importance. Firstly, resistant cells survive at the expense of sensitive ones under antibiotic selection pressure and grow up to become the dominant component of the flora. Secondly, once this occurs, further penetration into the sensitive gut flora of other animals, and possibly man, may occur by cross-infection. Both of these factors are an inevitable sequel to the medical, veterinary and agricultural uses of antibiotics. There is no doubt that the continuing use of antibiotics has exerted a considerable selection pressure in favour of antibiotic resistance in commensal and pathogenic bacteria both in man and animals. Therapeutic and sub-therapeutic usages, as in prophylaxis or growth promotion in animals, exert this selection pressure.

Selection of antibiotic-resistant organisms in animals

Workers in different countries have demonstrated close correlation between the extent of antibiotic usage and the incidence of antibiotic-resistant *E. coli* in the intestinal flora of domestic animals.

Many surveys have dealt mainly with problems arising from the continuous feeding to animals of antimicrobial drugs to obtain growth promotion (Smith, 1966, 1971a, b; Walton, 1966b; Smith and Halls, 1966; Bulling and Stephan, 1971; Loken, Wagner and Henke, 1971; Mercer *et al.*, 1971; van den Heever, 1972; Søgaard, 1973; Burton *et al.*, 1974; Linton, Howe and Osborne, 1975; Wierup *et al.*, 1975). Mercer *et al.* (1971), for example, demonstrated that 80% of *E. coli* strains isolated from pigs and calves fed antimicrobial drugs carried resistance to one or more drugs, whereas the populations in herds not being fed antibiotics fell to 16% or below.

The incidence of drug resistance among *E. coli* in healthy animals can be ascribed also to the use of antibiotics in therapy or in the prevention of infectious disease (Søgaard, 1973). Patterns of antibiotic resistance have been related to the usage of a particular drug. For instance, in countries where neomycin is widely used in the treatment of calves, the frequency of occurrence of resistant strains of *E. coli* to this drug is high (Loken, Wagner and Henke, 1971) compared with other countries, e.g. Sweden, where the drug is used much less (Wierup, 1975). The ever increasing range of R determinants in *S. typhimurium* strain type 29 in the well documented outbreak of 1963–1969 correlated closely with the pattern of drugs used throughout the period (Anderson, 1968b).

Persistence of antibiotic-resistant E. coli *in animals*

The persistence of drug resistance in the animal gut has been related also to the pattern of usage. This includes both the route and the duration of administration. In dairy herds, administration by the intramammary route over short periods of time in the treatment of mastitis, or as a prophylactic at the end of the lactation period, had little or no effect on drug resistance in *E. coli* in the herd nor in its environment (Rollins *et al.*, 1973). Also in pigs (Edwards, 1961), calves (Edwards, 1962) and poultry (Rollins *et al.*, 1973), where antibiotics were given by the oral route over short periods of time, it was shown that the high initial levels of drug resistance which arose in the gut flora soon decreased. However, in contrast, on farms where antibiotics were fed continuously at sub-therapeutic levels, the incidence of resistant enteric organisms and frequency of occurrence of multiple resistance was greater, and persisted long after the selection pressure was removed. Linton *et al.* (1975) demonstrated this in pigs and calves following the feeding of tetracycline whilst no selection for resistance was demonstrated by the non-antibiotic growth promoters nitrovin and quindoxin (*Figure 26.1*). The *E. coli* flora in two calves over a period of 104 days is traced in *Figure 26.2* (Linton, unpublished). One calf received 100 ppm tetracycline in food for 30 days, the other none. Up to 10 colonies, isolated on antibiotic-free bile lactose agar, were examined from each sample of faeces. Each was O-serotyped and their resistance to at least one antibiotic was determined. The numbers of resistant *E. coli* present in both calves before the period of medication constituted a significant proportion of the gut flora. This is a common feature in many calves at the present time. In the untreated calf these gradually decreased with time, only occasional peaks of dominance being recorded. In the treated calf, the sensitive flora became increasingly suppressed, and the resistant strains rapidly reached 100% of the *E. coli* flora; these persisted at this high level for the 24 days post-treatment period up to the time of slaughter. The selection of specific resistant O-serotypes and their persistence in the calf gut are also illustrated in *Figure 26.2*.

In summary, after short exposures to antibiotics, as in therapy, resistant organisms which are selected and form the dominant faecal flora are usually replaced by sensitive strains and the flora reverts to a dominantly sensitive one. The greatest selection pressure in favour of drug resistance occurs where antibiotics are administered over long periods of time by the oral route. This also favours the persistence of resistant strains long after the selection pressure has been removed. The effect of continuous exposure therefore stabilizes the resistant organisms to become part of the 'normal' flora of the gut. The situation

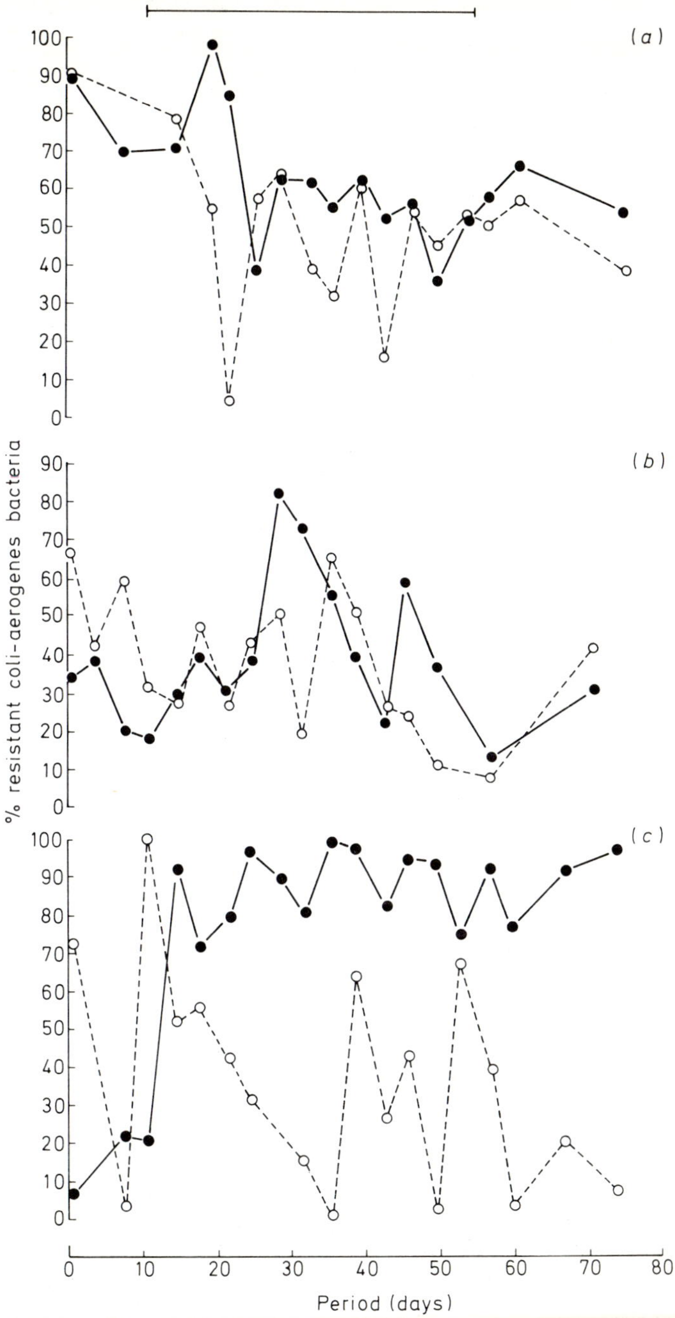

Figure 26.1 The effects on the intestinal coli-aerogenes bacteria of continuously feeding for 6 weeks (a) quindoxin, (b) nitrovin or (c) tetracycline to pigs at levels of 100 ppm of diet. The average percentage of strains resistant to tetracycline in each group of 4 pigs is plotted against time (●); ○ = values obtained for the control pigs. The period of medication is indicated by the solid bar. (From Linton, A.H., Howe, Katherine and Osborne, A.D. (1975). J. appl. Bact., **38**, *255)*

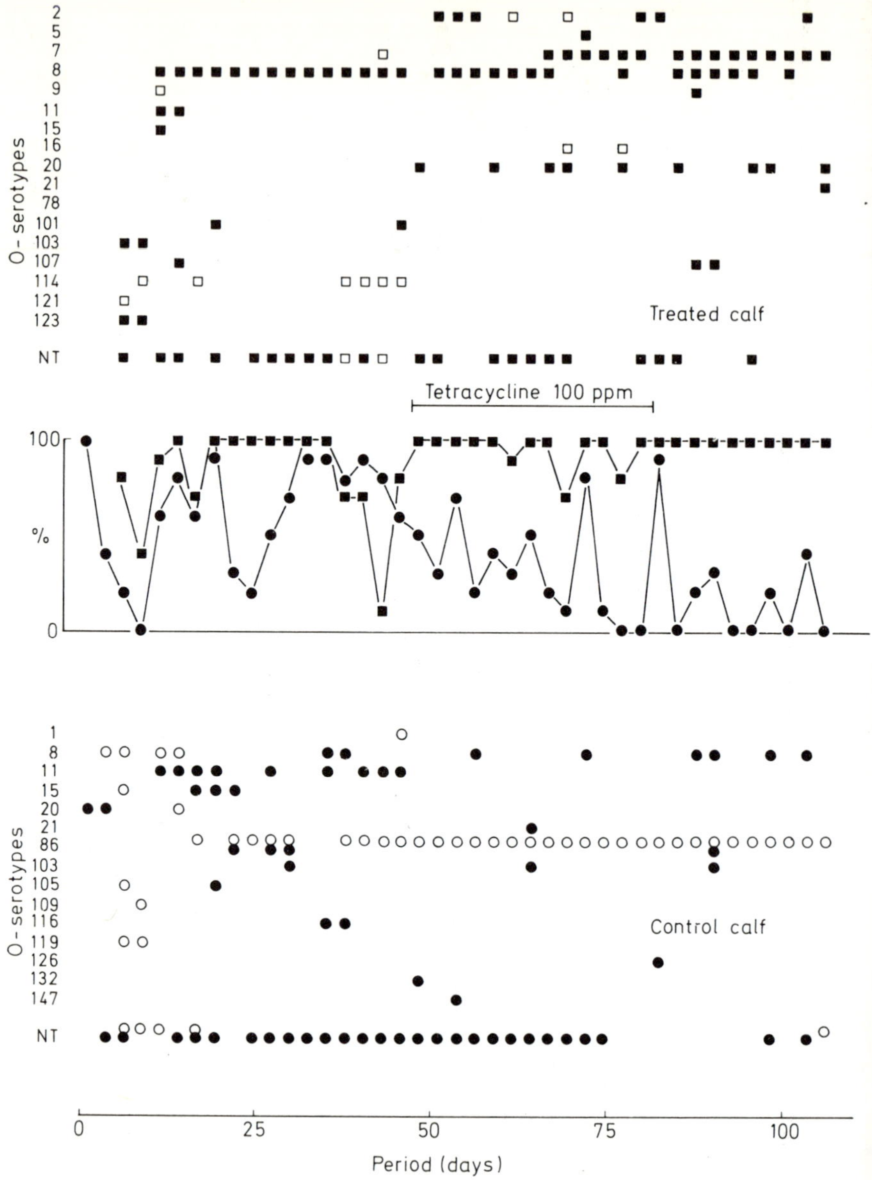

Figure 26.2 The effect of continuous feeding of tetracycline (30 days) on O-serotypes of E. coli *and the percentage of antibiotic-resistant* E. coli *in the faeces of a calf compared with an untreated animal,* ■, ● *= Antibiotic-resistant serotypes;* □, ○ *= antibiotic-sensitive serotypes*

that is commonly found in pigs and calves at the present time suggests that the continuous medication of these animals over many years has built up a resistant flora, doubtless passed on from one generation to the next, in which resistant serotypes have become stabilized in, and often saturate, the gut flora.

Selection of antibiotic-resistant bacteria in man

Antibiotics have been shown also to change the intestinal *E. coli* flora in man (Hartley, 1975). Their effects depend on the route of administration (oral or parenteral), the mode of action of the antibiotic (bactericidal or bacteriostatic) and the degree of absorption of the antibiotic from the upper gastrointestinal tract. Oral administration of antibiotics, which are poorly absorbed from the upper gastrointestinal tract generally have the greatest effect on the faecal flora. For instance, studies in man have shown that oral therapy with tetracycline, a drug which is incompletely absorbed from the gastrointestinal tract (McVay, 1952), results in an increase in the number of tetracycline-resistant bacteria in the faecal flora (Knothe, 1963; Sompolinsky, Yaron and Alkan, 1967; Guinée, Ugueto and Van Leeuwen, 1971; Datta *et al.*, 1971; Linton *et al.*, 1972; Hirsh, Burton and Blenden, 1973). Administration of sub-therapeutic doses was also found to select for resistant *E. coli* (Goldberg *et al.*, 1961).

Persistence of antibiotic-resistant E. coli *in man*

Meevootisom and Sawyer (1973) observed that a sensitive faecal flora was restored one week after completion of low-dosage tetracycline therapy; others demonstrated the re-establishment of sensitive *E. coli* 2–5 weeks after therapeutic courses of tetracycline (Datta *et al.*, 1971; Koonkhamlert and Sawyer, 1973). In certain individuals or groups, tetracycline-resistant *E. coli* were found to persist in large numbers for much longer periods of time after therapy (Gage, Gunther and Spaulding, 1961; Sompolinsky, Yaron and Alkan, 1967; Hirsh, Burton and Blenden, 1973; Jonsson, 1974). Datta *et al.* (1971) found that the change of the predominant *E. coli* population from sensitive to resistant or back from resistant to sensitive, was accompanied by a change of serotype. Hartley and Richmond (1975) studied the persistence of specific O-serotypes of *E. coli* in man after the antibiotic selection pressure had been removed. They concluded that persistence of an R-plasmid carrying strain is not a property of the plasmid so much as of the bacterium itself. Some strains of *E. coli* are better colonizers of the human gut than others, irrespective of whether they are sensitive or resistant to antibiotics. A preponderance of antibiotic-sensitive *E. coli* has been found in the human gut (Ewing and Davis, 1961; Guinée, 1963; Hartley *et al.*, 1975). Certain O-serotypes are found more frequently than others and their prevalence is doubtless a measure of their ability to colonize the human gut. The range of O-serotypes which carry R-plasmids is more limited; some are relatively common but others are rare. These observations may explain why a few resistant *E. coli* persist after removal of antibiotic selection pressure. The majority of resistant *E. coli* which are not good colonizers, are rapidly replaced by a sensitive flora but a few resistant strains may persist if they possess the relatively unique virtue of being able to colonize the gut in competition with the sensitive flora.

Another possibility must be considered. If R-plasmids should be transformed to a sensitive recipient which is a good colonizer, then the resultant resistant strain may persist for a long time.

It is encouraging to note the rarity of R-factors in O-serotypes most commonly colonizing the human gut in the absence of a selection pressure. This situation, however, could rapidly change if extensive and indiscriminant use of antibiotics is practised.

The Ecology of Antibiotic-Resistant *E. coli* in Man and Animals

ANTIBIOTIC-RESISTANT *E. COLI* IN MAN AND HIS ENVIRONMENT

Although antibiotics are used in the treatment of domiciliary patients, the most extensive use of antibiotic therapy is concentrated in hospitals. This is reflected in the high levels of R-plasmid carrying commensal and pathogenic bacteria in hospitalized patients (Salzmann and Klemm, 1966; Datta, 1969; Cooke *et al.*, 1971; Lebek, 1972). There is no doubt that when patients leave hospital carrying large numbers of resistant *E. coli*, under certain circumstances, by close contact or indirectly by food handling, these will be passed to other people.

The number of resistant *E. coli* in non-hospitalized people not receiving antibiotics is usually very low. Datta (1969) found less than 25% but Wiedemann, Knothe and Holzer (1970) concluded that the resistant enterobacterial flora rarely exceeded 1.0% and, in the majority of people fell below 0.01%. Nevertheless, a number of surveys indicate that over 50% of healthy adults and children excrete these in detectable but small numbers (Datta, 1969; Moorhouse, 1969; Linton *et al.*, 1974). A study of pooled sewage from residential housing estates and separately from hospitals in the same areas, made possible a comparison between the two types of population on a much broader basis than could be achieved by the examination of limited numbers of individual faecal samples (Linton *et al.*, 1974). The results confirmed that sewage from hospitals contained a much higher proportion of resistant R-factor carrying strains with multiple resistance than were found in domestic sewage.

However, when the total volume of sewage from hospitals and domestic sources reaching the Bristol sewage works was computed, it became clear that more than 90% of R-factors in pooled sewage from the whole city were probably derived from people living outside hospital. This conclusion was reached despite the fact that in normal healthy people resistant coliform bacilli can be only regularly detected by plating dilutions of faeces onto media incorporating antibiotics as selective agents. Grabow and Prozesky (1973) also demonstrated high levels of R-plasmid carrying bacteria in sewage in S. Africa and concluded that this may be of prime importance in the spread of resistant bacteria. They suggested that this could occur by the sprinkling of crops irrigated with contaminated water.

Enormous numbers of R-factor bearing coliforms are often discharged into rivers or the sea. Smith (1970b) found that the incidence of resistant *E. coli* was low in fresh water flowing through rural areas, highest through urban areas and less in samples taken in the lower parts of urban areas not receiving sewage. He concluded that most fresh water contamination is from human sources and hence could provide a source of R-factors for animals in their drinking water, rather than a significant recycling to man.

In sea water Smith (1971a) and Anson (1976) found that coliform bacilli do not survive for more than a few days and therefore effluent into the sea reaches an end point relative to the epidemiology of resistant bacteria (*Figure 26.3*).

Most available evidence suggests that water would need to be grossly polluted with sewage, to the level of being obnoxious, before infection with enteric pathogens occurs (Report, 1959; Regnier and Park, 1972). The evidence suggests, therefore, that contaminated river or coastal waters do not constitute a significant source of antibiotic-resistant bacteria for man.

THE POTENTIAL FLOW OF ANTIBIOTIC-RESISTANT *E. COLI* FROM ANIMALS TO MAN

In the final analysis the anxiety engendered by the continuing problem of drug resistance is that as time proceeds, the usefulness of antibiotics in the treatment of disease in both animals and man will decline. The situation in the animal field is of greater significance if resistant organisms in animals can also colonize man and thereby superimpose a continuing and additional load to the reservoir already present in man. The significance of the potential flow of R-factors from animals to man, as opposed to the recycling by cross-infection within the human population, is much disputed. But, if animals are a source of these organisms for man, then the use or misuse of antibiotics in animals becomes a subject of vital importance in the future therapy of human infectious disease.

The recommendations of the Swann Committee (Report, 1969b) restricting the use of antibiotics in veterinary practice were based on the assumption that resistant bacteria from animal sources pose a definite risk to human health or, more particularly, the treatment of human disease in the long term. Whilst this view was accepted by most workers, the evidence for it was not conclusive at the time the Swann Report was published. Further evidence in support of the recommendation has emerged since, but more is needed.

Despite extensive investigations into the incidence of antibiotic-resistant *E. coli* in domestic animals and man, many questions remain unanswered. For instance, how important is the resistant animal reservoir for man and, if it does constitute a hazard, what are the main routes by which these organisms reach man? In an attempt to answer some of these questions an extensive research programme has been underway at Bristol over the past years. Part of this work is in the process of being published (Howe and Linton, 1976; Howe, Linton and Osborne, 1976a, b) but much is incomplete. An attempt will therefore be made to summarize the main findings and to appraise the present position.

Assuming that animals constitute a source of resistant *E. coli* for man, the possible flow of these organisms between animals, and between the animal reservoirs and man are summarized (*Figure 26.3*). The most probable routes by which resistant *E. coli* reach man are:

(1) by direct contact;
(2) by handling raw meat;
(3) by eating inadequately cooked meat, or its products, or other foods eaten uncooked which may be contaminated from raw meat in the kitchen.

Each of these will be considered in detail later but it was assumed that the most important route was *via* the food chain. It was therefore decided to survey the principal animals which provide meat for human consumption. These include sheep, cattle, calves, pigs and poultry.

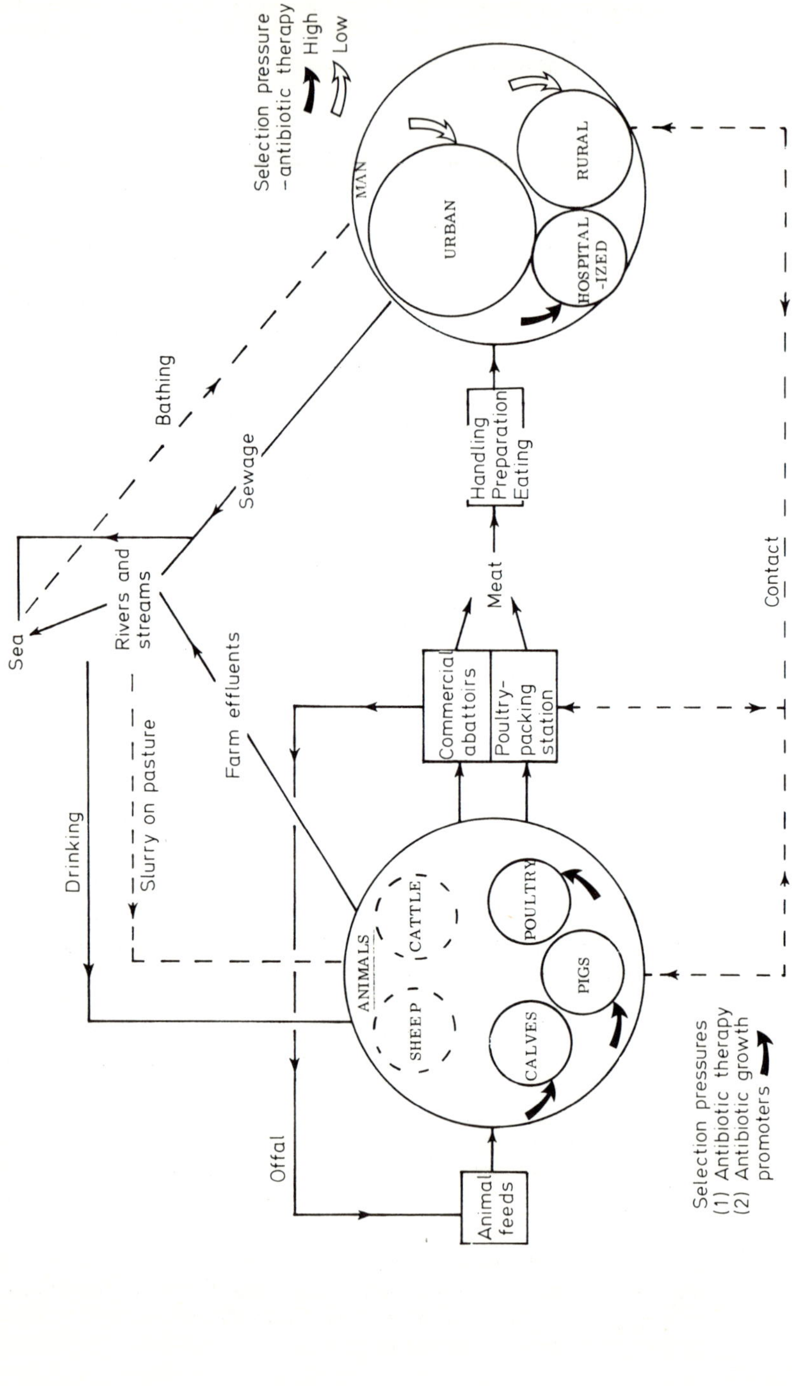

Figure 26.3 E. coli *flow chart between animals and man*

The following investigations were carried out:

(1) The principal reservoirs of resistant gut organisms in meat animals were identified and quantified.

(2) The level of carcass contamination with gut organisms at slaughter was determined.

(3) *Escherichia coli* in the gut of normal meat animals and on carcasses at slaughter were compared with those found in the normal human gut and in certain human diseases.

For cross-infection studies to be set on a sound basis, it was necessary to distinguish 'animal' from 'human' strains or to conclude, with reasonable certainty, that they could not be distinguished. We have used the dual characters of antibiotic-resistance patterns and O-serotyping by an agglutination test using a microtitre technique (Howe and Linton, 1976). Evidence of similarity between biochemically confirmed *E. coli* found in animals and man, and in the animal gut flora and on their carcasses, rested upon these two characters. In this way the various animals constituting the potential reservoirs of drug-resistant *E. coli* for man were identified, and the situation in animals was compared with that found in man using data obtained by similar means (Hartley *et al.*, 1975).

Identifying the animal reservoir

Presumptive coliform counts. Many workers have investigated the occurrence of antibiotic-resistant coliform bacilli in animals (e.g. Mitsuhashi, Hashimoto and Suzuki, 1967; Smith, 1967; Kelly, Moorhouse and Collins, 1971; Stephan and Bulling, 1971; Guinée, 1972; Walton, 1972; Renault *et al.*, 1973; Larsen and Nielsen, 1975; Wierup, 1975), but few attempts have been made to quantitate the resistant gut flora and to identify the animal species carrying the greatest numbers. To do this we determined first the presumptive coliform counts in faeces taken from the principal meat animals, sampled both on farms and at abattoirs. The counts were determined on antibiotic-free medium. The average of these counts were then compared with similar counts made using the same decimal dilutions cultured on media containing tetracycline or ampicillin. The proportion of coliforms resistant to at least these two antibiotics were thus determined. The average results for representative numbers of each of the animal species, including man, are presented in *Table 26.1.*

As reported in the literature (Smith, 1961; Smith and Crabb, 1961; Larsen and Larsen, 1972), considerable variations in total numbers of coliforms occur between the animal species. This was most marked in adult cattle in which often no coliforms could be detected and in the same animal for many days, only to appear from time to time and then in very low numbers (Howe, Linton and Osborne, 1976a). In calves, and other animals including sheep and pigs, covering a wide age range, and in poultry, the numbers of coliforms were of a high order (Linton, Howe and Osborne, 1975). In contrast, counts on antibiotic-containing media showed marked differences. Resistance to tetracycline and ampicillin were not detected in sheep and cattle.

Proportions of antibiotic-resistant E. coli. Although antibiotic resistance may be carried by coliforms in general, *E. coli* as a distinct species was studied for a

Table 26.1 The reservoir of resistant coliform bacilli in sheep, cattle, calves, pigs and poultry compared with man

Animal species	*Description of source*	*Nature of specimens*	*Number examined*	*Number of animals*	*Presumptive coliform counts* ($\log_{10}$ g^{-1}) *on* *BLA*	*BLA+T*	*BLA+A*
Sheep	Abattoir	Faeces	60	60	6.7	0	0
Cattle	Farm	Faeces	402	6	1.7	0	0
	Abattoir	Faeces	8	8	5.5	0	0
Calves	Farm	Rectal swabs	400	400	–	–	–
	Farm	Faeces	40	8	7.2	4.9	4.9
	Abattoir	Faeces	102	46	8.8	8.4	N.D.
Pigs	Farm	Faeces	43	43	6.8	5.3	2.6
	Abattoir	Faeces	16	16	7.0	6.1	4.3
Poultry	Farm	Faeces	154	12	8.2	7.2	N.D.
	Abattoir	Abdominal swabs	152	152	–	–	–
	Frozen birds	Abdominal fluids	31	31	2.5 ml^{-1}	2.3 ml^{-1}	N.D.
Man		Faeces	51	51	7.2	0.4	0

BLA = bile lactose agar;
BLA+T = bile lactose agar + tetracycline (25 μg ml^{-1});
BLA+A = bile lactose agar + ampicillin (25 μg ml^{-1}).
N.D. = not done.

number of reasons. It includes animal and human pathogens but, more particularly, serotyping as a method of strain identification could be used in *E. coli* as a valuable tool in cross-infection studies.

Up to a maximum of ten colonies of coliform bacilli were picked from each of the series of plates used for the presumptive coliform counts, both from the antibiotic-free and the antibiotic-containing media. Each isolate was tested biochemically (Eijkman at 44°C and Indole at 44°C, *see* Reports, 1956, 1969a) to identify *E. coli*. All strains of *E. coli* were O-serotyped by an agglutination test using a microtitre technique (Howe and Linton, 1976) and their sensitivity or resistance to a range of antibiotics determined (Linton, Howe and Osborne, 1975).

The numbers of *E. coli* resistant to at least one of eight antibiotics tested were compared with the total number of isolates from each animal species. This comparison was only valid between isolates grown on antibiotic-free medium in which no selection pressure for resistance to antibiotics was exerted. The results are shown in *Table 26.2*. In adult cattle, even by daily sampling for

Table 26.2 The reservoir of resistant *E. coli* in sheep, cattle, calves, pigs and poultry compared with man

Animal species	*Description of source*	*Nature of specimens*	*Proportion of resistant* E. coli *on BLA* *No. of colonies*	*% resistant*
Sheep	Abattoir	Faeces	460	0.02
Cattle	Farm	Faeces	735	0
	Abattoir	Faeces	78	0
Calves	Farm	Rectal swabs	3 882	63.0
	Farm	Faeces	380	37.6
	Abattoir	Faeces	1 012	99.6
Pigs	Farm	Faeces	650	54.2
	Abattoir	Faeces	142	63.4
Poultry	Farm	Faeces	1 493	82.7
	Abattoir	Abdominal swabs	1 505	93.0
	Frozen birds	Abdominal fluids	169	89.3
Man		Faeces	510	9.4

100 days, no resistant *E. coli* were found. The rarity of resistance in adult cattle is supported by the observations of Larsen and Larsen (1972) who found only four resistant *E. coli*, not plasmid-carrying, in 150 samples from different cattle. Of 600 isolates from sheep, only one colony was resistant and this was to sulphonamides alone. In calves the findings were quite different. In a county-wide survey of calves on 400 separate farms, 63% of *E. coli* were resistant to at least one antibiotic whilst in veal calves intensively reared, 99.6% were resistant (Howe and Linton, 1976; Howe, Linton and Osborne, 1976b). Pigs and poultry yielded similarly high percentages of resistant *E. coli* ranging from 44.2 to 92.6%.

From these quantitative assessments it would appear that sheep and adult cattle do not constitute a reservoir of antibiotic-resistant *E. coli*. On the other hand, calves, pigs and poultry carry significantly large reservoirs of these organisms.

The 'richness' of resistant reservoirs in meat animals. Having identified the potential reservoirs of drug resistance, the distribution of R-determinants for a wide range of clinically useful antibiotics was determined. This was done for each of the *E. coli* isolates from the various animal species. The percentages of all isolates from each animal species, in which each R-determinant was found, are presented in *Table 26.3*. Resistance to sulphonamides, streptomycin and

Table 26.3 Percentage of *E. coli* carrying various R-determinants

Animal species	*Nature of source*	*Number of resistant isolates studied*	*R-determinants* Su	S	T	A	C	Ne	Fz
Sheep	Abattoir	1	1*	0	0	0	0	0	0
Cattle	Abattoir	0	0	0	0	0	0	0	0
Calves	Farm	2 445	89	83	47	36	14	4	3
	Abattoir	1 008	82	82	99	16	4	3	11
Pigs	Farm	352	73	57	56	5	0	0	0.4
	Abattoir	90	87	57	63	3	0	0	1
Poultry	Farm	1 235	97	24	60	0	0	N.D.	N.D.
	Abattoir	1 400	97	29	28	0	4	N.D.	N.D.
Man		48	88	21	63				

*A single colony.
N.D. = not done.
All *E. coli* isolated on antibiotic-free medium.

tetracycline were found in the highest proportions of isolates from calves, pigs and poultry. Ampicillin-resistance was followed in descending order by resistance to chloramphenicol, neomycin and furazolidone but these were found less frequently and were more common in isolates from calves. It is known that tetracycline-resistance is always carried on plasmids in naturally occurring isolates (Franklin, 1967). The wide distribution of this R-determinant in strains of *E. coli* from these three meat animals must indicate high levels of plasmid carriage, even though their ability to be transferred was proved in only a representative sample of all isolates.

A further analysis of the data indicated the number of R-determinants present in each isolate. In *Table 26.4* the percentages of all isolates carrying different numbers of R-determinants showed that whilst the majority carried one, two or three R-determinants, some *E. coli* from calves and pigs carried up to six in individual isolates.

From these observations it is clear that not only is drug resistance common in calves, pigs and poultry but each reservoir is 'rich' in the range of R-determinants it contains.

The diversity of O-serotypes of resistant E. coli *in the various animal reservoirs.* The significance of the animal reservoirs as potential sources of resistant bacteria for man may depend in the last analysis on how readily animal strains are able to colonize the human gut. The factors which decide this are virtually unknown for man but the O-serotype of the strains may be significant. Adhesion to the gut

Table 26.4 Percentage of *E. coli* isolates carrying different numbers of R-determinants

Animal species	*Nature of source*	*Number of resistant isolates studied*	*Number of R-determinants* 1	2	3	4	5	6
Sheep	Abattoir	1	1*	0	0	0	0	0
Cattle	Abattoir	0	0	0	0	0	0	0
Calves	Farm	2 445	11	40	22	17	9	1
	Abattoir	1 008	10	12	55	19	4	0.5
Pigs	Farm	352	39	28	33	0.5	0	0
	Abattoir	90	33	24	41	1	0	0
Poultry	Farm	1 235	36	40	24	0	0	0
	Abattoir	1 400	53	34	13	0	0	0
Man		48	17	54	29	0	0	0

*A single colony.
All *E. coli* isolated on antibiotic-free medium.

wall may be associated with specific surface structures which include the O-antigens. All *E. coli* isolates from animal sources were O-serotyped and their diversity within each animal species determined. The overall findings are summarized later (*Table 26.10*). In addition to the diversity of serotypes within individual animals, it was also evident that the range of O-serotypes in the gut flora of meat animals was very extensive and not greatly dissimilar from that of man.

Should the O-serotype be linked with the ability of strains of *E. coli* to colonize the human gut, the greater the diversity of O-serotypes in the animal the greater the chances of gut colonization occurring. In man it is a rare event to isolate more than one resistant serotype from a single faecal specimen, even using selective procedures. In animals, using antibiotic-free media for isolation, multiple O-serotypes were found in single samples from calves, pigs and poultry (*Table 26.5*). The animal reservoir is therefore not only 'rich' in R-determinants but also 'diverse' in O-serotypes and thus presents a potentially greater hazard for man.

Table 26.5 Percentage of samples containing different numbers of resistant *E. coli* O-serotypes

Animal species	*Nature of source*	*Number of samples examined*	*Number of O-serotypes per faecal sample* 0	1	2	3	4	5	6	7	8
Sheep	Abattoir	60	98	2	0	0	0	0	0	0	0
Cattle	Farm and abattoir	410	100	0	0	0	0	0	0	0	0
Calves	Farm	440	22	38	28	8	2	2	0.3	0	0
	Abattoir	102	0	0	7	19	33	19	17	4	1
Pigs	Farm	43	12	17	16	23	14	8	6	2	2
	Abattoir	16	6	0	13	19	19	13	19	6	6
Poultry	Farm	169	0	14	7	7	44	7	14	0	7
	Abattoir	152	0	11	25	20	17	8	8	8	3
Man		51	90	6	2	2	0	0	0	0	0

All *E. coli* isolated on antibiotic-free medium.

Routes of cross-infection from animals to man

Having identified the reservoirs of antibiotic-resistant *E. coli* in animals, the routes by which these may reach man were considered (*Figure 26.3*). It was thought that these were mainly limited to: (1) contact between animals and man, and (2) animal foods eaten by man.

(1) Contact. There is evidence that healthy humans in contact with animals show a higher incidence of antibiotic-resistant bacteria in their 'normal' flora than others (Smith and Crabb, 1961; Wells and James, 1973; Fein *et al.*, 1974; Linton *et al.*, 1974). Levy, Fitzgerald and Macone (1976) demonstrated cross-infection of a genetically marked strain of *E. coli* from infected chickens to humans in contact with the birds. Whilst this may be of importance to the individual, the number of people having direct contact with animals must be very small compared with the whole human population and this route is, therefore, judged to be of little general importance.

(2) Animal foods. Animal products, like milk (usually pasteurized) and eggs (usually sterile) are unlikely to be significant. On the other hand, the handling and ingestion of meat is likely to be of general importance. Guinée, Ugueto and van Leeuwen (1970) found a higher incidence of resistant *E. coli* in kitchen personnel (presumably due to the handling of raw meat) compared with office personnel. Other workers (Cooke *et al.*, 1970; Shooter *et al.*, 1970) reported that raw meat brought into hospital kitchens was an important source for the transmission of coliforms from food to patients. Dorn *et al.* (1975) studied 14 families eating home-killed beef and pork and concluded that handling of contaminated meat was the main route by which antibiotic-resistant organisms reached man from animals.

(*a*) *Carcass contamination – red meat.* For organisms found on raw meat to be of animal origin the carcass most probably would be contaminated with gut flora at slaughter (Moorhouse, O'Grady and O'Connor, 1970). Walton (1970) demonstrated that 52% and 83% of bovine and porcine carcasses respectively slaughtered at commercial abattoirs were contaminated with *E. coli*. Babcock, Berryhill and Marsh (1973) in the U.S.A. showed that of 98 dressed beef isolates, 79.6% were resistant to at least one antibacterial agent. The demonstration of resistant *E. coli* on beef carcasses was contrary to our experience but it was not certain that the strains examined by these workers came from the gut flora. Others have reported heavy contamination of meat products with *E. coli* (Moorhouse, O'Grady and O'Connor, 1969; Walton and Lewis, 1971).

The presence of antibiotic-resistant *E. coli* in the animal gut and on the carcass is not proof of identity. In the reports quoted above, the carcass contamination may have come from the gut contents but this is not certain. We have sought to establish this relationship by using the shared characters of antibiotic-resistance and O-serotype. Paired samples of rectal contents, and swabs taken from defined areas of the carcass surface, were examined from cattle, sheep, pigs and calves (*Table 26.6*). Under conditions of slaughter at the abattoir of the Meat Research Institute, the amount of contamination by *E. coli* was negligible, indicating that under conditions of good hygienic practice no contamination need occur (*Table 26.7*). However, animals slaughtered at commercial abattoirs

Table 26.6 Carcass contamination with tetracycline-resistant coliforms

Species	*Number of carcasses examined*	*Number contaminated*		*Bacterial count*			
		with coliforms	*with resistant coliforms*	*Total coliforms Mean*	*Range* ($\log_{10}$ 100 cm^{-2})	*Resistant coliforms Mean*	*Range* ($\log_{10}$ 100 cm^{-2})
Veal calves	46	46	46	1.2	0–5.8.	1.1	0–5.8
Pigs	16	16	16	2.7	0–4.8	*see* footnote*	
Beef	12	11	0	1.4	0–4.3	0	
Sheep	60	45	0	2.3	0–5.4	0	
Poultry	31	31	31	2.5**	1.0–6.4**	2.3**	1.0–6.0**

*The number of tetracycline-resistant coliforms was not determined quantitatively but they were numerous.
**Data quoted per ml of fluid from frozen birds on thawing.

were invariably contaminated with numerous O-serotypes of *E. coli*. In the case of sheep and adult cattle the carcass contamination was by antibiotic-sensitive strains suggesting that most, if not all, must have come from the antibiotic-sensitive gut flora and not from the abattoir environment which most probably would have included resistant strains. The carcasses of pigs and calves invariably demonstrated the presence of resistant strains. Frequently the resistant O-serotypes on the carcasses were identical with those isolated from the rectal contents of the same animal suggesting that direct contamination of the carcass had occurred from the gut of the same animal. Cross-contamination was shown to occur between carcasses on the same slaughter line, by the same *E. coli* O-serotypes found in the gut flora of at least one of the animals (*Table 26.8*). Frequently *E. coli* found on the carcasses were not found in the gut contents of the group of animals being slaughtered on the same day. It may be that these were present but failed to be detected in the gut flora or, more probably, may have arisen from the abattoir environment on the instruments or hands of the slaughtermen. Cross-contamination from other animal species was a strong possibility since different animals were slaughtered by the same men but in different parts of the abattoir.

A summary of both antibiotic-sensitive and resistant *E. coli* O-serotypes found in animals and on carcasses at slaughter are presented in *Table 26.9*. A large proportion of all O-serotypes were found both in faeces and on carcasses within each animal species providing strong evidence that carcass meat is frequently contaminated with gut organisms under conditions of practice at commercial abattoirs.

(*b*) *Carcass contamination – white meat.* Poultry presents a different problem. On the scale demanded by commerce it is impossible to slaughter chickens without getting substantial levels of contamination (Schothorst, Northolt and Kampelmacher, 1976). Even under laboratory conditions it was not possible to prepare birds without contamination with gut organisms (Howe, unpublished work). This may, in part, be due to the anatomical difficulties in evisceration. A large proportion of birds are frozen but, after thawing, fluids from the abdominal cavity were found to contain as many as 10^6 resistant *E. coli* per ml (the average of 31 table birds examined was $10^{2.3}$ *E. coli* ml^{-1}). Kim and Stephens (1972)

Table 26.7 The O-serotypes of *E. coli* detected in Group A pigs before and at the time of slaughter

Pig reference	1							2							3							4						
O-serotype	F_1	F_2	F_3	*1*	*2*	*3*	*C*	F_1	F_2	F_3	*1*	*2*	*3*	*C*	F_1	F_2	F_3	*1*	*2*	*3*	*C*	F_1	F_2	F_3	*1*	*2*	*3*	*C*
2							–							S							–							–
4							–						S	–				R			–							–
8	S/R	S	S	S	S	S/R	–		S	S	S	S	S	–			S/R	R	S/R	S	–	S	S	S/R	R	S	S/R	–
9			R		R	S	R							R							–						S	–
10							–							–							–						R	–
23							–							–							–			S				–
26							–							–							–	S						–
29							–			R			R	–	R		R				–			R	R		R	–
34							–							–						R	–							–
36							–							–							–				R			–
38				S			–							–						R	–							–
53							–						S	–							–							–
60							–							–							–						R	–
70			R				–							–							–							–
73				R			–							–							–							–
76							–		S					–							–							–
83							–							–							–				S	S/R	S/R	–
95			R				–							–							–							–
100	S						–				S	S	S	–			S		S		–							–
101							–							–							–						R	–
109							–					S		–							–							–
114							–							–							–				R			–
115							–		S					–							–							–
117							–							–							–				R			–
120							–		S					–							–							–
132							–							–						R	–							–
138		S					–							–		S					–		S					–
143				R			–							–							–							–
145							–							–				S			–							–
153							–							–							–			S			R	–

F_1 = Faecal sample taken 50 days before slaughter;
F_2 = Faecal sample taken 30 days before slaughter;
F_3 = Faecal sample taken after slaughter.

1 = Caecal contents taken after slaughter;
2 = colon contents taken after slaughter;
3 = colon/rectum contents taken after slaughter;

Table 26.8 Antibiotic-sensitive and resistant O-serotypes of *E. coli*, isolated from the rectal contents and carcasses from pigs 9–12, slaughtered at a commercial abattoir

Pig reference	*9*		*10*		*11*		*12*	
O-serotype	*Faeces*	*Carcass*	*Faeces*	*Carcass*	*Faeces*	*Carcass*	*Faeces*	*Carcass*
1				S	R		R	S/R
2					R			
4		S		S		S		
8	R							S
9		R	R		R			
16		R				R		
17								R
22				S				
23				R				
27	R							
28				S				
38						R		
40								S
41	R	R						
46				R				
49				S				
51			R					
60			R					
80							R	
87								S
88			R					
91		S		R		S		
93								S
100						S		
101		R						
102	S			S		S		S
104	R							
107								S
108					R			
112 ab	R							
115		S		S	R		S/R	S
126								S
134		R			R			
141			R	R	R	R		R
146				S				
147			R		S			
149	R			S			R	
153			R					

S = Antibiotic-sensitive; R = antibiotic-resistant.

also found that the greatest number of *E. coli* isolates from 'ready-to-cook' broilers were obtained from the fluid and from the abdominal cavity.

(3) *Handling of meat in the kitchen.* Since carcasses have been shown to be contaminated regularly with gut coliforms it is inevitable that antibiotic resistant strains reach the kitchen on raw pork, veal and poultry meats. Little raw meat is consumed in this country and it might be assumed that the process of cooking forms a complete barrier to the flow of these organisms to man. Meat foods have been shown to be the commonest sources of salmonellae infections for man in

Table 26.9 Frequency of occurrence of *E. coli* O-types in faeces and on carcasses at slaughter

	O-antigen types of E. coli *in*				
	Faeces only	*Carcass only*	*Faeces and carcasses*	*Total in faeces*	*% faecal O-types on carcasses*
Resistant					
Sheep	1	2	0	1	0
Cattle	0	0	0	0	0
Calves	25	6	32	57	56
Pigs	49	7	32	81	39.5
Poultry	33	51	37	70	52.9
Sensitive					
Sheep	25	17	36	61	59
cattle	7	23	3	10	30
Calves	0	6	0	0	0
Pigs	25	15	15	40	37.5
Poultry	6	6	1	7	14.3

Number of animals studied: sheep 60; cattle 8; calves 36; pigs 24; poultry 40.

this country (Lee, 1974) and it is to be expected that resistant *E. coli* will reach man by the same route. Poultry is particularly suspect since the larger proportion of salmonellae outbreaks have been traced to this meat. This may be due to inadequate thawing of carcasses prior to cooking which results in the centre of the carcass not reaching pasteurization temperatures in the cooking process (Noah, 1975). A more likely route is the contamination of the kitchen surfaces, implements and hands of the cook during the handling of the raw meat. Other foods in the kitchen, eaten uncooked or not requiring further cooking, may thereby become contaminated with resistant *E. coli*. People, other than the kitchen staff eating these foods may thereby become infected by these organisms. The evidence available at present strongly suggests that the handling of contaminated raw meat is the most important route by which *E. coli* reaches man.

A COMPARISON BETWEEN RESISTANT *E. COLI* OF ANIMAL AND HUMAN ORIGIN

Earlier the question was raised as to the possibility of distinguishing between *E. coli* from animal and human sources. Shooter *et al.* (1974) found that 64% of *E. coli* from abattoir sources could not be typed, and the results of Bettelheim *et al.* (1974) also suggested that non-typeable *E. coli* strains are abundant in the animal population; the distribution of O-types however was not stated. They concluded that their results indicated differences in serotype distribution of *E. coli* in man and animals and that the flow of *E. coli* from animals to man may be limited in the general population. This could be either because serotypes from animals are not generally reaching the human population to any great extent, or because they are not able to establish well in the human bowel. We have demonstrated heavy contamination of carcass meats and suggested the strong probability that humans are regularly exposed to animal strains. This is in agreement with Walton (1970), but he later concluded that although resistant enteric bacteria are present on freshly slaughtered carcasses in large numbers, they are not transferred to retail meat and meat products in numbers that could increase the intestinal resistance problem already present in humans (Walton and Lewis, 1971). He considered that his study indicated a serious pollution of foods by humans. This may in part be true for red meats but it cannot apply to poultry which are sealed in polythene bags until they reach the kitchen. The next question to answer is are 'animal' strains able to implant in the human bowel? Smith (1969) concluded that animal strains were poorer than human strains at colonizing the alimentary tract but this conclusion was reached after studying only one subject with very few strains. Cooke *et al*. (1970) reported patients excreting serotypes present also in their food and suggested that many of the strains of *E. coli* entered the kitchen in raw meat and poultry and other foodstuffs. They were also able to produce readily temporary colonization of the human gut with animal strains (Cooke, Hettiaratchy and Buck, 1972) and concluded that there was probably no great difference between the persistence in the bowel of human and animal strains.

Qualitative similarities

In our studies a wide range of O-serotypes of *E. coli* have been found in animals and we have compared these with those found in the human gut (Hartley *et al.*, 1975). *Table 26.10* presents the data for O-serotypes of resistant *E. coli* isolated from the rectal contents of calves, pigs and poultry. Since these were isolated on antibiotic-free media and are therefore unselected, they comprised the majority strains in the faecal flora of the animals examined. The proportion of animals from which each O-serotype was isolated is roughly quantified in this table; resistant *E. coli* from humans are also included. A direct comparison is not possible since the human resistant strains were isolated on antibiotic media and therefore comprised minority strains. It is clear that many O-serotypes are common to man and to one or more of the three animal species examined. Based on O-serotyping alone it is therefore not possible to distinguish 'animal' and 'human' gut strains of *E. coli.*

What of strains from human infections? In a recent survey 180 isolates were examined from urinary tract infection U.T.I. (Petrocheilou and Richmond, 1976) and their antibiotic sensitivity or resistance and O-serotypes were determined. These results are summarized in *Table 26.11.* A large proportion of the O-serotypes isolated from U.T.I. have also been isolated from human gut floras but 14 resistant O-serotypes were not isolated by Hartley *et al.* (1975). It is quite possible that as the survey in man is extended these 14 strains also will be found. However, these 14 O-serotypes have been isolated from the gut contents of calves, pigs and poultry in our survey. This does not prove animal origin but the possibility is suggested.

Quantitative differences

Although a similar range of resistant O-serotypes were found in man and the various animal species investigated, the proportion of resistant to sensitive isolates was much higher in animals than in man (*Table 26.1*). It was rare to isolate

Table 26.10 Relative incidence of resistant *E. coli* O-serotypes in three animal species compared with man

O-serotype	*Man (86)**	*Calves (400)**	*Pigs (53)**	*Poultry (62)**	*O-serotype*	*Man (86)**	*Calves (400)**	*Pigs (53)**	*Poultry (62)**
1	4.7	+	++	++	69	–	–	+	+
2	5.8	+	+++	+	70	–	–	–	+++
3	–	+	–	+++	71	1.2	–	+	+
4	1.2	+	–	+++	73	–	+	–	+
5	4.7	+	++	++	75	2.3	+	+	+
6	5.8	+	–	+	76	1.2	+	+	+
7	3.5	+	+	+	77	5.8	+	–	–
8	16.3	+++	+++	+++	78	1.2	+	++	–
9	18.6	++	++	+++	79	–	–	–	+
10	–	–	+	–	80	–	–	–	+
11	2.3	+	+	–	81	2.3	–	–	–
12	1.2	+	+	–	82	1.2	–	–	–
13	–	+	–	+++	83	5.8	–	–	+++
15	1.2	+	+	++	84	–	+	+	–
16	2.3	+	+	–	85	1.2	–	–	–
17	1.2	+++	–	+	86	7.0	++	+	–
18	4.7	+	–	–	88	1.2	+	+	+
19	2.3	–	+	+	89	2.3	–	–	–
20	8.1	+	+	+	90	–	+	–	–
21	4.7	++	++	+++	91	–	–	–	+
23	3.5	+	–	–	93	–	–	+	+
24	–	–	+	+	95	1.2	–	+	+
25	7.0	+	–	++	96	–	–	–	+++
26	–	++	+	+	98	–	–	+	–
27	3.5	–	+	+	99	1.2	+	–	–
28	1.2	–	–	–	100	–	–	+	–
29	–	–	+	–	101	10.5	+	+++	+
30	1.2	–	+	–	102	–	–	+	–
32	–	+	–	–	103	1.2	+	–	+
34	–	+	–	+	104	–	–	+	+
35	1.2	–	–	–	105	–	–	–	+
36	–	+	–	–	106	1.2	–	–	–
37	1.2	–	–	–	107	1.2	+	++	++
38	–	–	+	+	108	1.2	+	++	+
39	1.2	–	–	+	109	2.3	+	++	–
40	–	+	++	++	110	–	+	–	–
41	–	–	+	–	111	–	+	–	–
42	1.2	–	–	–	112ab	–	–	+	+
44	–	–	–	+++	113	1.2	+	–	+
45	–	+	–	+	114	–	–	–	+++
49	–	–	+	+	115	1.2	–	+	–
50	1.2	+	–	–	116	1.2	–	–	–
51	1.2	–	+	–	117	–	+	–	–
55	1.2	–	–	–	118	–	+	+	++
57	1.2	–	–	–	119	–	–	–	+
59	–	–	–	+	120	–	–	–	+
60	–	–	+	–	123	2.3	++	–	+
61	1.2	–	–	–	125	–	+	–	–
63	1.2	–	–	–	126	–	+	–	–
64	2.3	–	+	–	127	–	+	+	–
65	–	–	+	+	128	–	+	–	++
68	1.2	+	–	–	130	5.8	–	–	+

Table 26.10 (continued)

131	2.3	+	–	++	140	1.2	–	–	–
132	1.2	+	–	+	141	–	–	+	+
133	–	–	+	+	143	–	–	+	–
134	2.3	–	+	–	145	–	+	–	–
135	–	–	–	+	149	1.2	–	+++	–
136	–	–	–	+	150	1.2	–	–	–
139	–	–	+	–	153	–	+	++	–

*Number of humans and animals examined.
+ = Below 5%; ++ = 5% to below 10%; +++ = above 10%.

Table 26.11 Comparison between the numbers of different O-serotypes of *E. coli* isolated from human faeces and human urinary tract infections (U.T.I.)

	Faeces only	*U.T.I. only*	*Faeces and U.T.I.*	*Total*
Antibiotic-sensitive	53	9	42	103
Antibiotic-resistant	39	14	26	81

Data from Dr. V. Petrocheilou.

resistant strains from man without the aid of selective media. The present position in animals may well be a consequence of the considerable antibiotic pressure exerted over many years in a variety of ways. The observations that a wide range of O-serotypes are resistant to antibiotics and that many of these are multiply resistant, indicate that R-plasmids have penetrated widely into the animal gut flora. The 'richness' and 'diversity' of O-serotypes in animals is greatly in excess of that currently found in man. The fact that the human flora is not saturated with resistant organisms is cause for some encouragement. It may indicate that the flow of resistant strains to man from animal sources is limited, but as we have shown, the potential risks are always there. To maintain the *status quo* in man it is essential to restrict the use of antibiotics as much as possible.

RESISTANT *E. COLI* AND HUMAN DISEASE

There has been much discussion about the possible hazards to human health of resistant *E. coli* in the gut (Smith and Armour, 1966; Lebek, 1972; Anderson, 1968b; Gruneberg, Leigh and Brumfitt, 1968; Report, 1969b; Datta, 1969; Richmond, 1972b). The presence of large numbers of resistant *E. coli* in the gut, even for long periods, may not cause any ill effects in the individual carrying them. If, however, the R-plasmids are transferred to an enteropathogen (e.g. *E. coli*, salmonella or *Shigella*) treatment of an infection by antibiotics is rendered more difficult. For instance, in 1972 strains of *S. typhi* carrying an R-plasmid mediating for resistance to chloramphenicol, caused an outbreak of 10 000 cases of typhoid fever in Mexico. It was considered that this was the consequence of the widespread and indiscriminant use of this drug which selected for resistance to itself in the gut flora. Chloramphenicol is the antibiotic of choice in the treatment of typhoid fever but the development of resistant *S. typhi* limited treatment to ampicillin and septrin, drugs not considered to be nearly as successful in treatment of this infection (Anderson and Smith, 1972). Strains of *S. typhi* carrying transferable chloramphenicol resistance have been isolated subsequently in India, Vietnam and Thailand (Anderson, 1974). Enteric infections by salmonella food-poisoning organisms and *Shigella*, which are usually limited to the alimentary tract, are rarely treated with antibiotics in man; their use often prolongs the period of excretion but, should a systemic infection with a resistant strain of salmonella arise, treatment may be rendered difficult.

Many enteropathogenic *E. coli* are multiply resistant and therapy may be seriously limited to such drugs as polymyxin, instead of neomycin and kanamycin the drugs of preference. In these infections antibiotic therapy may not be indicated or necessary but in neonatal infections which may prove fatal, as in the Middlesborough outbreak, the limited choice of antibiotics may prove extremely serious (Anderson, 1968c).

The treatment of nosocomial infections, frequently caused by resistant enteric bacteria, may limit the choice of the antibiotic used; the resistance spectrum is not so wide as to render treatment impossible but is more complicated (Anderson, Datta and Shaw, 1972). A small number of cases of neonatal meningitis has been reported by *E. coli* resistant to kanamycin (McCracken, 1971). However, few strains have been found resistant to gentamycin the antibiotic of choice.

Urinary tract infections are by far the commonest infection caused by *E. coli.* Sulphonamide therapy is the drug of choice. However, a high proportion of infections by sulphonamide-resistant strains are being reported (Gillespie *et al.*, 1971, Shaw *et al.*, 1973). This observation is of interest in the light of the large numbers of sulphonamide-resistant *E. coli* found in animals and poultry (*Table 26.3*). Resistance is not a serious problem in these infections since a choice of other agents is available but sulphonamides cannot be used.

In summary, the main difficulty in the treatment of human infections with resistant *E. coli* is to limit the choice of antibiotic for therapy. Generally the resistance spectrum is not so wide as to render treatment impossible. The alternative treatment however may be more costly and could necessitate the choice of an antibiotic having additional and undesirable side effects. The majority of non-systemic enteric infections in man should not need antibiotic therapy and therefore no immediate problem arises with infections by resistant strains. R-factor mediated resistance may cause grave problems in the treatment of a limited number of conditions, particularly neonatal enteritis, meningitis and systemic salmonella infections and enteric fevers.

An Appraisal of the Hazards and Advantages of Antibiotics

The very large reservoirs of antibiotic-resistant *E. coli* in certain farm animals and in poultry must reflect antibiotic use. It was hoped that after the Swann recommendations were implemented, prohibiting the use of clinically useful antibiotics for growth promotion, the incidence of antibiotic resistance in farm animals would decline. This has not been realized (Smith, 1975). There is in fact little indication that the overall sales of antibiotics for veterinary use has decreased as a consequence of the Swann report and it is probable that farm animals are receiving just as much antibiotic at the present time ostensibly for different purposes. In addition to their continued use therapeutically large amounts are being used prophylactically. As a consequence of intensive methods of husbandry, the prophylactic use of antibiotics to counteract some of the disease risks involved, is vital. Such use builds up reservoirs of resistant organisms equally as well as antibiotics used for growth promotion. The prophylactic use of sulphonamides to prevent coccidiosis (Heller and Smith, 1973) is largely responsible for the high proportion of *E. coli* in poultry being resistant to this chemotherapeutic agent. Synthetic agents, which do not select for antibiotic resistance (Linton, Howe and Osborne, 1975) are being successfully used in growth promotion and possibly similar agents should be developed for prophylaxis.

The situation in animals also has its parallels in man. Antibiotic therapy establishes resistant populations in the gut of man and this is particularly so in hospitals where antibiotics are widely used. Cross-infection with resistant bacteria in hospitals is a constant hazard to patients especially those undergoing surgery. Fortunately, cross-infection with resistant organisms is rarely experienced outside hospital where the majority of people live. Nevertheless people, even outside hospitals whether receiving antibiotics or not, carry at least a minority of resistant *E. coli* in their gut. These may be of little importance in the healthy individual but should infection occur with *E. coli*, such as in women with a predisposition for urinary tract infection, the chances of the strain being resistant are increased. The gut flora in man is not as saturated with R-plasmids as in the flora of pigs, calves and poultry. However, since the use of antibiotics will inevitably select for resistance and these could be of significance to the individual sooner or later, the use of antibiotics must be scrupulously regulated.

Human infections with resistant organisms may present difficulties in therapy and therefore the resistant flora in man must be restricted as far as possible. The question therefore arises as to the importance of the animal reservoir for man. Any cross-infection ultimately derived from farm animals will be additive to that already cycling by cross-infection in man himself. Resistant *E. coli* in farm animals and in poultry cannot be distinguished from those regularly colonizing the human gut and causing infections in man. It seems highly probable that substantial numbers of *E. coli* are able to reach man by way of the food chain. This route has been well established for salmonella and the evidence strongly indicates a similar truth for *E. coli.* It is therefore essential that every attempt must be made to reduce the total load of resistant *E. coli* for man. This must involve the scrupulous use of antibiotics both in man and in animals for whatever purpose. The evidence to date confirms the views of the Swann Committee prohibiting the use of antibiotics of clinical importance for growth promotion in animals, and possibly this prohibition should be extended to their use for prophylaxis and generally to reduce their use for all non-therapeutic purposes.

Acknowledgments

The author wishes to acknowledge numerous helpful discussions with Professor Mark Richmond, Keith Linton, Christine Hartley, Kay Howe, Dudley Osborne and Vasso Petrocheilou. The combined research of this group, together with the expert technical assistance of Helen Clements, Barbara Handley and their colleagues has made possible this appraisal of a broad and contentious subject. The work was supported by grants from the Medical and Agricultural Research Councils.

References

ANDERSON, E.S. (1968a). *Ann. Rev. Microbiol.*, **22**, 131

ANDERSON, E.S. (1968b). *Brit. Med. J.*, **3**, 333

ANDERSON, E.S. (1968c). *Brit. Med. J.*, **1**, 293

ANDERSON, E.S. (1974). *J. Hyg., Camb.*, **74**, 289

ANDERSON, E.S., DATTA, N. and SHAW, E.J. (1972). *Brit. Med. J.*, **3**, 82

ANDERSON, E.S. and SMITH, H.R.(1972). *Brit. Med. J.*, **3**, 329

ANDERSON, J.D. (1974). *J. med. Microbiol.*, **8**, 83

ANDERSON, J.D., GILLESPIE, W.A. and RICHMOND, M.H. (1973a). *J. med. Microbiol.*, **6**, 461

ANDERSON, J.D., INGRAM, L.C., RICHMOND, M.H. and WIEDEMANN, B. (1973b). *J. med. Microbiol.*, **6**, 475

ANSON, A. (1976). Ph.D. Thesis, Bristol

BABCOCK, G.F., BERRYHILL, D.L. and MARSH, O.H. (1973). *Appl. Microbiol.*, **25**, 21

BETTELHEIM, K.A., BUSHROD, A.M., CHANDLER, E., COOKE, E.M., O'FARRELL, S. and SHOOTER, R.A. (1974). *J. Hyg., Camb.*, **73**, 467

BULLING, E. and STEPHAN, R. (1971). *Zbl. Vet. Med. B.*, **18**, 449

BURTON, G.C., HIRSH, D.C., BLENDEN, D.C. and ZEIGLER, J.L. (1974). In *The Normal Microbial Flora of Man*, p. 241. Symposium No. 3. Soc. Appl. Bacteriol. Eds Skinner, F.A. and Carr, J.G. Academic Press, London and N.Y.

COOKE, E.M., HETTIARATCHY, I.G.T. and BUCK, A.C. (1972). *J. med. Microbiol.*, **5**, 361

COOKE, E.M., SHOOTER, R.A., BREADON, A.L. and O'FARRELL, S.M. (1971). *Lancet*, **2**, 8

COOKE, E.M., SHOOTER, R.A., KUMAR, P.J., ROUSSEAU, S.A. and FOULKES, A.L. (1970). *Lancet*, **1**, 436

DATTA, N. ,(1969). *Brit. Med. J.*, **2**, 407

DATTA, N., FAIERS, M.C., REEVES, D.S., BRUMFITT, W., ORSKOV, F. and ORSKOV, I. (1971). *Lancet*, **1**, 312

DORN, C.R., TSUTAKAWA, R.K., FEIN, D., BURTON, G.C. and BLENDEN, D.C. (1975). *Am. J. Epidemiol.*, **102**, 319

EDWARDS, S.J. (1961). *J. Comp. Path.*, **71**, 243

EDWARDS, S.J. (1962). *J. Comp. Path.*, **72**, 420

EWING, W.H. and DAVIS, B.R. (1961). CDC Publication, Communicable Disease Centre, Atlanta, p. 1

FEIN, D., BURTON, G., TSUTAKAWA, R. and BLENDEN, D.C. (1974). *J. inf. Dis.*, **130**, 274

FRANKLIN, T.J. (1967). *Biochem. J.*, **105**, 371

GAGE, P., GUNTHER, C.B. and SPAULDING, E.H. (1961). *Bacteriol. Proc.*, p.117

GARDNER, P. and SMITH, D.H. (1970). *N. Engl. J. Med.*, **282**, 161

GILLESPIE, W.A., LEE, P.A., LINTON, K.B. and ROWLAND, A.J. (1971). *Lancet*, **2**, 675

GOLDBERG, H.S., GOODMAN, R.N., LOGUE, J.T. and HANDLER, F.P. (1961). *Antimic. Ag. Chemo.*, **p. 80**

GRABOW, W.O.K. and PROZESKY, O.W. (1973). *Antimic. Ag. Chemo.*, **3**, 175

GRUNEBERG, R.N., LEIGH, D.A. and BRUMFITT, W. (1968). In *Urinary Tract Infection*, p. 68. Eds O'Grady, F. and Brumfitt, W. Oxford University Press

GUINEE, P.A.M. (1963). Ph.D. Thesis, Utrecht

GUINEE, P.A.M. (1972). *Ann. N.Y. Acad. Sci.*, **182**, 40

GUINEE, P.A.M., UGUETO, N.R. and LEEUWEN, N. VAN (1970). *Appl. Microbiol.*, **20**, 531

GUINEE, P.A.M., UGUETO, N.R. and LEEUWEN, W.J. VAN (1971). *Ned. T. Geneesk*, **115**, 998

HARTLEY, C.L. (1975). Ph.D. Thesis, Bristol

HARTLEY, C.L., HOWE, K., LINTON, A.H., LINTON, K.B. and RICHMOND, M.H. (1975). *Antimicrob. Ag. Chemo.*, **8**, 122

HARTLEY, C.L. and RICHMOND, M.H. (1975). *Brit. Med. J.*, **4**, 71

HEEVER, L.W. VAN DEN (1972). *J.S. Afr. Vet. Ass.*, **43**, 71

HELLER, E.D. and SMITH, H.W. (1973). *J. Hyg., Camb.*, **71**, 771

HIRSH, D.C., BURTON, G.C. and BLENDEN, D.C. (1973). *Antimic. Ag. Chemo.*, **4**, 69

HOWE, K. and LINTON, A.H. (1976). *J. appl. Bact.*, **40**, 317

HOWE, K., LINTON, A.H. and OSBORNE, A.D. (1976a). *J. appl. Bact.*, **40**, 331

HOWE, K., LINTON, A.H. and OSBORNE, A.D. (1976b). *J. appl. Bact.*, **41**, 37

JONSSON, M. (1974). *Scand. J. inf. Dis.*, **6**, 339

KASUYA, M. (1964). *J. Bact.*, **88**, 322

KELLY, W.R., MOORHOUSE, E.C. and COLLINS, J.D. (1971). *J. Irish Med. Assoc.*, **64**, 29

KIM, T.K. and STEPHENS, J.F. (1972). *Poultry Science*, **51**, 1165

KNOTHE, V.H. (1963). *Deut. Med. Wochenschr.*, **88**, 1469

KOONKHAMLERT, C. and SAWYER, W.D. (1973). *Antimic. Ag. Chemo.*, **4**, 198

LACEY, R.W. (1975). *J. Antimicrob. Chemother.*, **1**, 25

LARSEN, H.E. and LARSEN, J.L. (1972). *Nord. vet. Med.*, **24**, 651

LARSEN, J.L. and NIELSEN, N.C. (1975). *Nord. vet. Med.*, **27**, 353

LEBEK, G. (1972). *1st Int. Symp. Infectious Antibiotic Resistance, Czechoslovakia*, p. 47. Eds Krcmery, V., Rosival, V. and Watanabe, T. Springer, Berlin

LEE, J.A. (1974). *J. Hyg., Camb.*, **72**, 185

LEVY, S.B., FITZGERALD, G.B. and MACONE, A.B. (1976). *Nature*, **260**, 40

LINTON, A.H., HOWE, K. and OSBORNE, A.D. (1975). *J. appl. Bact.*, **38**, 255

LINTON, K.B., LEE, P.A., RICHMOND, M.H., GILLESPIE, W.A., ROWLAND, A.J. and BAKER, V.N. (1972). *J. Hyg., Camb.*, **70**, 99

LINTON, K.B., RICHMOND, M.H., BEVAN, R. and GILLESPIE, W.A. (1974). *J. med. Microbiol.*, **7**, 91

LOKEN, K.I., WAGNER, L.W. and HENKE, C.L. (1971). *Am. J. vet. Res.*, **32**, 1207

McCRACKEN, G.H.(1971). *J. Ped.*, **78**, 942

McVAY, L.V. (1952). *J. clin. Investig.*, **31**, 27

MEEVOOTISOM, V. and SAWYER, W.D. (1973). *J. Med. Assoc. Thai.*, **56**, 732

MERCER, H.D., POCURULL, D., GAINES, W., WILSON, S. and BENNETT, J.V. (1971). *Appl. Microbiol.*, **22**, 700

MITSUHASHI, S., HASHIMOTO, H. and SUZUKI, K. (1967). *J. Bact.*, **94**, 1166

MOORHOUSE, E.C. (1969). *Brit. Med. J.*, **2**, 405

MOORHOUSE, E.C., O'GRADY, M.F. and O'CONNOR, H. (1969). *Lancet*, **2**, 50

MOORHOUSE, E.C., O'GRADY, M.F. and O'CONNOR, H. (1970). *Lancet*, **2**, 664

NOAH, N.D. (1975). *Brit. Med. J.*, **4**, 714

PETROCHEILOU, V. and RICHMOND, M.H. (1976). *Antimic. Ag. Chemo.*, **9**, 1

REGNIER, A.P. and PARK, R.W.A. (1972). *Nature*, **239**, 408

RENAULT, L., RAYNAND, J.P., BRETHAAU, H., AYCARDI, J., ROUX, J. and FERRANDO, R. (1973). *Rec. Med. Vet.*, **149**, 637

REPORT (1956). *Report of the coli-aerogenes (1956).* Sub-Committee of the Society for Applied Bacteriology

REPORT (1959). *J. Hyg., Camb.*, **57**, 435

REPORT (1969a). *The Bacteriological Examination of Water Supplies*, No. 17, 4th edn, H.M.S.O., London

REPORT (1969b). *Swann Committee.* Report of the Joint Committee on the Use of Antibiotics in Animal Husbandry and Veterinary Medicine. H.M.S.O., London

RICHMOND, M.H. (1972a). In *The Molecular Basis of Antibiotic Action,* Gale, E.F., Cundliffe, E., Reynolds, P.E., Richmond, M.H. and Warring, M.J. John Wiley, London

RICHMOND, M.H. (1972b). *J. appl. Bact.*, **35**, 155

ROLLINS, L.D., POCURULL, D.W., MERCER, H.D., NATZKE, R.P. and POSTLE, D.S. (1973). *J. Dairy Sci.*, **57**, 944

SALZMANN, T.C. and KLEMM, L. (1966). *Antimicrob. Ag. Chemo.*, **p.212**

SALZMANN, T.C. and KLEMM, L. (1968). *Proc. Soc. exp. Biol. Med.*, **128**, 392

SCHOTHORST, M. VAN, NORTHOLT, M.D. and KAMPELMACHER, E.H. (1976). *J. Hyg., Camb.*, **76**, 57

SHAW, E.J., PURSELL, R.E., DATTA, N. and BRUMFITT, W. (1973). *J. med. Microbiol.*, **6**, 451

SHOOTER, R.A., COOKE, E.M., O'FARRELL, S.M., BETTELHEIM, K.A., CHANDLER, M.E. and BUSHROD, F.M. (1974). *J. Hyg., Camb.*, **73**, 245

SHOOTER, R.A., COOKE, E.M., ROUSSEAU, S.A. and BREADEN, A.L. (1970). *Lancet*, **2**, 226

SIEGAL, D., HUBER, W.G. and DRYSDALE, S. (1974). *Antimic. Ag. Chemo.*, **8**, 538

SIEGAL, D., HUBER, W.R. and ENLOE, F. (1974). *Antimic. Ag. Chemo.*, **6**, 697

SMITH, D.H. and ARMOUR, S.E. (1966). *Lancet*, **2**, 15

SMITH, H.W. (1961). *J. appl. Bact.*, **24**, 235

SMITH, H.W. (1966). *J. Hyg., Camb.*, **64**, 465

SMITH, H.W. (1967). *N.Z. Vet. J.*, **15**, 153

SMITH, H.W. (1969). *Lancet*, **1**, 1174

SMITH, H.W. (1970a). *J. med. Microbiol.*, **3**, 165

SMITH, H.W. (1970b). *Nature*, **228**, 1286

SMITH, H.W. (1971a). *Nature*, **234**, 155

SMITH, H.W. (1971b). *Adv. vet. Sci.*, **15**, 67

SMITH, H.W. (1975). *Nature*, **258**, 628

SMITH, H.W. and CRABB, W.E. (1961). *J. path. Bact.*, **82**, 53

SMITH, H.W. and HALLS, S. (1966). *Brit. Med. J.*, **1**, 266

SMITH, M.G. (1975). *J. Hyg., Camb.*, **75**, 363

SOGAARD, H. (1973). *Acta. Vet. Scand.*, **14**, 381

SOMPOLINSKY, D., YARON, V. and ALKAN, W.J. (1967). *Am. J. Proctocol.*, **18**, 471

STEPHAN, V.R. and BULLING, E. (1971). *Berl. Münch. Tierärztl Wschr.*, **84**, 30

WALTON, J.R. (1966a). *Nature*, **211**, 312

WALTON, J.R. (1966b). *Lancet*, **2**, 1300

WALTON, J.R. (1970). *Lancet*, **2**, 561

WALTON, J.R. (1972). *Ann. N.Y. Acad. Sci.*, **182**, 358

WALTON, J.R. and LEWIS, L.E. (1971). *Lancet*, **2**, 255

WELLS, D.M. and JAMES, O.B. (1973). *J. Hyg., Camb.*, **71**, 209

WIEDEMANN, B. (1972). In *Bacterial Plasmids and Antibiotic Resistance*, p. 75. Eds Krčméry, V., Rosival, L. and Watanabe, T. Springer, Berlin

WIEDEMANN, B., KNOTHE, H. and HOLZER, P. (1970). *Zbl. Bakt. (Orig.)*, **212**, 97

WIERUP, M. (1975). *Nord. vet. Med.*, **27**, 77

WIERUP, M., LARSSON, K., HOLTENIUS, P., JACOBSSON, S.O. and MANSSON, I. (1975). *Nord. vet. Med.*, **27**, 253

27

ANTIBIOTIC RESISTANCE IN BACTERIA AND ASSOCIATED PROBLEMS IN FARM ANIMALS BEFORE AND AFTER THE 1969 SWANN REPORT

H. WILLIAMS SMITH
Houghton Poultry Research Station, Huntingdon

At the first Antibiotics in Agriculture Symposium, information was presented (Smith, 1962) indicating that the incidence of antibiotic resistance in bacteria pathogenic for farm animals had increased to a point at which it was complicating the therapy of disease in these animals. Although the therapeutic use of antibiotics was partly responsible, there was clear-cut evidence that the continuous feeding for growth promotional purposes of diets containing antibiotics was responsible for a high proportion of it. This applied particularly in the case of the very high incidence in pigs and poultry of penicillin- and tetracycline-resistant *Staphylococcus aureus* and tetracycline-resistant *Clostridium welchii* and pathogenic *Escherichia coli.* The feeding of tetracycline-containing diets, too, was profoundly influencing the ecology of the non-pathogenic *E. coli* that inhabit the alimentary tract of pigs and chickens in that the tetracycline-sensitive forms that had previously formed the bulk of these *E. coli* were being replaced by tetracycline-resistant forms. The effect on the national pig herd of Britain had become such that in 1957 a survey indicated that practically *all* the *E. coli* in the faeces of 36% of bacon pigs and 18% of market pigs were tetracycline-resistant (Smith and Crabb, 1957). Although this was of considerable ecological interest it was obviously not, at the time, of veterinary or medical interest. However, the gradual realization of the importance of the discovery by Japanese workers in 1959 of transmissible antibiotic resistance altered all that because it became apparent that the tetracycline-resistant non-pathogenic *E. coli* harboured by pigs and poultry fed tetracycline-containing diets might, in fact, constitute an enormous reservoir of tetracycline resistance, potentially transmissible to pathogenic *E. coli* and salmonellae and which might 'spill-over' from the animal community to the human community. These possibilities were made more likely by the finding in 1967 that the tetracycline resistance in most of the non-pathogenic *E. coli* in the alimentary tracts of pigs and poultry fed tetracycline-containing diets was indeed of the transmissible type – the tetracycline resistance was transmitted from 22 of 30 strains from pigs in different tetracycline-fed herds and from 27 of 30 strains from chickens in different tetracycline-fed flocks (Smith, 1971). A survey performed at about the same time on pathogenic strains of *E. coli* isolated from human beings or animals suffering from generalized infections or diarrhoea, too, revealed a high incidence of antibiotic resistance (*Table 27.1*). Many of these strains were multiply resistant, implying that the use of any one of the antibiotics to which they were resistant, particularly, for example, as a feed antibiotic would be expected to increase their number in the

Table 27.1 Incidence of antibiotic resistance in strains of *E. coli* isolated from diseased human beings and domestic animals (from Smith, 1966)

	Source					
Strains	*Human beings*	*Pigs* *1960–62*	*Pigs* *1965*	*Calves*	*Lambs*	*Chickens*
Number examined	70	70	70	100	25	35
% Resistant to:						
Tetracyclines	36.6	28.6	38.6	50.0	8.0	17.1
Streptomycin	35.3	11.4	40.0	52.0	8.0	2.9
Sulphonamides	33.0	8.6	22.9	57.0	12.0	17.1
Chloramphenicol	14.3	7.1	7.1	15.0	0	0
Ampicillin	18.6	0	0	14.0	4.0	0
Neomycin	4.3	0	7.1	5.0	0	0
Furazolidone	1.4	0	7.1	7.0	0	0
Polymyxin	0	0	0	0	0	0
Nalidixic acid	0	0	0	0	0	0
% Resistant to:						
One or more antibiotics	42.7	28.6	61.4	65.0	12.0	28.6
Two or more antibiotics	36.7	11.3	32.5	56.0	12.0	5.8
Three or more antibiotics	28.2	8.5	21.2	45.0	8.0	2.9
Four or more antibiotics	21.2	7.1	7.1	25.0	0	0
Five or more antibiotics	9.9	0	0	5.0	0	0
Six antibiotics	2.8	0	0	4.0	0	0

The pig strains were classified according to the period in which they were isolated. Results for cephalosporin C were the same as those for ampicillin, and those for kanamycin and framycetin the same as those for neomycin.

environment. The results for the pig strains were a good illustration of the general situation that was developing as a consequence of the continued use of antibiotics, i.e. a doubling of the proportion of resistant strains between 1960–62 and 1965 with the presence in the 1965 collection of strains resistant to two antibiotics, neomycin and furazolidone, to which all the strains in the 1960–62 collection were sensitive. In the 1960–62 collection, tetracycline resistance was the most common form of resistance, probably a reflection of the common use of tetracycline as feed additives for nutritional purposes. Nearly all of the tetracycline, chloramphenicol and neomycin resistance in the pathogenic human and animal strains was transmissible. So was the ampicillin resistance in two-thirds of the strains and most of the streptomycin and sulphonamide resistance in the multiply-resistant, but not in the singly-resistant, strains; it was not possible to transmit the furazolidone resistance of any of the strains. Also in Britain, Anderson (1965) and Anderson and Lewis (1965) demonstrated a great increase in the incidence of antibiotic resistance in *Salmonella typhimurium* from 1961 onwards until during the period December 1964 to February 1965, 61% of 450 strains of *S. typhimurium* examined were resistant to one or more antibiotics. At least 18 phage types of the organisms were represented amongst the resistant strains and a minimum of 14 patterns of antibiotic resistance was found. Some strains were resistant to as many as five antibiotics, these including ampicillin, streptomycin, tetracyclines, chloramphenicol, neomycin and sulphonamides. Resistance was most common among strains of phage type 29, a type considered to be bovine in origin. Of 4700 strains of *S. typhimurium* they received between December 1964 and October 1965, 1700 (36%) belonged to phage type 29; 1660 (97.6%) of these type 29 strains were resistant to one or more antibiotics. Originally sensitive to all antibiotics, resistance to streptomycin and sulphonamides appeared in type 29 strains received in 1963. Tetracycline resistance was added early in 1964. By June 1964, most strains of type 29 they examined were resistant to streptomycin, tetracycline and sulphonamides. Within a few months, ampicillin resistance was added to this pattern. Of the 1700 strains of type 29 received between December 1964 and October 1965, 500 were of human and 1200 of animal origin; the great majority of the animal strains had been isolated from calves. Evidence was presented indicating that the antibiotic resistance of these 1700 strains, which was mainly transmissible, had been acquired when the strains were resident in the calf population. A high incidence of resistance among strains of *S. typhimurium* that had been isolated from diseased calves in Britain was also reported by Stevens, Gibson and Hughes (1967); practically all the strains of phage type 29 they examined were resistant to tetracyclines, streptomycin and sulphonamides. The feeding of antibiotic-containing diets to calves for growth promotional purposes has never been permitted in Britain so this was not the reason for the antibiotic resistance reported by these workers. It is highly probable that the reason was the indiscriminate use of antibiotics in the prevention and treatment of calf diseases. It is significant in this respect that the sharp increase in incidence recorded by Anderson and Lewis (1965) coincided with the rapid devlopment of the intensive system of calf rearing in Britain, a system that involved the congregating together of large numbers of young calves from many different sources and in which antibiotics were used on a massive scale in attempting to combat the resulting high incidence of calf morbidity, *one* of the causal agents being salmonellae. Nevertheless, these observations, those on pigs and chickens fed antibiotic-containing diets and others (for review *see* Smith, 1971 and Appendix of U.S. Task Force Report, 1972) together with the fears of the possible implications of the then newly discovered transmissible resistance were largely responsible for the British Government setting up a committee of enquiry in 1968 under the Chairmanship of Sir Michael Swann. The main recommendation of their report, commonly referred to as the Swann Report, was that the antibiotics used as feed additives for growth promotion should be those that have little or no application as therapeutic agents in man or animals and that do not produce cross-resistance with antibiotics that are used for this purpose. This recommendation was implemented by the British Government in March 1971. The subject was also investigated by the Task Force of the Foods and Drugs Administration in the U.S.A. which reported in 1972, and by the World Health Organization which reported in 1974. Unlike the Swann Report the Task Force's report has not been implemented. Since the publication of this well documented report, numerous additional scientific papers on antibiotic resistance in animals have appeared that confirm and amplify the findings of those referred to in its appendices and in the review by Smith (1971). They include the papers of Aden *et al.*

(1969); Bulling and Stephan (1972); Bulling, Stephan and Sebek (1973); Fein *et al.* (1974); Guinée *et al.* (1972); Heever (1972); Hariharan, Barnum and Mitchell (1974); Kelly, Moorhouse and Collins (1971); Lakhotia and Stephens (1973); Larsen and Larsen (1975); Linton, Howe and Osborne (1975); Loken, Wagner and Henke (1971); Manten *et al.* (1971); Marsik, Parisi and Blenden (1975); Pohl *et al.* (1974); Pocunull, Gaines and Mercer (1971); Sato *et al.* (1975); Siegal, Huber and Enloe (1974); Smith (1970b); Sokol, Koppel and Mikula (1969); Sojka *et al.* (1972); Stephan and Bulling (1973); Swiderski and Lackowicz (1974); Vogd *et al.* (1973); and Wierup (1975). Several interesting facts emerge from these studies with regard to antibiotic-resistant strains of salmonellae isolated from domestic animals. These include the much higher incidence of such strains in the North American Continent, where antibiotics are used on a large scale, than in Europe, where they are used in a more restricted manner. In N. America this high incidence applies to salmonellae isolated from most species of domestic animals whereas in Europe a fairly high incidence is found in salmonellae isolated from calves and a low incidence in other domestic animals. In all surveys by far the highest incidence is found in *S. typhimurium*, although in some parts of Europe antibiotic resistance is also common in *Salmonella panama*. In Canada, Hariharan, Barnum and Mitchell (1974) found over 36% of 108 isolates of *S. typhimurium* from animals to be chloramphenicol-resistant; the incidence of such strains in surveys from other countries is low.

The Transfer of R-Factors in the Alimentary Tract of Domestic Animals

Although enormous populations of non-pathogenic *E. coli* with transmissible antibiotic resistance (R^+) become dominant in the alimentary tract of animals given antibiotics, especially as feed additives, the point of crucial importance is whether, and to what extent, their antibiotic resistance can be transferred to other enterobacteria, and especially to pathogenic enterobacteria. Efforts to transmit resistance experimentally in the alimentary tract of man and of laboratory animals have been largely unsuccessful unless the normal bacterial flora is modified by using gnotobiotic animals or by resorting to the selective use of antibiotics. Greater success has been achieved in domestic animals. Walton (1966), for example, demonstrated transfer by giving R^+ *E. coli* to chickens immediately after hatching when their alimentary tracts were sterile. Prospective recipient *E. coli* or *S. typhimurium* organisms were given 6 hours later, before food or water were made available. Later, Smith (1970b) achieved transfer, sometimes in epidemic form, in chickens with a normal alimentary flora. This was performed by giving cultures of R^+ *E. coli* to groups of chickens in their drinking water for the first 3 days of life. On the fourth day, they were given cultures of a smooth antibiotic-sensitive *S. typhimurium* strain, the prospective recipient strain, by mouth. Six days later they were killed and their faeces and livers were examined for the presence of recipient organisms that had acquired the R-factors of the prospective donor *E. coli* strain. Some of the results of attempts to transfer R-factors from different strains of *E. coli* to a strain of *S. typhimurium*, a strain known to be both a good recipient of R-factors *in vitro* and a good colonizer of the alimentary tract of chickens, are summarized in *Table 27.2*. The best *in vivo* donors were those that were best at donating *in vitro* and best at colonizing the alimentary tract (e.g. F21); no transfer was

Table 27.2 The transfer of R-factors in chickens from different strains of *E. coli* to *S. typhimurium* of phage type 36 (from Smith, 1970b)

Donor E. coli	*R-factor possessed*	*Ability to transmit R-factor* in vitro	*Ability to colonize chicken faeces*	*No. of 17 chickens whose faecal* S. typhimurium *had acquired the R-factor of the donor*
F21	T	Good	Good	16 (15)
F20	T	Poor	Good	0
B63	SSuCT	Moderate	Poor	0
F14	ASSuNTC	Poor	Poor	0

A = Ampicillin; S = streptomycin; Su = sulphonamides; N = neomycin; T = tetracyclines; C = chloramphenicol.
*The figures in brackets are the number of chickens in which all the *S. typhimurium* in their faeces had acquired R-factors.

detected when the donors were poor in either one or both of these respects (e.g. F20, B63 or F14). In chickens in which a high rate of transfer had occurred, it was common to find R^+ *S. typhimurium* organisms in the liver in addition to in the faeces, indicating that *S. typhimurium* organisms, after acquiring the R-factors of the *E. coli* in the alimentary tract, had then invaded the body. Viable counts performed on caecal contents of some of these chicks revealed that *S. typhimurium* organisms that had acquired R-factors outnumbered R^+ *E. coli*, thus providing additional evidence that the R-factor transfer observed was indeed taking place *in vivo* and not on the culture medium employed for its detection. *Table 27.3* compares the results of transferring the R-factor of the good *E. coli in vitro* donor, F17, to a selection of different strains of salmonellae. In view of the findings of the surveys referred to earlier, that the highest incidence of R-factors is found in *S. typhimurium*, it is not surprising that *S. typhimurium* strains were found to be the best salmonella recipients in these experiments. It is noteworthy, again in relation to these surveys, that the best recipient belonged to phage type 29, a type commonly isolated from calves. When diets containing antibiotics were fed at the same time as the transfer experiments were

Table 27.3 The transfer of R-factors from *E. coli* F17 to salmonella strains (from Smith, 1970b)

Recipient strain	*Ability to acquire R-factors* in vitro	*Ability to colonize chicken faeces*	*No. of 17 chickens with R+ recipient organisms in their faeces*
S. typhimurium phage type 29	Good	Good	16 (10)
S. typhimurium phage type 36	Good	Good	13 (7)
S. thompson	Poor	Good	3 (2)
S. arizonae	Poor	Good	0
S. anatum	Good	Poor	0
S. montivideo	Poor	Poor	0
S. gallinarum	Poor	Poor	1 (0)

The transmissible resistance pattern of F17 was ASNT. For other details *see Table 27.2.*

being performed, the usual outcome was a great increase in transfer rate if the donor organisms contained a resistance determinant for the antibiotic that was being fed and when this was the case and streptomycin or ampicillin were fed, the only *S. typhimurium* organisms found either in the faeces or livers of the chickens were resistant to these antibiotics.

Transfer can also be demonstrated *in vivo* by giving only prospective recipient organisms, antibiotics being administered at the same time to select out R^+ donor organisms present naturally in the environment in small numbers. An example of transfer achieved in this manner is demonstrated in *Table 27.4* (Smith and Tucker, 1975a). In this particular experiment groups of 40 chicks were given *S. typhimurium* orally and then fed continuously on diets containing 100 mg kg^{-1} of ampicillin. This profoundly depressed the concentration of *E. coli* in the alimentary tract of the chicks – two days after the commencement of the experiment they were only found in the faeces of one of them but the particular *E. coli* isolated possessed an R-factor determining resistance not only to ampicillin but also to streptomycin, sulphonamides, chloramphenicol, tetracyclines and spectinomycin (ASSuCTSp). At the next faecal examination, seven days later, and subsequently, high concentrations of *E. coli* were found in all the chicks in this group and practically all of them possessed the ASSuCTSp R-factor. A substantial depression of *S. typhimurium* had also occurred in the faeces of the chicks at 2 days. Much higher concentrations were found at 9 days, when ampicillin-resistant forms were detected for the first time. A high proportion of the *S. typhimurium* organisms isolated from these chicks at this, and at subsequent examinations, possessed the ASSuCTSp R-factor, R^+ *E. coli* and R^+ *S. typhimurium* were also found in the faeces of chicks in similarly designed experiments but in which streptomycin, chloramphenicol, tetracyclines or spectinomycin was administered instead of ampicillin. Many of these organisms possessed the ASSuCTSp R-factor, the whole experiment demonstrating that such organisms can become dominant in the alimentary tract of chicks infected experimentally with *S. typhimurium* and then exposed to any *one* of these five antibiotics. Furthermore, the R-factors were found in the *E. coli* populations of individual chicks before they were found in their *S. typhimurium* populations. It seems logical, therefore, to assume that very small numbers of *E. coli* possessing these R-factors were present in the alimentary tract of the chicks at the start of the experiment or gained access to it some time afterwards. There they ultimately achieved dominance owing to the selection pressure provided by the antibiotic-containing food. Later they transferred their R-factors to the *S. typhimurium* organisms in their alimentary tracts. These R^+ *S. typhimurium* organisms, in turn, came to dominate their sensitive counterparts, again owing to the selection pressure provided by the antibiotic-containing food.

Assessment of the Effect of the Swann Report

THE PERSISTENCE OF TETRACYCLINE-RESISTANT *E. COLI* IN THE PIG POPULATION

The main and immediate consequence of the implementation of the Swann Report by the British Government in March 1971 was the cessation of the then

Table 27.4 The isolation of *E. coli* and *S. typhimurium* from the faeces of groups of chickens experimentally infected with *S. typhimurium* and then fed a diet containing 100 mg kg^{-1} of ampicillin (from Smith and Tucker, 1975a)

Time* (days)	*Percentage of 40 chickens from which* E. coli *was isolated when fed a diet containing:* ampicillin >++	>50	>1	no antibiotic >++	>50	>1	S. typhimurium *was isolated when fed a diet containing* Ampicillin >+	>50	D	T	No antibiotic >+	>50	D	T
0	65	100	100 (0)	65	100	100 (0)	29	64	97	100 (0)	18	71	97	100 (0)
2	0	3	3 (3)	65	100	100 (0)	0	35	93	100 (0)	28	86	100	100 (0)
9	64	97	100 (94)	61	100	100 (0)	23	59	89	100 (40)	5	59	100	100 (0)
15	40	100	100(100)	73	100	100 (0)	16	39	82	100 (60)	15	44	100	100 (0)
21	57	100	100(100)	48	100	100 (0)	0	10	60	97 (63)	8	18	70	97 (0)
28	55	100	100(100)	35	100	100 (0)	0	10	41	69 (70)	3	16	61	84 (0)
35	67	100	100(100)	48	100	100 (0)	0	10	30	57 (80)	0	3	43	65 (0)
41	40	100	100(100)	25	100	100 (0)	0	3	7	34 (95)	3	19	24	43 (0)
Medicated food replaced by ordinary food on day 46														
48	62	100	100(100)	40	100	100 (0)	0	17	27	47 (95)	0	8	11	21 (0)
56	70	100	100(100)	15	100	100 (0)	0	0	7	7(100)	0	3	5	13 (0)

*After the commencement of feeding medicated diets, 3 days after orally infecting the chickens when 3 days old with *S. typhimurium.*
T = *S. typhimurium* isolated by selenite enrichment or by direct culture (D). 1 or 50 = 1 or 50 colonies of *S. typhimurium* or *E. coli* grew on the culture plate used for this purpose; + = culture plate covered by mainly discrete colonies; ++ = covered by semi-confluent colonies.
The figures in brackets are the percentage of positive faecal specimens in which were detected organisms with an R-factor determining resistance to ampicillin, streptomycin, sulphonamides, chloramphenicol, tetracyclines and spectinomycin.

common practice of feeding pigs and table poultry on diets containing tetracyclines for the purpose of growth promotion. This had no obvious impact on the nutritional status of these animals, probably because other growth promoting antibiotics such as bacitracin, virginiamycin, nitrovin and flavomycin soon became available. It might, however, have been expected to have had an impact on the ecology of the enormous populations of tetracycline-resistant *E. coli* known to be present in the pigs and poultry of Britain at that time, because these *E. coli* owed their upsurge to dominance largely to the widespread use of tetracyclines as feed additives during the previous 17 or so years. This subject has been investigated by Smith (1973, 1975) who monitored the incidence of antibiotic-resistant *E. coli* in the faeces of pigs exposed for sale in Chelmsford market from 1956 to 1975. On each occasion, individual faecal specimens from 100 pigs in different pens were examined; this ensured that a high proportion of the pigs had come from different farms. The results are summarized in *Table 27.5*; those for examining a selection of the strains for transmissible tetracycline resistance are shown in *Table 27.6*. It is probable that the substantial amount of tetracycline-resistant *E. coli* found in the 1956 survey was mainly the consequence of the first few years of use of tetracyclines as feed additives and the much greater amount in the 1970 survey the consequence of their continued use. If these results are typical of the position in Britain as a whole, then in 1970 the dominant *E. coli* organisms in the pig population were tetracycline-resistant ones, usually possessing conjugation ability and, as such, potentially able to transmit plasmids other than those coding for tetracycline resistance. In the four years since prohibition, the *amount* of tetracycline-resistant *E. coli* in the pig population might have decreased slightly but the incidence of pigs excreting these organisms (100% in 1975) had not. The failure of prohibition to achieve a greater impact, also noted on individual pig farms (*Table 27.6*), may be because during the long period in which the *E. coli* in the pig population had been exposed to tetracyclines, resistant strains had emerged which were now able to compete on equal terms with sensitive strains. The decrease since 1970 in the proportion of tetracycline-resistant strains whose resistance was transmissible (*Table 27.7*) suggests that, in a comparatively tetracycline-free environment, possession of a mechanism for transmitting tetracycline resistance is, in general, disadvantageous. The continued veterinary use of tetracycline could also have contributed to the failure. The veterinary use of streptomycin and sulphonamides was undoubtedly responsible for a substantial amount of the streptomycin and sulphonamide resistance arising during the study period because these two antibiotics have never been used in pigs as feed additives. The use of either antibiotic could have contributed to this situation because of 144 streptomycin-resistant strains isolated from different pigs in the 1972–75 surveys, 127 were also sulphonamide-resistant, probably because streptomycin and sulphonamide resistance are commonly linked on the same plasmid. The use of these antibiotics could also have made some contribution to the survival of tetracycline-resistant *E. coli* because 63 of the 144 strains previously mentioned were tetracycline-resistant, and 28 of 146 strains which had been selected because they were tetracycline-resistant were also streptomycin-resistant. The use of streptomycin was probably largely responsible for the finding of *E. coli* organisms resistant to the comparatively rarely used spectinomycin, all of 27 spectinomycin-resistant

Table 27.5 Antibiotic sensitivity of *E. coli* in faecal specimens of pigs (from Smith, 1975)

Antibiotic	*Year when specimens were collected*	*% of specimens in which the* E. coli *were:* *All resistant*	*Resistant & sensitive*	*Nearly all sensitive*	*All sensitive*
Oxytetracycline	1956	18	13	22	47
	1970	64	22	7	7
	1972	36	41	16	7
	1973	23	62	13	2
	1974	25	53	18	4
	1975	41	52	7	0
Streptomycin	1956	0	0	2	98
	1970	15	45	20	20
	1972	7	42	30	21
	1973	10	58	22	10
	1974	8	54	24	14
	1975	13	55	25	7
Sulphonamides	1956	2	2	4	92
	1970	12	32	18	38
	1972	5	41	29	25
	1973	10	58	22	10
	1974	13	48	21	18
	1975	14	51	26	9
Chloramphenicol	1956	0	0	0	100
	1970	0	3	2	95
	1972	0	1	3	96
	1973	0	8	19	73
	1974	0	4	30	66
	1975	0	0	8	92
Ampicillin	1970	1	20	15	64
	1972	0	12	18	70
	1973	0	24	35	31
	1974	0	20	48	32
	1975	2	16	51	31
Neomycin	1970	1	1	5	93
	1972	0	1	1	98
	1973	0	5	7	88
	1974	1	0	7	92
	1975	1	2	5	92
Furazolidone	1970	1	3	4	92
	1972	1	1	6	92
	1973	0	4	13	83
	1974	0	0	2	98
	1975	0	0	1	99
Spectinomycin	1972	3	20	26	51
	1973	1	23	34	42
	1974	1	16	31	52
	1975	0	4	43	53
Polymyxin, trimethoprim and sodium nalidixate	1972 1973 1974 1975	0	0	0	100

Table 27.6 Persistence of tetracycline-resistant *E. coli* among the faecal flora of pigs after the withdrawal of tetracycline feeding (from Smith and Crabb, 1957)

		Number of 10 faecal specimens in which the E. coli *were:*				
Farm number	*Time*	*All resistant*	*Largely resistant*	*Mainly resistant*	*Nearly all sensitive*	*All sensitive*
1	Before withdrawal	10	0	0	0	0
	7 months after withdrawal	1	6	2	1	0
2	Before withdrawal	8	2	0	0	0
	7 months after withdrawal	8	2	0	0	0
3	Before withdrawal	10	0	0	0	0
	7 months after withdrawal	9	1	0	0	0
4	Before withdrawal	10	0	0	0	0
	7 months after withdrawal	10	0	0	0	0

The feeding of diets containing tetracyclines had been practised on these farms for 2 years.

strains isolated from different pigs also being streptomycin-resistant, a consequence of the fact that one form of plasmid-determined streptomycin resistance is mediated through an adenylating enzyme that inactivates spectinomycin in addition to streptomycin. That no *E. coli* organisms resistant to trimethoprim, polymyxin or nalidixic acid were isolated in any of the surveys was probably a reflection of the very low degree of exposure of the pig population to these antibiotics.

The failure of prohibition of the growth promotion use of tetracyclines to markedly reduce the amount of tetracycline-resistant *E. coli* in the pig population stresses the fallacy of assuming that the ecological changes brought about largely by the persistent and widespread use of antibiotics can be reversed simply by resorting to a policy of withdrawal. It serves also to emphasize the need of strict adherence to the main recommendation of the Swann Report when the use of *new* antibiotics is being considered.

Table 27.7 Incidence of transmissible resistance in *E. coli* strains isolated at different times (from Smith, 1975)

Resistance studied	*Year of isolation*	*No. of resistant strains examined*	*% whose resistance was transmissible*
Tetracycline	1970	30	73
	1972	30	60
	1974	50	32
	1975	50	36
Streptomycin	1970	0	0
	1972	28	46
	1974	50	28
	1975	50	40

THE EFFECT OF DIETS CONTAINING PERMITTED ANTIBIOTICS ON SALMONELLA EXCRETION

Following the prohibition of the use of 'therapeutic' antibiotics as feed additives for growth promotion in Britain in 1971, other antibiotics were permitted to be used for this purpose. These included bacitracin, virginiamycin, nitrovin and flavomycin.

Although these antibiotics are not active against enterobacteria, they are active against many of the other bacteria that inhabit the alimentary tract. Consequently their use as feed additives might disturb the ecological balance in the alimentary tract in favour of the enterobacteria, particularly the salmonellae. The results of an experiment to investigate this possibility are summarized in *Table 27.8*. Groups of 45 chicks were infected with *S. typhimurium* three days after they were put on a diet containing 10 or 100 mg kg^{-1} of different permitted antibiotics, and the concentration of *S. typhimurium* organisms in their faeces estimated at different times afterwards. Tylosin was included in this investigation because it is used in some countries for growth promotion. The amount and duration of excretion of these organisms by the groups fed flavomycin, tylosin and nitrovin was much greater than by the group fed antibiotic-free diet, this being especially so in the case of both groups fed the tylosin-containing diets and the group fed the diet containing 100 mg kg^{-1} of nitrovin. The amount of *S. typhimurium* organisms excreted by groups fed virginiamycin and bacitracin was only slightly greater than that in the group fed antibiotic-free diets (the results for the 100 mg kg^{-1} level of these antibiotics are not shown in the table). These experiments were repeated on several occasions. In the groups fed diets containing bacitracin or virginiamycin, the amount of *S. typhimurium* organisms they excreted were, at the most, only slightly greater than that excreted by the groups fed antibiotic-free diets. All four groups fed diets containing 100 mg kg^{-1} of nitrovin excreted much greater amounts – an example of the quantitative extent of this excretion is given in *Table 27.9*; so did some, but not all of the groups fed diets containing flavomycin, tylosin or 10 mg kg^{-1} of nitrovin, the differing results obtained with the same antibiotic only being noted when the tests with that antibiotic were performed on different occasions. These differing results may well be a reflection of differences in the resident alimentary bacterial flora of the chickens employed on the different occasions. Because chickens are an important source of food poisoning for human beings, it is apparent then that in assessing the suitability of an antibiotic for growth promotion use account should be taken of its effect on salmonella excretion. With this in mind it is suggested that consideration be given to enlarging the main recommendation of the Swann Report by stating that, apart from satisfying the criteria already laid down, antibiotics used for growth promotion should also not favour the colonization of the alimentary tract by salmonellae.

Acknowledgment

I am grateful to Mrs. Margaret Webster for her help with the preparation of this manuscript.

Table 27.8 The isolation of *S. typhimurium* from the faeces of groups of experimentally infected chickens fed diets containing 10 or 100 mg kg^{-1} of different antibiotics (from Smith and Tucker, 1975b)

Time (days)*	*Virginiamycin* (10 mg kg^{-1})		*Bacitracin* (10 mg kg^{-1})		*Flavomycin* (10 mg kg^{-1})		*Flavomycin* (100 mg kg^{-1})		*Tylosin* (10 mg kg^{-1})		*Tylosin* (100 mg kg^{-1})		*Nitrovin* (10 mg kg^{-1})		*Nitrovin* (100 mg kg^{-1})		*No antibiotics*	
	D	T	D	T	D	T	D	T	D	T	D	T	D	T	D	T	D	T
5	94	100	97	100	97	100	94	100	97	100	97	100	94	100	97	100	91	100
14	88	97	86	100	90	100	73	97	97	100	79	100	94	100	91	97	94	97
21	30	67	36	71	80	93	58	88	88	91	57	78	78	100	76	93	50	73
28	48	69	20	40	50	97	38	69	64	97	32	63	49	85	65	86	27	31
35	0	11	14	43	46	86	47	75	54	90	25	44	45	94	52	85	4	8
42	14	17	4	16	42	88	55	88	70	100	63	94	82	89	83	100	8	8
49	0	0	0	28	38	78	41	77	80	100	57	94	23	65	70	97	4	4
56	0	7	0	7	15	40	28	60	67	97	57	94	20	50	65	97	0	0
63	0	4	7	14	7	75	36	55	76	96	50	88	20	48	97	97	0	4
70	4	7	0	0	7	7	10	40	83	90	73	94	0	29	25	71	0	0
77	0	0	0	0	3	3	3	7	66	86	53	97	0	0	37	75	0	0
84	0	0	0	0	14	14	3	7	40	82	79	96	0	4	4	35	0	0
91	0	4	0	0	0	0	0	7	11	32	41	58	0	0	8	35	0	0
98	0	0	0	0	0	0	0	3	11	18	4	18	0	0	8	32	0	0
105	0	0	0	0	0	0	3	7	7	7	0	10	0	0	4	28	0	0
112	0	0	0	0	0	0	0	3	7	7	4	4	0	0	4	4	0	0

Column heading: *% of chickens from which* S. typhimurium *was isolated when fed diets containing:*

*After the chickens were infected when 3 days old, antibiotic-containing food was fed from day 1.
D = *S. typhimurium* isolated by direct culture; T = by direct culture or following enrichment in selenite broth. At the commencement of the experiment each group consisted of 45 chickens.

Table 27.9 Concentration of *S. typhimurium* organisms in the faeces of chickens fed diets containing 100 mg kg^{-1} of nitrovin or no antibiotic (from Smith and Tucker, 1975b)

Time (days)	*% of chickens whose faeces had the following concentrations of* S. typhimurium *when fed diets containing:* Nitrovin (100 mg kg^{-1}) *>+*	*>50*	*D**	*T**	*No antibiotics >+*	*>50*	*D*	*T*
5	9	56	98	100	9	41	97	97
10	8	67	98	98	3	50	89	97
19	5	36	83	98	2	19	83	91
26	13	79	95	100	0	7	45	76
33	19	48	89	97	2	2	19	40
40	2	31	75	85	0	0	13	28
47	0	28	60	90	0	0	3	13
54	3	16	52	90	0	2	3	6
61	0	4	32	57	0	0	0	2
68	0	10	40	78	0	0	2	5
75	0	2	30	52	0	0	2	2
82	0	2	16	65	0	2	5	5
89	0	8	20	31	0	0	3	3
96	0	4	11	24	0	0	2	3
103	0	0	9	17	0	0	2	3
110	0	2	8	15	0	0	2	3
117	0	0	2	3	0	0	2	2

*T = *S. typhimurium* isolated by selenite enrichment or direct culture. D = isolated by direct culture; 50 = 50 colonies of *S. typhimurium* grew on the culture plate used for this purpose; + = the culture plate was covered with discrete colonies.
For other details and abbreviations *see Table 27.7.*

References

ADEN, D.P., REED, N.D., UNDERDAHL, N.R. and MEBUS, C.A. (1969). *App. Microbiol.,* **18**, 961
ANDERSON, E.S. (1965). *Nature,* **208**, 1016
ANDERSON, E.S. and LEWIS, M.J. (1965). *Nature,* **206**, 579
BULLING, E. and STEPHAN, R. (1972). *Zent. Vet. Med.,* **19B**, 268
BULLING, E., STEPHAN, R. and SEBEK, V. (1973). *Zent. Bakter. Parasit. Inf. und Hyg.,* **225**, 245
FEIN, D., BURTON, G., TSUTAKAWA, R. and BLENDEN, D.C. (1974). *J. inf. Dis.,* **130**, 274
GUINEE, P.A.M., FRIK, J., UGUETO, N.R., LEEUWEN, W.J. VAN and KOL, P.J. VAN (1972). *Tidj. Diergen.,* **97**, 705
HARIHARAN, H., BARNUM, D.A. and MITCHELL, W.R. (1974). *Can. J. comp. Med.,* **38**, 213
HEEVER, L.W. VAN DEN (1972). *J. S.A. Vet. Ass.,* **43**, 71
KELLY, W.R., MOORHOUSE, E.C. and COLLINS, J.D. (1971). *Irish Vet. J.,* **26**, 49
LAKHOTIA, R.L. and STEPHENS, J.F. (1973). *Poultry Sci.,* **52**, 2266
LARSEN, H.E. and LARSEN, J.L. (1975). *Nord. Vet. Med.,* **27**, 65
LINTON, A.H., HOWE, K. and OSBORNE, A.D. (1975). *J. appl. Bact.,* **38**, 255
LOKEN, K.I., WAGNER, L.W. and HENKE, C.L. (1971). *Am. J. vet. Res.,* **32**, 1207

MANTEN, A., GUINEE, P.A.M., KAMPELMACHER, E.H. and VOGD, C.E. (1971). *Bull. W.H.O.,* **45**, 85

MARSIK, F.J., PARISI, J.T. and BLENDEN, D.C. (1975). *J. inf. Dis.,* **132**, 296

POCUNULL, D.W., GAINES, S.A. and MERCER, H.D. (1971). *App. Microbiol.,* **21**, 358

POHL, P., THOMAS, J., LAUB, R. and ROBAEYS, G. VAN (1974). *Ann. Med. Vet.,* **118**, 252

SATO, G., FURUTA, Y., KODAMA, H., IWAO, T. and OKA, M. (1975). *Am. J. vet. Res.,* **36**, 839

SIEGAL, D., HUBER, W.G. and ENLOE, F. (1974). *Antimicrob. Agents and Chemother.,* **6**, 697

SMITH, H. WILLIAMS (1962). In *Antibiotics in Agriculture,* p. 374. Proc. Uni. Nottingham, 9th Easter School in Agricultural Science 1962. Butterworths, London

SMITH, H. WILLIAMS (1966). *J. Hyg.,* **64**, 465

SMITH, H. WILLIAMS (1970a). *J. med. Microbiol.,* **3**, 165

SMITH, H. WILLIAMS (1970b). *J. med. Microbiol.,* **3**, 181

SMITH, H. WILLIAMS (1971). *Adv. vet. Sci. comp. Med.,* **15**, 67

SMITH, H. WILLIAMS (1973). *Nature,* **243**, 237

SMITH, H. WILLIAMS (1975). *Nature,* **258**, 628

SMITH, H. WILLIAMS and CRABB, W.E. (1957). *Vet. Record,* **69**, 24

SMITH, H. WILLIAMS and TUCKER, J.F. (1975a). *J. Hyg.,* **75**, 275

SMITH, H. WILLIAMS and TUCKER, J.F. (1975b). *J. Hyg.,* **75**, 293

SOJKA, W.J., SLAVIN, G., BRAND, T.F. and DAVIES, G. (1972). *Br. Vet. J.,* **128**, 189

SOKOL, A., KOPPEL, Z. and MIKULA, L. (1969). *J. Hyg., Epidemiol., Microbiol., Immunol.,* **13**, 347

STEPHAN, R. and BULLING, E. (1973). *Zent. Bakter. Parasit. Inf. Hyg.,* **225**, 257

STEVENS, A.J., GIBSON, E.A. and HUGHES, L.E. (1967). *Vet. Record,* **80**, 154

SWANN REPORT (1969). Report of the Joint Committee on the use of antibiotics in animal husbandry and veterinary medicine. Cmnd 4190. H.M.S.O., London

SWIDERSKI, M. and LACKWICZ, T.M. (1974). *Acta Microbiol. Pol.,* **6A**, 152

U.S. TASK FORCE REPORT (1972). *The Use of Antibiotics in Animal Feeds.* Foods and Drugs Administration, U.S. Department of Health, Education and Welfare, Rockville, Maryland

VOGD, C.E., GUINEE, P.A.M., MANTEN, A. and VALKENBURG, J.J. (1973). *Antonie van Leeuwenhoek, J. Microbiol. Ser.,* **39**, 321

WALTON, J. (1966). *Nature, Lond.,* **211**, 312

W.H.O. REPORT (1974). *The Public Health Aspects of Antibiotics in Feed Stuff.* W.H.O., Copenhagen

WIERUP, M. (1975). *Nord. Vet. Med.,* **27**, 77

LIST OF PARTICIPANTS

Basler, Dr. W.	Ciba-Geigy AG, Switzerland
Brander, Prof. G.C.	Research Division, Beecham Pharmaceuticals, Walton Oaks, Dorking Rd, Tadworth, Surrey RH3 7AJ
Braude, Dr. R.	National Institute for Research in Dairying, Shinfield, Reading, Berks RG2 9AT
Bushby, Dr. S.R.M.	Wellcome Research Lanoratories, Research Triangle Park, 27709, North Carolina, U.S.A.
Buswell, Mr. J.F.	Research Division, Beecham Pharmaceuticals, Walton Oaks, Dorking Rd, Tadworth, Surrey RH3 7AJ
Coleman, Dr. K.	Research Division, Beecham Pharmaceuticals, Walton Oaks, Dorking Rd, Tadworth, Surrey RH3 7AJ
Corry, Dr. Janet	Metropolitan Police Forensic Science Laboratory, 109 Lambeth Road, London SE1 7LP
Doyle, Mr. F.P.	Director of Research, Beecham Pharmaceuticals, Brockham Park, Betchworth, Surrey
Drysdale, Dr. A.D.	B.P. Nutrition (U.K.) Ltd, Witham, Essex
Greenwood, Dr. D.	Department of Microbiology, University of Nottingham, City Hospital, Nottingham NG5 1PH
Harris, Miss Anne M.	Microbiology Division, Glaxo Research Ltd., Greenford UB6 0HE
Haxton, Miss Jane	Ministry of Agriculture, Fisheries and Food, (Food Science Division), Great Westminster House, Horseferry Road, London SW1
Hendy, Mr. P.G.	Glaxo Laboratories Ltd. (Veterinary Advisory Department), Greenford UB6 0HE

Hibbitt, Dr. K.G.	Institute for Research on Animal Diseases, Compton, Newbury, Berks
Howie, Sir James William	Knockmalloch, Newtonmore, Invernesshire, Scotland
Linton, Dr. A.H.	Department of Bacteriology, Medical School, University of Bristol, Bristol BS8 1TD
Lipińska, Dr. Ewa	Institute of Dairy Industry, Warsaw, Poland
Martin, Mr. B.	21 Hill Street, Kilmarnock, Ayrshire, Scotland
Martin, Dr. C.K.A.	Gesellschaft für Molekularbiologische Forschung mbH, Stöckheim über Braunschweig, West Germany
McCracken, Mrs Ann	Veterinary Research Laboratories, Stormont, Belfast BT4 3SD, Northern Ireland
Muggleton, Dr. P.W.	Microbiology Division, Glaxo Research Ltd., Greenford UB6 0HE
O'Grady, Prof. F.	Department of Microbiology, Medical School, City Hospital, Nottingham NG5 1PH
Palmer, Mr. G.H.	Research Division, Beecham Pharmaceuticals Ltd., Walton Oaks, Dorking Rd, Tadworth, Surrey RH3 7AJ
Palmer, Mr. V.M.	Research Laboratory, A. Guinness, Sons & Co., St. James's Gate Brewery, Dublin 8, Eire
Pearson, Dr. J.K.L.	Veterinary Research Laboratories, Department of Agriculture, Stormont, Belfast BT4 3SD, Northern Ireland
Ralovich, Dr. B.	Institute of Microbiology, University Medical School, Pécs, Hungary
Rosen, Dr. G.D.	Consultant, London
Seaman, Dr. A.	Department of Applied Biochemistry and Nutrition, Faculty of Agricultural Science, University of Nottingham, Sutton Bonington, Loughborough, Leics.
Shahamat, Mr. M.	Department of Microbiology, University of Tehran, Iran

Smith, Dr. H. Williams	Houghton Poultry Research Station, Huntingdon, Cambs PE17 2DA
Stockdale, Dr. H.	Fermentation Division, Shell Research Ltd., Sittingbourne, Kent
Sutherland, Mr. R.	Research Division, Beecham Pharmaceuticals, Brockham Park, Betchworth, Surrey
Syrett, Mr. R.F.	Microbiology Department, Ministry of Agriculture, Fisheries and Food, Newcastle-upon-Tyne NE1 2YA
Uvarov, Miss O.	British Veterinary Association, 7 Mansfield Street, London W1
Walton, Dr. J.R.	Veterinary Field Station, University of Liverpool, Wirral, Leahurst, L64 7TE
Webster, Mr. W.R.	Veterinary Services Branch, Department of Primary Industries, Brisbane, Australia
Welsby, Mr. D.	Kerry Co-op. Creameries Ltd, Listowel, Eire
White, Mr. G.	Wellcome Research Laboratories, Berkhamsted, HP4 2QE
Wilson, Dr. C.D.	Ministry of Agriculture, Fisheries and Food, (A.D.A.S.), Weybridge, Surrey
Witter, Prof. L.D.	Departments of Food Science and Microbiology, University of Illinois, Urbana, Illinois, U.S.A.
Wood, Mr. L.V.	Department of Applied Biochemistry and Nutrition, Faculty of Agricultural Science, University of Nottingham, Sutton Bonington, Loughborough, Leics.
Woodbine, Dr. M.	Department of Applied Biochemistry and Nutrition, Faculty of Agricultural Science, University of Nottingham, Sutton Bonington, Loughborough, Leics.
Wubishet, Mr. A.	College of Agriculture, Addis Ababa University, Ethiopia
Zwart Voorspuij, Dr. A.J.	Municipal Hospital, Dordrecht, The Netherlands

ORGANISM INDEX

Actinoplanes sp, 18
Aeromonas sp, 183–5, 187
Agrobacterium radiobacter, 35, 42
Aspergillus fischeri var. *glaber*, 275, 276, 278–83
flavus, 268
oryzae, 109
parasiticus, 109

Bacillus spp, 44
anthracis, 203
cereus, 109
var. *mycoides*, 36, 42, 240
circulans, 45
coagulans, 42, 115
polymyxa, 109
pumilus, 35, 42
stearothermophilus, 37, 42, 108, 112–5
var. *calidolactis*, 314
subtilis, 35–7, 44, 45, 105, 113
Bacterium anitratum (Acinetobacter calcoaceticus), 37
Bacteroides spp, 33, 317
fragilis, 34
Bordetella bronchiseptica, 39, 41
Brucella spp, 34
abortus, 70
Byssochlamys fulva, 275–7, 279–82
nivea, 275–9, 282, 283

Candida spp, 35
Citrobacter freundii, 70
Cladosporium spp, 37, 116
Clostridium botulinum, 36, 37, 41, 42, 45, 103, 111, 136
butyricum, 107, 115
nigrifaciens, 42
oedamatiens, 45
pasteurianum, 114, 115
perfringens (welchii), 32, 45, 70, 111, 136, 203, 261, 344
putrefaciens, 46
sporogenes, 36, 42, 45
thermosaccharolyticum, 42
Corynebacterium bovis, 203
diphtheriae, 39, 70

Corynebacterium (*cont.*)
pyogenes, 199, 203, 208, 217, 220, 235
renale, 43, 44, 201
Cytophaga spp, 34

Eimeria tenella, 65
Entamoeba histolytica, 40
Enterobacter aerogenes, 33, 34, 37–9, 70, 76
Erysipelothrix rhusiopathiae, 29, 30, 34, 70, 199–201
Escherichia coli, 8, 14, 33, 36, 37, 39, 40, 42, 43, 46, 58, 70, 72, 73, 75–7, 82–7, 94–7, 133, 134, 136, 183, 186, 187, 189, 190, 199–201, 205, 207, 208, 215, 218, 223, 235, 237, 251, 253, 259–63, 297–300, 313, 339, 344, 345, 347–53

Fusobacterium nucleatum, 36

Haemophilus spp, 70, 72
influenzae, 58, 70, 72, 73
parahaemolyticus, 208
Hansenula beyerinckii, 183, 190, 191

Klebsiella aerogenes, 14, 72
pneumoniae, 8, 70, 72

Lactobacillus acidophilus, 120, 122
casei, 64, 117
helveticus, 117, 122
Leptospira canicola, 201
Listeria monocytogenes, 30, 33, 44

Microbacterium thermosphactum, 34, 157–73
Micrococcus flavus, 112
luteus, 32
Micromonospora spp, 18
Monascus spp, 268
Moraxella lacunata, 70
Mycobacterium tuberculosis, 38, 40, 44, 70, 292
Mycoplasma spp, 34
gallisepticum, 200
suispneumoniae, 34

Neisseria gonorrhoeae, 70
meningitidis, 70
Neurospora crassa, 275, 283
Nocardia asteroides, 40, 70

Paecilomyces spp, 268
Pasteurella septica, 70
Plasmodium berghei, 65
gallinaceum, 65
Propionibacterium shermanii, 117, 118, 120
Proteus spp, 6, 33, 41, 43, 70, 76
mirabilis, 203
morganii, 96
vulgaris, 43, 66, 69, 72
Pseudomonas acidovorans, 37
aeruginosa, 34, 36–41, 46, 54, 59, 60, 70, 92–4, 98, 182, 251
fluorescens, 135
Pythium irregulare, 35
vexans, 35

Rhizobium spp, 34
Rhizopus nigricans, 35

Saccharomyces cerevisiae, 36, 37
pastorianus, 38
Salmonella spp, 33, 46, 111, 200, 201, 229, 354
anatum, 133, 348
arizonae, 37, 348
dublin, 229–31
gallinarum, 348
montivideo, 348
panama, 347
paratyphi, 39
senftenberg, 133
thompson, 348
typhi, 43, 70, 337, 338
thyphimurium, 36, 46, 70, 72, 208, 251, 316, 345–50, 354–6
Sarcina lutea, 36, 39, 112, 240, 242, 314
Serratia marcescens, 14, 36
Shigella spp, 38, 39, 43, 70, 337
flexneri, 36
sonnei, 72, 96
Staphylococcus aureus, 8, 14, 32, 37–40, 42, 43, 46, 62, 70, 72, 73, 111, 135, 139–56, 182, 183, 185, 187, 188, 199, 203, 222, 235–7, 246, 247, 249, 251, 252, 344
Streptococcus agalactiae, 33, 70, 199, 203, 218, 219, 222, 224, 235, 245–7
cremoris, 33, 117
diacetilactis, 117
dysgalactiae, 203
epidermidis, 240
equi, 201
faecalis, 8, 33, 36, 38–40, 58, 66, 70, 74, 77, 89–91, 201, 203
faecium, 33, 35, 133
lactis, 33, 103, 108–10, 112, 117–9
(mutants), 122
pneumoniae, 70, 72
pyogenes, 33, 40, 44, 70, 72
sanguis, 36
thermophilus, 33, 117, 122
uberis, 33, 203, 223
Streptomyces spp, 9, 13

Treponema hyodysenteriae, 207, 208
pallidum, 38
Trichophyton mentagrophytes, 37

Veillonella parvula, 36
Vibrio comma (cholerae), 70
costicolus (costicola), 34

Zygosaccharomyces nadsonii, 41
soya, 36

AUTHOR INDEX

Abou-Donia, M.M., 76, 81
Abd-el-Malek, Y., 139, 156
Abraham, E.P., 39
Abranches, P., 182, 195
Acar, J.F., 71, 79
Acred, P., 309, 314
Adair Doris, M., 40
Adams, D.M., 32, 136, 137, 175, 192
Adams, E.W., 245, 246, 254
Aden, D.P., 347, 356
Ades, G.L., 138
Ahmed, F.I.K., 36
Ahmed, Z., 43
Alder, V.G., 38
Alderton, G., 136, 137
Alexander, M., 137
Alford, J.A., 42, 46, 50
Alkan, W.J., 321, 343
Allen, A.R., 109, 126
Allwood, M.C., 132, 137, 138, 176–9, 192, 193, 195
Alper, T., 36
Altemeier, W.A., 222, 226
Ambanelli, G., 45
Amiel, J.L., 78, 81
Amyes, S.G.B., 75, 79
Anagnostopoulos, G.D., 133, 137
Anatskaya, A.A., 112, 113, 130
Anderson, A.A., 37
Anderson, E.S., 315, 317, 318, 337, 338, 340, 345, 346, 356
Anderson, J.C., 253, 254
Anderson, J.D., 73, 79, 316, 340
Anderson, J.M., 137
Andrassay, Eva, 41, 42
Andrews, W.H., 137
Andriole, V.T., 92, 98
Angelotti, R., 32
Anghern, P., 73, 74, 79, 81, 177, 192
Angier, R.B., 64, 79, 81
Anson, A., 322, 340
Apirion, D., 138, 180, 193
Arioli, V., 18, 23
Armour, S.E., 337, 342
Aronson, A.L., 222, 226
Arret, B., 240, 244
Arvilommi, H., 77, 81
Asan, T., 45
Ashwood-Smith, M.J., 180, 192
Asscher, A.W., 38
Attwell, R.W., 105, 126
Auerbach, Helen, 38
Aycardi, J., 325, 342

Babcock, G.F., 330, 340
Bahler, M.E., 44
Bailey, F.J., 110, 126
Baillie, M., 42
Baird-Parker, A.C., 32, 33, 42, 45, 137, 240, 244
Bajetta, E., 44, 50, 99
Baker, B.R., 67, 79
Baker, V.N., 321, 341
Baldini, P., 45
Ball, A.P., 76, 79
Barach, J.T., 32, 136, 137, 175, 192
Baran, W.L., 41
Baranova, I.P., 110, 126
Barber, M., 218, 226
Barber, R.S., 124, 126
Bardie, F., 222, 227
Barduta, Z., 111, 112, 122, 124, 127
Barker, J., 75, 79
Barnes, Ella M., 34
Barnett, M., 69, 72, 79, 229, 231
Barnum, D.A., 347, 356
Barr, F.S., 39, 42
Barrington, G.P., 270, 271
Basford, F.R., 65, 79
Batchelor, F.R., 39, 96, 99, 302–4
Bayer, M.E., 180, 192
Bean, P.G., 42
Beare-Rogers, J.L., 137
Beecham Research Laboratories, 39
Beerens, H., 178, 194
Beeuwkes, H., 39
Belitz, H.D., 109, 130
Belkropp, R.A., 141, 156
Bendall, M.J., 75, 80
Benedict, C.D., 138
Benedict, E.D., 138
Beng-thong Ho, 67, 79
Benians, M., 246, 247, 249–51, 254
Bennett, J.V., 317, 342
Berdy, J., 15, 17, 23

Beretta, G., 18, 23
Berryhill, D.L., 330, 340
Bertelsen, S., 230, 231
Bettelheim, K.A., 334, 340, 342
Bevan, R., 322, 330, 341
Bijok, E., 120, 129
Bille, N., 207–9
Billings, C.E., 40
Birch-Anderson, A., 94, 99
Bird, R.G., 259, 264
Birdsell, D.C., 180, 192
Birn, K.J., 222, 228
Bishop, A., 65, 79
Bissonnette, G.C., 137
Bissonnette, G.K., 137
Black, C.A., 139, 140, 156
Blanchard, C.J., 40
Blenden, D.C., 317, 321, 330, 340, 341, 347, 356, 357
Bliss, E.A., 177, 192
Blobel, H., 252, 254
Bloom, J., 94, 99
Blumberg, P.M., 94, 99
Boag, K., 157, 173
Board, R.G., 157, 173
Bockemühl, J., 33
Bodansby, M., 109, 126
Bogatko, J., 124, 129
Bogert, A.B., 138
Bogoroditskaya, V.P., 111, 130
Böhni, E., 72, 77, 79
Bokma, L.H., 43, 47, 56, 295
Bolin, H.R., 46, 50
Bonadonna, G., 44, 49, 50
Bondi, A., 177, 192
Bonet-Maury, P., 40
Boothe, J.H., 64, 79, 81
Boots Co., 43
Borg, A.I.F., 41
Borovsky, M.P., 39
Boswell, P.A., 32
Botstein, D., 137
Bottone, E.J., 176, 192
Boucher, R.M.G., 36, 37, 44
Boyd, B.L., 65, 80
Boyle, F.P., 46, 50
Boylen, C.W., 137
Bradley, S.G., 38
Brambilla, Cristina, 44, 49, 50
Bramley, A.J., 251, 255
Brand, T.F., 347, 357
Brander, G.C., 199, 205, 209, 220, 222, 226, 227
Brandman, Z., 176, 192
Brasamilino, E., 44, 49, 50
Braswell, J.R., 180, 192
Bratlie, O., 220, 226
Braude, R., 124, 126
Breadon, A.L., 321, 340, 342
Brecka, A., 110, 129
Breeze, A.S., 176, 177, 192, 193
Brethau, H., 325, 342
Bridges, B.A., 138, 180, 192
Briggs, A., 36
Brock, T.D., 35
Brooker, B.E., 250, 255
Bross, I., 38
Brours, M.F.J., 41
Brown, A.G., 98
Brown, G.M., 67, 76, 79, 81
Brown, M.R.W., 37, 175, 182, 192, 193
Brownlee, G., 29, 40
Brownlie, J., 251, 252, 254
Brugnatelli, Luise, 44, 49, 50
Brumfitt, J., 17, 23
Brumfitt, W., 92, 98, 321, 337, 338, 340, 341
Brzin, Bronka, 37, 51
Buchanan, R.L., 46, 51
Buck, A.C., 335, 340
Buckley, Helen R., 35
Bullin, C.H., 75, 81
Bulling, E., 317, 325, 340, 343, 347, 356
Bultz, J.K., 36
Burchall, J.J., 67–9, 79, 80
Burman, L., 94, 99
Burman, N.P., 33
Burns, J., 36
Burroughs, R., 267, 271
Burton, G., 330, 340, 347, 356
Burton, G.C., 317, 321, 330, 340, 341
Bushby, M.B., 73, 79
Bushby, S.R.M., 29, 41, 65–7, 69–74, 77, 79–81, 229–31
Bushrod, A.M., 334, 340, 342
Busta, F.F., 132, 133, 137, 138, 151, 156, 180, 182, 195
Buswell, J.F., 307
Butterworth, D., 98
Bywater, R.J., 311, 314

Cabenca-Silva, C., 182, 195
Calbert, H.E., 114, 126
Calia, F.M., 92, 99
Calinescu, S., 111, 112, 122, 124, 127
Calcott, P.H., 179, 194
Calnan, J.S., 230, 231
Cameron, J., 38, 40
Campanini, M., 107, 114, 115, 129
Campbell, C.K., 35
Campbell, J.N., 242–4
Camper, N.A., 35
Cantrell, H.F., 35
Cappel, R., 92, 98
Carleton, J., 176, 177, 193
Carmen, P.E., 43
Carrington, H.C., 65, 79
Carroll, D.E., 37
Carson, A.W., 157, 173

Casenio, J., 122, 130
Caserio, G., 175, 192
Casolari, A., 45, 107, 114, 115, 129
Cassara, A., 114, 115, 129
Cattan, A., 78, 81
Cawston, W.C., 69, 80
Červenka, J., 116, 128
Chabbert, Y.A., 71, 79
Chambers, G., 223, 227
Chandler, M.E., 177, 192, 334, 340, 342
Chapman, G.H., 32
Chapman, H.R., 143, 156
Charlson, R., 37
Chausler, W.J., 141, 156
Cheeseman, G.C., 104, 128
Chen, J.K., 136, 137
Chen, M., 137
Cheng, C.M., 137
Cheng, K.J., 261, 264
Chisholm, G.D., 230, 231
Chitu, M., 175, 193
Chudyk, R.V., 35
Ciegler, A., 41
Clara, J., 43
Clark, D.S., 182, 195
Clark, P.C., 182, 195
Clarke, D.A., 41
Clarke, J.H., 268, 271
Clarkson, J.B., 43
Claydon, T.J., 136, 137
Claypool, L., 109, 126
Clegg, L.F.L., 138, 175, 181, 182, 191, 194, 195
Cline, M.J., 252, 255
Coates, M.E., 124, 126
Cohen, S.N., 35
Cole, C.B., 245–7, 252, 254
Cole, M., 97, 98
Coleman, N., 65, 80
Coleman, Virginia R., 39, 47, 52, 53, 89, 98
Collins, J.D., 224, 227, 325, 341, 347, 356
Collins-Thompson, D.L., 133, 137, 157, 172, 173, 182, 193
Comber, K.R., 309, 314
Combs, Jean, 38
Conney, A.H., 43, 47, 51
Cook, A.M., 178, 192
Cooke, E.M., 322, 330, 334, 335, 340, 342
Cooke, W.B., 35
Cooney, J.J., 37
Cooper, E.A., 37
Coronelli, C., 18, 23
Corry, J.E.L., 132, 133, 137, 174, 175, 182, 192
Costerton, J.W., 261, 264
Cosulich, D.B., 64, 81
Cota-Robles, E.H., 180, 192
Covell, N.D., 109, 126
Crabb, W.E., 325, 330, 342, 344, 353, 357
Craig, W.A., 222, 227
Crawford, D.C., 41
Crichton, T.C., 82, 88
Crisley, F.D., 32
Cross, T., 105, 126
Crowshaw, B., 176, 192
Crowther, A.F., 65, 79
Cruickshank, R., 33, 34
Cullen, G.A., 246, 254
Cummings, D.J., 73, 79
Cundliffe, E., 47, 52, 179, 193
Curd, F.H.S., 65, 79
Curran, H.R., 36, 37, 175, 192
Curtis, N.A.C., 96, 99
Cuthbert, W.A., 139, 140, 156

Dabbah, R., 138
Dakin, J.C., 41, 42
Daniel, L.J., 66, 79
Darland,, G.K., 35
Darrell, J.H., 69, 72, 74, 80
Datta, N., 75, 78, 80, 321, 322, 337, 338, 340
Davey, D.G., 65, 79
Davidson, I., 140, 156
Davies, G., 347, 357
Davies, J., 20, 23
Davies, R., 137, 175, 180, 193, 196
Davis, B.R., 321, 340
Davis, I., 47, 51
Davitiyananada, D., 229, 231
Dawes, E.A., 180, 193
Dawson, M.H., 47, 53
Dean, A.C.R., 118, 126
Deasey, P.B., 36
Debusscher, L., 92, 97, 98
Deigh, Rosalyn, A., 39, 91, 98
Delena, M., 44, 49, 50
Delorenzo, W.F., 74, 80
De Maine, J.B., 59, 63, 91, 99
Demeter, K.J., 122, 126
Denerley, H., 270, 271
Derrick, Christine, M., 46, 55
Der Vartanian, M.E., 37
Despierres, M., 33
De Voe, I.W., 180, 195
De Vor, H., 183, 194
Devriese, L.A., 75, 80
Dhala, S.A., 34
Dietzler, D.N., 137
Diggs, C.D., 137
Dinerman, A.A., 111, 126
Ditchett, P.J., 175, 195
Dobrzanski, W.T., 109, 110, 128
Dodd, F.H., 205, 209, 218–20, 227
Dolczalek, J., 124, 129
Dolidze, G.G., 122, 127
Domanska, M., 110, 122, 128
Donefer, E., 270, 271
Donelly, C.E., 139, 140, 156
Dorn, C.R., 330, 340

Dowdell, M.J., 157, 173
Dowding, J., 20, 23
Doyle, F.P., 3
Dring, G.J., 109, 127, 137
Drysdale, A.D., 265, 271
Drysdale, S., 315, 342
Dudani, A.T., 110, 112, 114, 128
Duguid, J.P., 33, 34
Duitschaever, C.L., 133, 137
Duncan, C.L., 138
Duran, L., 114, 126
Durban, E., 42
Durlinger, L., 39
Durst, J., 33
Dyett, E.J., 157, 173

Eagon, R.G., 138
Edel, W., 182, 193
Edwards, S.J., 33, 218, 222, 223, 227, 232, 238, 318, 340
Edwards, V.M., 138
Eelderink, I., 183, 194
Efimova, W.A., 112, 113, 130
Egorov, N.S., 110, 112, 126
Ehret, J., 92, 98
Eickhoff, T.C., 92, 98
Eisenthal, R., 38
Eisman, P.C., 37
El-Badavi, S.M., 110, 126
Elek, S.D., 47, 55
El-Gendy, S.M., 110, 126
Elion, G.B., 64, 65, 71, 80
Elliker, P.R., 181, 183
Elliot, J.I., 270, 271
Elliott, R.P., 36, 182, 193
Elsley, F.W.H., 270, 271
Elson, S., 97, 98
Emaldi, G.C., 122, 130
Emerson, M.R., 275, 283
Enloe, F., 315, 342, 347, 357
Epps, N.A., 174, 193
Erlich, H., 137
Erwin, D.G., 137
Etchells, J.L., 41
Evans, Florence L., 41
Evans, F.R., 36, 37, 175, 192
Evans, J.M., 32, 220, 228, 235, 236, 238
Ewing, W.H., 321, 340
Eyles, D.E., 65, 80
Ezekiel, D.H., 138

Fabian, F.W., 148, 156
Fabri, F., 115, 128
Fabri, J., 115
Faiers, M.C., 321, 340
Falco, E.A., 64, 65, 67, 80, 81
Falkow, S., 48, 51
Fallon, R.J., 34
Fan, C.L., 180, 193
Fannin, S.L., 222, 227
Farias, R.N., 133, 137
Farkas, J., 41, 42, 45, 115, 128
Farr, J., 109, 128
Faull, W.B., 223, 227
Fay, J.P., 42, 133, 137
Feigelson, P., 37
Fein, D., 330, 340, 347, 356
Feindt, E., 33
Ferguson, A.R., 32
Ferone, R., 66, 69, 80, 81
Ferrando, R., 325, 342
Ferrer, A., 82, 88
Fewins, B.G., 139, 140, 156
Filipkowski, S., 124, 129
Fincher, M.G., 245, 254
Findus (report), 115, 126
Finegold, S.M., 33, 34
Finland, M., 41, 97, 99, 222, 227
Fisher, Jane C., 296, 297–302
Fitzgerald, C.P., 37
Fitzgerald, G.B., 330, 341
Flores, J., 114, 126
Florestano, H.J., 44
Floris, M., 38
Flowers, R.S., 32, 136, 137, 175, 192
Fogh, B., 47, 52
Forray, A., 33
Forte, C., 177, 192
Foster, J.W., 177, 194
Foulkes, A.L., 330, 335, 340
Fowle, A.S.E., 58, 62
Fowler, G.G., 105, 112, 114, 115, 126, 130
Francis, D.W., 137
Frank, M.M., 252, 254
Frank, R., 37
Franklin, T.J., 48, 52, 179, 193, 328, 340
Frazier, W.C., 181, 193
Freame, Barbara, 45
Freeman, M., 66, 81
Freunsgaard, K., 76, 80
Frik, J., 347, 356
Fryer, J.J., 180, 193
Fryer, T.F., 141, 156
Fullbrook, P.D., 97, 98
Fung, D.Y.C., 137
Funke, H., 220, 227
Furr, J.R., 179, 193
Furuta, Y., 347, 357

Gabis, D.A., 182, 193
Gage, P., 321, 340
Gaines, S.A., 347, 357
Gaines, W., 317, 342
Gale, E.F., 47, 52, 179, 193
Gallant, J., 137
Gardner, G.A., 34, 157, 173
Gardner, P., 34, 317, 341

Garrod, L.P., 40, 47, 48, 52, 69, 72, 74, 80, 212, 216, 230, 231
Gaske, M.A., 137, 175, 182, 193
Gastaldi, C., 139, 156
Geldreich, E.E., 138
Gennari, M., 175, 192
Gialdroni-Grassi, G., 40
Gibbs, B.M., 111, 115, 116, 126
Gibson, E.A., 346, 357
Gibson, T., 139, 156
Gilbert, R.J., 177, 195
Gillespie, W.A., 38, 316, 321, 322, 330, 338, 340, 341
Gillett, A., 223, 227
Goddard, A.E., 37
Goel, M.C., 114, 126
Goepfert, J.M., 133, 138
Goff, J.H., 136, 137
Goldberg, H.S., 47, 52, 321, 341
Goldblith, S.A., 175, 182, 195
Goldin, M., 38
Goldstein, F., 71, 79
Goldstein, I.M., 252, 254
Gomez, R.F., 132, 137, 180, 191, 193
Gontzea, J., 111, 112, 122, 124, 127
Goodman, R.N., 321, 341
Goodwin, L.G., 65, 80
Goresline, H.E., 35
Gori, E., 38, 39
Gorman, S.P., 177, 193
Gould, G.W., 105, 106, 126, 127, 137
Gould, W.A., 46, 55
Grabow, W.O.K., 322, 341
Grace, M.E., 72, 80
Graham, P.H., 34
Granberry, W.D., 37
Grant, E., 180, 192
Grassi, C., 40
Gray, R.J.H., 135, 137, 175, 182, 193
Grecz, W., 42
Green, A.F., 29
Green, E., 223, 227
Greenberg, J., 65, 80
Greenman, R.L., 220, 228
Greenwood, D., 60–3, 82, 85, 87, 88, 94, 98
Greer, D.O., 218, 219, 224, 227
Gregory, Margaret E., 112, 113, 127
Greineder, D.K., 252, 255
Griffiths, R.P., 137
Grigg, G.W., 138
Griffin, T.K., 219, 227
Grindey, G.B., 48, 52
Gross, E., 103, 104, 111, 126, 127
Gross, V.J., 267, 271
Grumbach, F., 38
Grunberg, E., 74, 77, 80
Grüneberg, R.N., 75, 76, 80, 337, 341
Gudkov, A.W., 110, 112, 117, 118, 120, 122, 127, 128
Guinée, P.A.M., 321, 325, 330, 341, 347, 357
Gunnison, Janet, B., 39, 46, 47, 52, 53, 89, 98, 301, 304
Gunther, C.B., 321, 340
Gupta, K.G., 107, 127

Hacking, A., 267, 271
Haight, R.D., 137
Hall, M.L.M., 157, 173
Hall, R.H., 104, 106, 114, 127
Halls, S., 317, 343
Hamada, M., 98, 99
Hamburger, M., 176, 177, 193
Hamdy, A.H., 40, 41
Hamilton, M.A., 137
Hamilton-Miller, J.H.M., 17, 23
Hamilton-Miller, J.M.T., 44, 96, 99
Hannawact, P., 138
Handford, P. Marian, 32
Handler, F.P., 321, 341
Hanscomb, G., 98
Hansen, I., 230, 231
Hara, S., 111
Harcourt, M., 176, 177, 193
Hardwick, A.G., 222, 228
Hargrove, R.E., 111, 127
Hariharan, H., 347, 356
Harmon, S.M., 32
Harper, G.J., 69, 80
Harper, J., 75, 81
Harper, K.A., 35
Harper, W.J., 107, 129
Harrewijn, G.A., 182, 194
Harrington, W.O., 41, 45, 46, 55
Harris, Anne M., 232, 236, 238
Harris, J.S., 82, 88
Harris, N.D., 180, 193
Harris, P.J., 34
Harrison, A.P., 180, 193
Harrison, G.F., 124, 126
Harrison, J., 261, 271
Harrison, W., 283
Hartley, C.L., 321, 325, 335, 341
Hartman, P.A., 33, 135–7
Hartman, P.S., 135–7
Hartsell, S.E., 175, 193
Harvey, R.J., 70, 80
Hashimoto, H., 325, 342
Hata, T., 97, 99
Hauschild, A.H.W., 32
Hawking, F., 65, 80
Hawley, H.B., 42, 109, 124, 127
Hayflick, L., 34
Hays, G.L., 115, 130
Healing, D., 75, 79
Heard, T.W., 208, 209
Heather, C.D., 175, 193
Hedrick, T.I., 179, 195
Heiniger, P.K., 182, 193

Heinemann, B., 105, 106, 109, 112, 113, 115, 126, 127, 130
Heinmets, F., 180, 193
Heldman, D.R., 179, 195
Heller, E.D., 339, 341
Hendricks, S.L., 141, 156
Hendry, G.S., 175, 193
Henke, C.L., 317, 318, 341, 347, 356
Henriksen, B., 230, 231
Henriques, E., 218, 227
Henry, Kathleen M., 112, 113, 127
Hensgens, C., 92, 98
Hentges, D.J., 36
Herbert, C.N., 246, 254
Hergott, J.A., 43
Hernandez, Briz S., 112, 114, 127
Hernandez, E., 114, 126
Herrell, W.E., 40
Herrfordt, L., 230, 231
Hettiaratchy, I.G.T., 335, 340
Hewitt, W.L., 39, 91, 98
Hibbitt, K.G., 245–7, 249–54
Higgs, T.M., 255
Higuchi, T., 6
Hill, A.W., 245, 253, 254
Hills, C.H., 41, 46, 55
Hilsheimer, R., 32
Hilson, G.R.F., 40
Hinshelwood, C., 118, 126
Hirsch, A., 124, 126
Hirsch, D.C., 317, 321, 340, 341
Hitchins, A.D., 175, 194
Hitchings, G.H., 41, 43, 47, 51, 64–72, 74, 80, 81, 87, 88, 230, 231
Hladikova, Z., 124, 129
Hoadley, A.W., 137, 180, 192
Hobby, Gladys L., 47, 48, 53
Hodges, H.G., 245, 254
Hoggarth, E., 65, 79
Höhne, K., 33
Holdowsky, S., 177, 193
Holtenius, P., 317, 343
Hommez, J., 75, 80
Holtrigter, B., 39
Holzer, P., 321, 343
Hood, J.D., 98
Hooper, M.C., 177, 195
Horner, K.J., 133, 137
Hornick, R.B., 92, 99
Howe, Katherine, 317, 318, 321, 323, 325, 327, 335, 339, 341, 347, 356
Howell, D., 222, 227, 312, 314
Huber, W.G., 315, 342, 347, 357
Huennekens, F.M., 66, 81
Hughes, A., 137, 175, 182, 193
Hughes, L.E., 346, 357
Hugo, W.B., 137, 176, 177, 179, 193
Huitson, J.J., 265, 271
Hull, R., 65, 80
Hulse, C., 34
Hunter, I.J., 76, 80
Hunter, P.A., 309, 314
Hurst, A., 104, 109–11, 115–7, 126, 127, 133, 137, 175, 182, 193
Hurt, W., 42
Hutchings, B.L., 64, 79, 81
Hutchison, J.G.P., 75, 79
Hylmar, B., 110, 114, 117, 118, 127, 129
Hymans, P.G., 183, 194

Iandolo, J.J., 136, 137, 151, 156, 175, 193
Iannini, P.B., 92, 98
Ienistea, C., 175, 193
Idziak, E.S., 174, 193
Ignatyev, A.D., 111, 124, 127
Impey, C.S., 34
Incze, K., 42
Inge, W.W., 222, 226
Ingram, L., 104, 109, 127
Ingram, L.C., 316, 340
Ingram, M., 41, 42, 45
Innes, A.G., 32
Irie, R., 132, 138
Ito, K.A., 136, 137
Iwai, Y., 97, 99
Iwao, T., 347, 357

Jackson, G.G., 94, 97, 99, 222, 227
Jackson, H., 138, 139, 156
Jacobs, S.E., 180, 193
Jacobsson, S.O., 317, 343
Jakubczyk, E., 110, 112, 118, 120, 123, 124, 127–30
James, O.B., 330, 343
Janssen, D.W., 133, 138
Jarchovska, H., 111, 128
Jarvis, B., 35, 45, 104, 109, 126, 128
Jarvis, S., 180, 195
Jasiorowski, H., 124, 128
Jawetz, E., 27, 39, 46, 47, 52, 53, 89, 90, 98, 99, 301, 304
Jay, J.M., 32
Jayne-Williams, D.J., 182, 193
Jefferies, L., 33
Jeffsoat, Joan, 104, 128
Jewell, Pamela, 40
Jezeski, J., 137, 139, 151, 156, 180
Jobanputra, R.S., 75, 78, 80
Johns, C.K., 139, 151, 156
Jones, Dorothy, 33
Jones, G.F., 270, 271
Jones, G.W., 246, 254
Jones, L.W., 107, 128
Jones, M.J., 65, 81
Jones, M.R., 205, 209, 220, 227
Jones, R.J., 39–41
Jones, Susan M., 30
Jongerius, E., 175, 194
Jonsson, M., 321, 341

Jordan, D.C., 133, 137
Jorgensen, N.A., 270, 271
Josephson, E.S., 65, 80
Jukič, N., 110, 129
Juven, B., 175, 194

Kabins, S.A., 48, 53
Kadison, E.R., 39
Käer, E., 43
Kagan, B.M., 222, 227
Kahan, F.M., 16, 22, 23
Kaindl, K., 35
Kalra, M.S., 110, 112, 114, 128, 130
Kaminski, S., 124, 129
Kamiryo, T., 94, 99
Kampelmacher, E.H., 182, 193, 331, 342, 347, 357
Kane, M.A., 252, 254
Kaplan, R., 138, 180, 193
Karlikanova, S.N., 112, 117, 118, 120, 128
Kass, E.H., 41
Kasuya, M., 316, 341
Katsube, Y., 252, 254
Katzer, B., 111, 128
Kautter, D.A., 32
Keefe, T.J., 222, 227
Keenan, D., 138
Keido, Y., 111
Kelley, L.M., 133, 138
Kelly, M.T., 92, 98
Kelly, W.R., 224, 227, 325, 341, 347, 356
Kennedy, C.R., 29, 40
Kenward, M.A., 182, 193
Kerr, A., 35, 42
Khan, I., 43
Khan, M.A., 30, 33
Kidson, A., 33, 34
Kim, T.K., 331, 341
Kimmelman, J.L., 30
King, Susan G., 45
Kirby, W.M.M., 59, 63, 92, 99
Kirshbaum, A., 240, 244
Kiss, I., 41, 115, 128, 130
Kiss, N., 115, 130
Kiss-Kurtz, N., 115, 128
Kissne, K. Natalia, 41
Kitchell, A.G., 41, 175, 192
Klastersky, J., 92, 97, 98
Klastrup, O., 221, 227
Klein, D.A., 133, 135, 138
Klein, M., 30
Klemm, L., 316, 321, 342
Knothe, V.H., 321, 322, 341, 343
Knox, R., 96, 99
Kny, L., 160, 173
Ko, K., 21, 23
Kobrina Yu, P., 116, 128
Koburger, J.A., 35
Koch, A.E., 69, 80
Koch, C., 252, 254
Kodama, H., 347, 357
Koelman, A., 40, 46, 54
Kohn, H.I., 82, 88
Koj, A., 254
Koji, M., 111
Kolar, J., 111, 128
Kolmer, J.A., 38
Kon, S.K., 112, 113, 124, 126, 127
Konieĉny, V., 111, 128
Koonkhamlert, C., 321, 341
Koopman, M.J., 175, 194
Koppel, Z., 347, 357
Kornblum, J., 177, 192
Korner, B., 76, 80
Korniewicz, A., 124, 128
Kosikowska, M., 110, 112, 118, 120, 124, 127–9
Kostenbauder, H.B., 177, 194
Kostritskaya, N.P., 114, 127
Kotsevalov, O., 47, 56
Kovacs, S., 242, 244
Kozak, W., 109, 110, 128
Kozakiewicz, Z., 268, 271
Kozlova, M.A., 116, 128
Kozlova, Yu, I., 110, 126
Kraft, A.A., 41
Kramer, Pamela A., 33
Krasz, A., 107, 114, 129
Kratky, F., 124, 129
Krikryl, F., 111, 128
Kropp, H., 16, 22, 23
Kruiswijk, J.T., 275, 283
Kruse, H., 109, 127, 133, 137
Kudryasheva, M.M., 114, 127
Kuila, R.K., 110, 128
Kulieva, I.P., 114, 115, 129, 130
Kull, K.C., 37
Kumar, P.J., 330, 335, 340
Kundrat, W., 122, 126
Kunin, C.M., 222, 227
Kunishige, E., 47, 52
Kurpiewska, W., 120, 129
Küster, E., 36
Kutoval, Kh.A., 114, 130
Kwiatowski, T., 44

Labuza, T.P., 137, 180, 193
Lacey, J., 267, 271
Lacey, R.W., 32, 73, 76, 79, 81, 317, 341
Lackcwicz, T.M., 347, 357
Lais, C.L., 137
Lakhotia, R.L., 347, 356
Lambert, H.P., 47, 48, 52
Lamikanra, A., 176, 178, 193
Lampen, J.O., 65, 81
Langerak, D.J., 41
Lanz, W.W., 135–7
Large, P.J., 180, 193

Lark, C., 178, 194
Lark, K.G., 178, 194
Larrsen, K., 317, 343
Larsen, H.E., 325, 327, 341, 347, 356
Larsen, H.J., 270, 271
Larsen, J.L., 207, 209, 325, 327, 341, 347, 356
Lascelles, A.K., 252, 254
Laub, R., 347, 357
Lawrence, T.L.J., 270, 271
Laxminarayana, H., 112, 114, 128
Lazarus, J.A., 38
Lazzarini, R.A., 137
Leakey, A., 75, 80
Leaman, Angela C., 296, 297, 299, 301, 302
Leaton, J., 173
Lebek, G., 75, 81, 321, 337, 340
Lechowich, R.V., 181, 194
Leckie, M.P., 137
Lee, A.C., 133, 138
Lee, J.A., 334, 341
Lee, P.A., 321, 338, 341
Lehman, J.J., 180, 193
Leigh, D.A., 92, 98, 337, 341
Le Louedec, C., 194, 217, 218, 220, 223, 227
Lemke, R.M., 182
Lenart Tulita, F., 48, 53
Lester-Smith, E., 40
Levi, A.A., 65, 79
Levine, M., 33
Levitov, A., 36
Levy, C., 247, 255
Levy, S.B., 330, 341
Lewis, E.L., 73, 76, 79, 81
Lewis, K.M., 139, 140, 156
Lewis, L.E., 300, 335, 343
Lewis, M.J., 345, 346, 356
Libudzisz, Z., 117, 127
Lillehoj, E.B., 41
Lilly, H.A., 33, 34, 42, 44
Lindgren, B., 31, 36
Linnett, P., 94, 99
Linnett, P.E., 108, 128
Linton, A.H., 208, 209, 315, 317, 318, 321, 323, 325, 327, 330, 335, 339, 341, 347, 356
Linton, K.B., 321, 325, 335, 338, 341
Lipinska, E., 110–2, 117, 118, 120–4, 127–30
Lipniewska, D., 110, 118, 129, 130
Litsky, W., 138
Little, T.W.A., 222, 228
Litvinova, M.N., 110, 112, 127
Livingstone, R.M., 270, 271
Llewellyn, G.G., 236, 238
Locatelli, C., 122, 126
Lockwood, J.L., 42
Loewe, S., 43
Logue, J.T., 321, 341
Loken, K.I., 317, 318, 341, 347, 356
Lokshina, R.V., 115
Lopez, A., 37
Lornian, V., 83, 88
Lovell, B.J., 65, 80
Lovell, R., 218, 227, 297
Lowbury, E.J.L., 33, 34, 39–41, 44
Lowry, R.J., 275, 283
Lubimova, L.A., 110, 112, 127
Luboshitzky, R., 38
Lucas, Mary B., 36, 37
Luedemann, G., 18, 23
Lund, F., 94, 99
Lux, R.E., 65, 81
Lyobe, S., 98, 99
Lyons, P.H., 139, 156

MacAdam, G.A., 176, 177, 192, 193
McCall, C.E., 97, 99
McCann, B., 114, 115, 126
McCleskey, C.S., 157, 173
McConnachie, E.W., 65, 79
McCracken, Ann, 239, 242–4
McCracken, G.H., 338, 341
McDonald, J.S., 245, 246, 254
McDonough, F.E., 111, 127
McDowell, G.H., 252, 254
McEvoy, I.J., 275, 283
McFarlane, A.S., 254
McFeters, G.A., 137
McIlton, C., 37
McIntosh, A.H., 175, 182, 195
MacKinnon, I.H., 177, 178, 194
Mackintosh, I.P., 60, 63, 82, 85, 88
McLaughlin, J.E., 94, 99
McLean, R.A., 42, 157, 173
MacLeod, R.A., 179, 194
McLeod, R.W., 145, 156
McParland, P.J., 219, 227
McVay, L.V., 321, 341
Mace, F.E., 35
Macone, A.B., 330, 341
Macris, B.J., 169, 173
Madsen, P.S., 222, 227
Maeda, K., 98, 99
Maehr, H., 15, 23
Mahoney, R.R., 109, 128
Maksimov, W.N., 110, 126
Mälkki, Y., 36
Mallman, W.L., 139, 156
Malovics, Helen, 33
Maltman, J.R., 179, 194
Maluszynska, G.M., 124, 129
Mann, M.E., 124, 126
Mansson, I., 317, 343
Manten, A., 46, 54, 301, 304, 347, 357
Markakis, P., 169, 173
Marmion, B.P., 33, 34
Marsh, O.H., 330, 340
Marshall, M., 220, 228

Marshall, M.J., 235, 238
Marshall, Valerie M., 46, 55
Marsik, F.J., 347, 357
Marth, E.H., 114, 126, 133, 138, 148, 156
Martin, B., 210
Martin, C.K.A., 15
Martin, J.P., 34, 282, 283
Maruyama, H.B., 138
Masachiro, S., 111
Maskell, R.M., 75, 81
Maslenikova, N.M., 111, 114, 115, 129, 130
Matelova, V., 110, 129
Mateyev, A., 114, 129
Mathe, G., 78, 81
Matosič, S., 110, 129
Matsen, J.M., 92, 98
Matsuhashi, S., 94, 99
Matsumae, A., 97, 99
Matsuyama, A., 36
Mattick, A.T.R., 143, 156
Mattingby, N.A., 111, 127
Mavromati, E., 111, 112, 122, 124, 127
Maxcy, R.B., 180, 194
May, J.E., 252, 254
Mayer, R.L., 37
Mebus, C.A., 347, 356
Meevootisom, V., 321, 341
Melchior, N.H., 94, 99
Melchiorre, B., 252, 254
Melling, J., 175, 192
Melmon, K.L., 252, 255
Mercer, H.D., 317, 318, 342, 347, 357
Mero, E., 33
Meyermann-Wisse, J., 46, 54, 301, 304
Michel, J., 38
Michener, H.D., 36, 37
Mickelson, M.N., 251, 255
Mikolajcik, E.M., 107, 129
Mikula, L., 347, 357
Miles, A.A., 34
Miller, G.H., 72, 81, 82, 88
Miller, J.K., 267, 271
Miller, L., 72, 81, 82, 88
Minks, J., 116, 128
Minor, T.E., 133, 138, 148, 156
Misato, T., 21, 23
Mitchel, R.E.J., 180, 194
Mitchell, H.K., 64, 81
Mitchell, W.R., 347, 356
Mitsuhashi, S., 98, 99, 325, 342
Mizen, L., 309, 314
Moats, W., 138
Moellering, R.C., Jr., 91, 92, 99
Moldovan, E., 111, 112, 122, 124, 127
Moncrief, F. Carolyn, 37
Mondale, L., 73, 79
Monroe, R.J., 41
Moore, T.D., 32
Moore, W.D., 69, 80
Moorhouse, E.C., 322, 325, 330, 341, 342, 347, 356
Moran, J.W., 136, 138
Moran, R.G., 48, 52
Morell, J.L., 103, 104, 108, 111, 127, 130
Morgan, R.F., 34, 180, 193
Morichi, T., 132, 138
Morris, A., 138, 177, 179, 194, 195
Morris, J.G., 180, 194
Morse, G.E., 220, 227, 245, 247, 251, 254, 254
Mossel, D.A.A., 42, 138, 174–6, 178, 182, 183, 191, 194
Mouton, R.P., 39, 40, 46, 54
Mowart, J.H., 64, 79, 81
Muggleton, P.W., 232
Muischnek, H., 43
Munkacsi, F., 36
Murphy, J.M., 245, 246, 254, 255
Murray, J.G., 223, 227
Musumeci, R., 44, 49, 50

Nakae, M., 97, 99
Nakagawa, Y., 133, 138
Nakayama, H., 138
Nakhla, L.S., 76, 81
Namiki, M., 36
Namiotkiewicz, H., 124, 129
Namiotkiewicz, J., 124, 129
Nass, C.A.G., 295, 301, 304
Natzke, R.P., 318, 342
Neal, P.M., 37
Neave, F.K., 141, 151, 156, 205, 209, 218, 220, 227, 252, 255
Nekhotenova, T.I., 115, 129
Nelson, F.E., 32, 35, 45, 133, 138, 175, 194
Nesselrooy-Van Zadelhof, C.F.M., 182, 194
Neu, H.C., 35, 94, 99
New, P.B., 42
Newbould, F.H.S., 219, 227, 252, 255
Newton, B.A., 176, 177, 194
Nichol, C.A., 66, 81
Nielsen, M.L., 230, 231
Nielsen, N.C., 207–9, 325, 341
Nies, A.S., 252, 255
Niven, C.F., 32
Noah, N.D., 334, 342
Norris, L.C., 66, 79
Nouws, J.F.M., 183, 194, 240, 244
Northolt, M.D., 182, 194, 331, 342
Nunheimer, T.D., 148, 156
Nyamubeya, B., 92, 98

Oberman, H., 110, 117, 129
O'Brien, J.J., 242–4
O'Connor, H., 330, 342
O'Farrell, S.M., 321, 334, 340
Ogawara, H., 98, 99
O'Grady, F., 47, 48, 52, 57, 58, 60–3, 82, 85, 88, 94, 97–9, 176, 194, 212, 216, 330, 342

Ohno, H., 97, 99
Oka, M., 347, 357
Okamura, S., 138
Okazaki, M., 133, 138
Okazawa, Y., 36
Okubadjo, O.A., 75, 81
Olexy, V., 97, 99
Oliver, C.W., 33
Oliver, M., 275, 283
Olsen, S.J., 219, 220, 222, 227
Omura, S., 97, 99
Openshaw, H.T., 65, 80
Oram, J.D., 251, 255
Ordal, Z.J., 31, 131, 135, 137–9, 151, 156–7, 172–3, 175, 181, 182, 191, 193
Orfanakis, M.G., 40
Orlova, N.Ya., 114, 130
Orskov, F., 321, 340
Osato, Y., 98, 99
Osborn, M.J., 66, 81
Osborne, A.D., 317, 318, 323, 325, 327, 339, 341, 347, 356
Osborne, C.D., 309, 314
Osborne, W.W., 33
Osipova, N.J., 111, 130
Osler, A.G., 252, 254
Ovcharova, T.P., 111, 114, 115, 129, 130

Pabis, E., 110, 129
Pablo, I.S., 175, 182, 195
Pacilio, J.C., 41
Packers, R.A., 33
Pagani, H., 18, 23
Paley, B., 175, 193
Palmer, G.H., 307
Palmer, V.M., 275, 283
Palumbo, S.A., 46, 50
Pape, G.S., 255
Parisi, J.T., 347, 357
Park, J.T., 94, 99
Park, R.W.A., 323, 342
Parker, B.N.J., 221, 222, 227
Patel, M., 45
Patel, N.K., 177, 194
Paterson, G.M., 110, 127
Pato, M.L., 76, 81
Patton, J., 157, 173
Paulton, R.J.L., 296, 297, 299–302
Payman, L.C., 65, 80
Payne, R.H., 75, 81
Payne, S.L., 138
Pearson, J.K.L., 217, 218, 220, 224, 227, 235, 238
Pechere, J.C., 77, 81
Peck, R.S., 47, 53
Pedersen, P.S., 221, 222, 227
Peelen-Knol, G., 242–4
Peeler, J.I., 32
Peeler, J.T., 32, 137
Pelhate, J., 268, 271
Pennington, J.H., 176, 194
Penny, R.H.C., 208, 209
Perault, R., 40
Percival, A., 92, 98
Perlman, D., 15, 23, 109, 126
Perry, W.L.M., 65, 80
Pesquera, T.I., 111, 114, 129
Peterkova, L., 110, 129
Peterson, W.H., 64, 81
Petrocheilou, V., 335, 342
Pezzani, G., 115, 126
Pickering, A., 255
Pierson, M.D., 138
Pietraszek, A., 124, 128
Pinder, R.M., 38
Piper, R., 82, 88
Pisano, F.D., 177, 194
Pisano, M.A., 36
Pittillo, R.F., 36, 37, 177, 194
Plastridge, W.N., 245, 254
Plommet, M., 217, 218, 220, 223, 227
Pocunull, D.W., 317, 318, 342, 347, 357
Pohl, P., 347, 357
Pollock, D.A., 218, 224, 227
Porretta, A., 107, 114, 129
Porta, A., 122, 126
Porter, J.N., 18, 23
Portoles, A., 39
Postgate, J.R., 132, 138, 180, 194
Postle, D.S., 318, 342
Potter, V.R., 67, 81
Prentice, G.A., 138
Price, C.W., 43
Prince, H.N., 74, 80
Prokop, V., 124, 129
Prozesky, O.W., 322, 341
Pugh, K.E., 235, 238
Pulay, G., 107, 114, 129
Pursell, R.E., 338, 342
Put, H.M.C., 176, 194, 275, 283
Pyanitsina, I.N., 110, 129

Raccach, M., 175, 194
Radaeva, J.R., 112, 113, 130
Radenbach, K.L., 44
Rajchert-Trzpil, M., 109, 110, 128
Ralovich, B., 33
Ramazanova, D.P., 114, 127
Rammel, C.G., 151, 156
Ramseier, H.R., 107, 120, 130
Randell, W.A., 43
Ranganathan, B., 110, 128
Rasmussen, F., 229, 231
Ratto, M.A., 138, 175, 182, 191–4
Ray, B., 132, 135, 136, 138, 175, 179–80, 182, 191, 194
Raynand, J.P., 325, 342
Read, R.B., 136, 138
Read, R.B. Jr., 182, 191, 194

Reading, C., 98
Reed, N.D., 347, 356
Reeves, C.B., 107, 129
Reeves, D.S., 94, 99, 321, 340
Regnier, A.P., 323, 342
Rehm, H.J., 37, 169, 173
Rehm, W.F., 229, 231
Reinbold, G.W., 33
Reiter, B., 46, 55, 139, 140, 143, 151, 156, 245–7, 250–2, 254, 255
Remington, J.S., 220, 228
Renault, L., 325, 342
Reyes, A.L., 182, 194
Reynolds, P.E., 47, 52, 179, 193
Rhoads, P.S., 40
Rhodes, Annette C., 45
Richards, R.M.E., 37, 38
Richards, T., 33, 145, 156
Richeson, E.M., 65, 80
Richmond, M.H., 47, 52, 96, 99, 179, 193, 316, 321, 325, 330, 335, 337, 340–2
Richter, J., 160, 173
Rickard, C.G., 245–6, 254
Ricks, G.R., 42
Riff, L.J., 94, 97, 99
Riggs, D.G., 311, 314
Riising, H.J., 208, 209
Ritter, P., 117, 130
Roberts, D., 157, 173
Roberts, D.H., 222, 228
Roberts, T.A., 42, 44–6, 55, 174, 175, 192, 194
Robertson, M.H., 43
Robinson, A.A.E., 223, 227
Robson, J.M., 38
Rodwell, V.W., 180, 193
Rogers, M.P., 41
Rogers, R.E., 157, 173
Rogerson, A.C., 138
Roguinsky, M., 220, 227
Rolinson, G.N., 92, 98, 99, 309, 314
Rollins, L.D., 318, 342
Rollo, I.M., 65, 80
Roman, A., 175, 193
Rose, C.D., 124, 126
Rose, F.L., 65, 79
Rose, R.E., 138
Rosenfeld, H., 37
Roslon, E., 121, 129
Rossi, Anna, 44, 49, 50
Rossini, L.J., 43
Roth, B., 65, 67, 81, 182, 194
Roth, L.A., 138, 175, 181, 191, 195
Roughley, R.J., 145, 156
Rousseau, S.A., 330, 335, 340, 342
Routien, J.B., 18, 23
Roux, J., 325, 342
Rowland, A.J., 321, 338, 341
Rowlands, G.J., 246, 254
Rowley, D., 254
Ruben, T.M., 115, 130
Rudavskaya, A.B., 114, 130
Ruf, R., 107, 130
Ruhl, D., 97, 98
Russell, A.D., 132, 137, 138, 175, 177, 179–82, 193–5
Russell, C., 36
Russell, E.J., 39, 90, 99
Russell, M.W., 250, 252, 255
Russell, P.B., 64, 65, 80

Saarimaa, H., 77, 81
Sabath, L.D., 39, 97, 99
Sachs, T., 38
Sahani, K.M., 111, 118, 130
Salzmann, T.C., 316, 322, 342
Sangiovanni, M., 38
Saraswat, D.S., 33
Sato, G., 347, 357
Satterlea, W., 92, 99
Sauberlich, H.E., 66, 81
Sauer, D.B., 266, 271
Sawicki, E., 36
Sawyer, W.D., 321, 341
Schaffner, C.P., 15, 23
Schalm, O.W., 222, 227, 251, 255
Schara, R.E. 41
Scheusner, D.L., 180, 182, 195
Schimpff, S., 92, 99
Schlumberger, J.R., 78, 81
Schmidt, C.F., 36
Schmidt, E.W., 46, 55
Schneider, M., 78, 81
Schneierson, S.S., 176, 192
Schoenbach, E.B., 177, 192
Schoene, E.S., 41
Schultze, W.D., 218–20, 222, 227
Schwarzenberg, L., 78, 81
Scott, E.M., 177, 193
Scurlock, A., 114, 127
Scwarz, L.H., 38
Seaman, A., 30, 33, 139, 275, 283, 296, 297, 299, 301, 302
Sebek, O.K., 20, 23
Sebek, V., 347, 356
Sedgewick, S.G., 138
Seeger, J., 115, 130
Seeliger, H.P.R., 33
Segner, N.P., 36
Seligman, S.J., 91, 98
Sellin, M.A., 73, 79
Semb, J., 64, 79, 81
Senesi, E., 122, 130
Serieys, F., 220, 227
Serpick, A., 92, 99
Sevag, M.G., 47, 51
Seydel, J.K., 72, 81, 82, 88
Shah, P.C., 251, 255
Shahidi, S.A., 32

Shalkop, W.T., 44
Sharpe, M.E., 139, 140, 143, 151, 156, 255
Shaw, E.J., 338, 340, 342
Shears, A.L., 253, 254
Shelley, D., 157, 172
Sherwood, M.B., 64, 80
Shibasaki, I., 133, 138
Shillinger, Yu.I., 111, 130
Shipp, C.R., 157, 173
Shkundova, Y.V., 110, 112, 114, 126, 130
Shooter, R.A., 321, 330, 334, 335, 340, 342
Shornikova, N.M., 115, 130
Shtenberg, A.J., 111, 124, 130
Siddiqui, M.A., 43
Sidhu, R., 107, 127
Siebeling, R.J., 37
Siegel, D., 315, 342, 347, 357
Sierra, G., 36, 44
Sigel, C.W., 72, 80
Sileva, M.W., 110, 112, 127
Silliker, J.H., 182, 193
Silverman, G.J., 175, 180, 182, 195
Silvestrova, O.I., 110, 126
Simmons, H.E., 222, 227
Simmons, N.A., 44
Simson, E., 75, 81
Singer, S., 71, 80
Sinskey, A.J., 132, 137, 175, 180, 182, 191, 193, 195
Sizer, D., 220, 228
Skaggs, B., 112, 130
Skaliy, P., 138
Skidmore, N.C., 35
Skold, O., 75, 81
Slavin, G., 347, 357
Smellie, J.M., 75, 80
Smith, A., 205, 209, 220, 227
Smith, B.A., 33
Smith, C.B., 40
Smith, D., 69, 80
Smith, D.H., 317, 337, 341, 342
Smith, D.K., 138
Smith, G., 275, 283
Smith, H.R., 338, 340
Smith, H.W., 47, 56, 75, 76, 199, 205, 209, 316, 317, 322, 325, 330, 335, 338, 339, 342–53, 355–7
Smith, J.T., 75, 79, 96, 99
Smith, M.G., 316, 343
Smolka, L.R., 133, 138
Smřeek, J., 43
Smulders, A.H.J.W., 240, 244
Snell, E.E., 64, 81
Snow, G.A., 48, 52, 179, 193
Søgaard, H., 317, 343
Sogn, L., 267, 271
Sojka, W.J., 297, 347, 357
Sokol, A., 347, 357
Solberg, M., 46, 51
Soltys, W., 110, 120, 122, 128, 129
Sompolinsky, D., 321, 343
Sonne, M., 90, 99
Sorrels, K.M., 174, 195
Soulides, D.A., 33
Soulides, E., 33
Sourander, L., 77, 81
Southworth, Jill M., 32
Spaulding, E.H., 321, 340
Speck, M.L., 132, 135–8, 174, 175, 179, 180, 182, 191, 194, 195
Spence, B.K., 219, 227
Splittstoesser, D.F., 283
Spratt, B.G., 94, 99
Stacey, K.A., 75, 81
Stacey, R.S., 38
Standiford, H.D., 59, 63, 91, 92, 99
Stankiewicz-Berger, H., 116, 130
Staudenbauer, W.L., 179, 195
Steel, K.J., 178, 192
Steigbigel, N.H., 97, 99
Steigbigel, R.T., 221, 228
Steinberg, R.A., 296, 304
Stella, V., 6
Stephan, R., 317, 325, 340, 343, 347, 356
Stephens, J.F., 331, 341, 347, 356
Stern, H., 47, 55
Stersky, A.K., 179, 195
Stevens, A.J., 346, 357
Stevens, Janet K., 33
Stewart, C.S., 270, 271
Stiles, M.E., 138, 139, 156, 175, 181, 182, 191, 194, 195
Stock, C.C., 41
Stocker, C.T., 41
Stokes, J.L., 33, 182, 195
Stokstad, E.L.R., 64, 79, 81
Stolley, P.D., 222, 227
Straka, R.P., 182, 195
Strandjev, A., 114, 129
Strominger, J.L., 94, 99, 108, 128
Strong, Dorothy H., 32
Strzalkowska, M., 111, 117, 124, 129
Stuart, D.G., 137
Stuart, M., 275, 283
Stuart, O.M., 245, 255
Stumbo, C.R., 105, 106, 109, 112, 113, 115, 126, 127, 130, 175, 195
Subbarrow, Y., 64, 79, 81
Sugihara, P.T., 33
Sulzbacher, W.L., 157, 173
Sussman, A.S., 275, 283
Sutherland, R., 12, 39, 89, 90, 92, 96, 99, 302–4, 309, 314
Sutter, Vera L., 33, 34
Suzuki, K., 325, 342
Svendsen, J., 207–9
Swain, R.H.A., 33, 34
Swaitek, A., 121, 129
Swann, M.M., 21, 23
Swartling, P., 31, 36

Swiderski, M., 347, 357
Swidler, G., 221, 228
Sykes, G., 175, 177, 195
Sylwestrowicz, H.D., 37
Szadkowska, M., 110, 112, 123, 128–30
Szazadus, I., 33

Takacs, J., 242, 244
Takahashi, I., 111, 139, 151, 156
Takahashi, S., 98, 99
Takako, T., 111
Takano, M., 132, 137
Tamburasev, G., 110, 129
Tamoni, G., 18, 23
Tancini, Gabrielle, 44, 49, 50
Tanguay, A.E., 138
Tanner, E.I., 41, 75, 81
Tapsall, J.W., 75, 81
Tatem, B.A., 92, 99
Tatsunori, K., 111
Taylor, W.W., 180, 193
Templeton, A.R., 42
Teply, M., 110, 117, 118, 127
Ter-Zakharyan Yu Z., 47, 55
Tesarkova, H., 110, 117, 118, 127
Testa, C., 175, 192
Thatcher, F.S., 182, 195
Then, R., 69, 73, 74, 79, 81, 177, 192
Thiemann, J.E., 18, 23
Thoma, R.W., 20, 23
Thomas, J., 347, 357
Thompson, J., 180, 195
Thompson, J.C., 35
Ticha, A., 111, 130
Tiemann, U., 109, 130
Timoney, R.F., 36
Todd, A.R., 65, 80
Todd, J.C., 222, 226
Tokmakova, V.N., 110, 130
Toma, C., 111, 112, 122, 124, 127
Tomaszewska, J., 118, 121, 129
Tombs, M.P., 104, 127
Tomlins, R.I., 132, 138, 179, 181, 191, 195
Tortora, G., 36
Traci, P.A., 138
Tramer, J., 104, 107, 112, 116, 128, 130
Treece, J.M., 247, 255
Trofimova, A.W., 112, 118, 120, 128
Trofimova, T., 110, 127
Tsuchido, T., 133, 138
Tsugo, T., 111, 114, 130
Tsutakawa, R., 330, 340, 347, 356
Tsutakawa, R.K., 330, 340
Tucker, J.F., 75, 76, 81, 349, 350, 355–7
Tuckey, S.L., 139, 156
Tupasi, T., 222, 227
Turco, G., 175, 192
Turner, W.H., 38
Turney, L.J., 41

Twedt, R.M., 137
Tybring, L., 94, 99
Tyrrell, E., 275, 283

Ugueto, N.R., 321, 330, 341, 347, 356
Umezawa, H., 97, 99
Underdahl, N.R., 347, 356
Ushakova, R.F., 116, 130
Utahara, R., 98, 99
Uvarov, O., 220, 228

Vaichulis, E.M.K., 177, 195
Valagussa, P., 44, 49, 50
Valkenburg, J.J., 347, 357
Van DenHeever, L.W., 317, 341, 347, 356
Van Den Boore, L., 92, 98
Van Den Bosch, L.L., 137
Vanderwerff, H., 64, 65, 80
Vanderzant, C., 175, 193
Van Doorne, H., 174, 183, 194
Van Kol, P.J., 347, 356
Van Leeuwen, N., 330, 341
Van Leeuwen, W.J., 321, 341, 347, 356
Van Leusdem, F.M., 182, 193, 240, 244
Van Robaeys, G., 347, 357
Van Rooyen, C.E., 92, 99
Van Schothorst, M., 182, 193, 240, 242–4, 331, 342
Van Uden, N., 182, 195
Vas, K., 41, 113–6, 128, 130
Vedros, N.A., 177, 195
Veronesi, U., 44, 49, 50
Vogd, C.E., 347, 357
Voris, L., 105, 106, 109, 112, 115, 126, 127, 130
Vuillemin, P., 27, 56

Wagner, L.W., 317, 318, 341, 347, 356
Wajid, K., 114, 130
Waksman, S.A., 27
Wald, E.R., 92, 99
Wallace, D.H., 41
Wallace, E.T., 76, 79
Waller, C.W., 64, 79, 81
Walker, H.W., 41
Walter, G., 180, 195
Walton, J.R., 259, 264, 316, 317, 325, 330, 334, 335, 343, 347, 357
Waring, M.J., 47, 52, 179, 193
Warke, G.M., 34
Warren, J.A., 174, 195
Warseck, M., 136, 138
Watanakunakorn, C., 90, 92, 99
Waters, M.E., 41
Waterworth, Pamela M., 69, 72, 74, 80, 230, 231
Watson, B.W., 60, 63, 82, 85, 88
Watson, D.J., 236, 238
Wawrzynczak, S., 124, 129

Wegner, K., 114, 130
Weil, A.J., 47, 56
Weinberg, A.N., 91, 92, 99
Weinberg, E.D., 138, 176, 177, 195
Weinstein, A.J., 92, 99
Weiser, H.H., 46, 55
Weiser, R., 38
Weissmann, G., 252, 254
Welch, A.D., 43, 66, 81
Wells, D.M., 330, 343
Welsby, D., 157
Wempe, E., 72, 81, 82, 88
Wennerstein, C., 92, 99
Werkheiser, W.C., 48, 52
Westgarth, D.R., 205, 209, 220, 227
Wheaton, E., 115, 130
White, G., 229, 231
White, H.R., 182, 194
White, R.J., 169, 130
Whitefield, M., 180, 193
Whittlestone, P., 34
Wiedemann, B., 316, 322, 340, 343
Widh, A., 75, 81
Wierup, M., 317, 318, 325, 343, 347, 357
Wilcox, H., 40
Wilkison, M., 283
Williams, L.E., 42
Williams, O.B., 181, 195
Williams, R.J., 64, 81
Williams, R.J.H., 42
Willoughby, E., 94, 99
Wilson, C.D., 218, 221, 222, 228
Wilson, C.R., 137
Wilson, E., 75, 81
Wilson, J.M., 175, 196
Wilson, L.L., 269, 271
Wilson, M.R., 208, 209
Wilson, S., 317, 342
Wimpenny, J., 38
Winsley, B.E., 37
Wise, E.M., 76, 81
Witter, L.D., 31, 131, 135–9, 151, 156, 157, 172, 173
Witting, D.A., 309, 314
Wittmann, H., 169, 173
Wix, A., 30
Wood, R.C., 66, 67, 81
Wood, R.L., 34
Wood, T.H., 35
Woodbine, M., 27, 29–31, 33, 34, 139, 156, 275, 283, 296
Woodcock, E., 138
Woods, D.D., 47, 51, 177, 195
Wright, C.L., 220, 227
Wright, H.B., 41
Wright, J.H., 196
Wu, S.Y., 133, 135, 138

Yadav, N.K., 107, 127
Yamaguchi, I., 21, 23
Yamazaki, S., 98, 99
Yanggita, T., 138
Yaron, V., 321, 343
Yates, A.R., 275, 283
Yazdany, S., 36
Young, J.L., 253, 254
Young, V.M., 92, 99
Yuce, K., 92, 99

Zajdel, J., 109, 128
Zebovitz, E., 32
Zeigler, J.L., 317, 340
Zieliński, W., 124, 128
Zimmerman, R.A., 36, 91, 99
Ziro, I., 111
Ziv, G., 221, 228, 311, 314
Zottola, F., 139, 156
Zwart Voorspuij, A.J., 43, 47, 56, 284, 295, 301, 304

SUBJECT INDEX

Acetaldehyde, 275–7, 280
Acetate, 275
Acetic acid, 36, 37, 41, 265, 276, 281
Acridin, 33
Acriflavine, 36, 37
Actidione, 34
Actinomycin C, 19
Actinomycin D, 19, 179
Additivity, 286
Adenine, 73
Adriamycin, 19, 45
Aflatoxicoses, 267
Agalactiae syndrome, 200
Ageing, 31
Alanine, 107
  racemase, 22
Albamycin T, 57
Aldehydes, 37, 178
Allergies, 218
Allopurinol, 64
Alveoli, mammary, 253
Amikacin, 15, 92
Aminobenzoic acid, 77, 177
Aminoglycosides, 3, 15, 21, 58, 89
6-Aminopenicillanic acid (6-APA), 3, 19
Amino salicylic acid, 44, 292
Aminosidin, 19
Amoxycillin, 9, 13, 16, 18, 89, 90, 307–11
Amphomycin, 19, 21
Amphotericin B, 19, 44
Ampicillin, 4, 6–8, 13, 14, 16, 29, 38–40, 43, 89, 203, 239, 297, 307
  resistance, 6, 345
Ampiclox LC, 313
Antagonism, 286
Antibiosis, 27
Antibiotic residue (milk), 23
Antifolates, 65
Antimicrobial proteins, 245
Antimycin A, 19
Antimycin D, 45
Apples, 115
Arsphenamines, 177
Ascorbic acid, 32, 42, 45
Ascospore activators, 275–83
Asparagus, 115
Aspirin, 3, 43
Atrophic rhinitis, 200
Aureofungin, 19
Aureomycin, 40
Azalomycin, 19
Azathioprine, 64
Azatryptophan, 37
Azetidinone, 13
Azide, sodium, 33, 34
Azidocillin, 16

Bacitracin, 19, 32, 34, 35, 38, 39, 42–4, 46, 109, 179
Bacitracin Zn, 21, 204, 259, 354
Bacon, 116
Bacterial endocarditis, 57
Bactofugation, 116, 117
Barley, 267
Basic fuchsin, 34
Beef, 330
Beets, 115
Benzoic acid, 37, 41
Benzoic acid Na, 46
Benzylalcohol, 37
Benzylalkonium, 36–8
Benzyl penicillin, 39, 44, 89
Bicyclomycin, 19
Bile salt, 34
Bismuth citrate, 33
Bismuth salicylate, 38
Bladder model, 82, 85
Blasticidin S, 19, 21
Bleomycin, 19, 44
Borsh, 115
Brilliant black reduction, 223
Brilliant green, 33, 182
Brocillin, 5
Bromodeoxyuridine, 36
Broxil, 5
Brucellosis, 58
Butter, 34
Butyric acid, 266
  iso-, 266

Calves, 323
  diarrhoea, 213
  enteritis, 201
  pneumonia, 201
  salmonellosis, 229, 316
  scours, 201
  septicaemia, 201
Candicidin B, 19
Capreomycin, 19
Capsule, 259
Carbadox, 204
Carbenicillin, 6, 7, 16, 18, 39, 59, 92
Carbomycin, 30, 40
Carbon dioxide, 31, 41, 157
Carboxypeptidase, 109
Carfecillin, 7
Carrot, 115
  puree, 115
Casein, 146, 252
Caseolysis, 145
Caseolytic, 146–8
Cationic
  detergents, 179
  proteins, 252
Cattle, 201, 323
Caviar, 115
Cefamandole, 16
Cefazolin, 10, 16
Cefoxitin, 16
Cefuroxime, 10, 16
Celbenin, 4
Cellocidin, 19
Cephacetrile, 16
Cephalexin, 10, 16, 94
Cephaloglycine, 10, 16
Cephalonium, 237
Cephaloridine, 10, 16
Cephalosporins, 3, 15, 16, 19, 39, 60, 203
Cephalosporin C, 9
Cephalosporin N, 9
Cephalothin, 10, 16
Cephamandole, 10
Cephamycin A, 10
Cephamycin B, 10
Cephamycin C, 10
Cephanone, 16
Cephapirin, 16
Cephapyrin, 10
Cephoxazole, 236, 237
Cephradine, 16
Cerates, 232
Cetrimide, 34
Chartreusin, 21
Cheese, 31, 103, 139
  Cheddar, 139, 145
  cottage, 143
  curd, 139
  Edam, 112, 116, 120, 122
  Emmental, 116, 122
Cheese (*cont.*)
  Gouda, 122
  processed, 105, 114
  Provolone, 122
  ripening, 122
  slurries, 139
  spreads, 114
  Stilton, 139
    blue, 143, 145, 149, 152
    white, 143, 149
  Tilsit, 121
Cherries, 115
Chicks, 316
Chilling, 37, 42
Chloral hydrate, 36
Chlorambucil, 44
Chloramphenicol, 18, 19, 34, 38–40, 43, 46, 109, 177, 179, 203, 239, 285, 291, 293, 295, 297, 337
  resistance, 345
Chlorbutol, 37
Chlorhexidine, 38, 179
Chlorine, 37
Chlorocresol, 36, 37
Chloromycetin, 34, 37, 40
Chloroquanine, 38
Chloroquine, 38
Chlortetracycline, 19, 21, 35, 39, 41, 42, 109
Chow-mein, 115
Chromomycin A_3, 19
Clavulanic acid, 13, 14
Clindamycin, 16
Clometicillin, 5
Cloxacillin, 4, 13, 39, 57, 60, 204, 220, 235, 236, 298, 307
  benzathine, 205
Coccidiosis, 65
Coccidiostats, 18
Codeine, 43
Cold, 41
  shock, 36
Coliform mastitis, 223
Colistin, 19, 34, 38–40, 44, 298
Combinations, 14, 47, 221
  anti-, 48
Complement
  units, 252
Components (three), 293, 295, 300
Corn, 115
Co-trimoxazole, 57
Cows, 270
Crab, 116
Cream
  long life, 31
  soups, 113
Cresols, 177
Crop(s), 322
  conservation, 265
Crystal violet, 33, 34, 136, 183

Cyclacillin, 16
Cycloheximide, 19, 21, 34, 35, 38, 42
Cyclophosphamide, 44, 45
Cyclopropenoid F.A., 41
Cycloserine, 12, 19, 22, 32, 38, 40, 41, 44, 59, 179
Cysteine, 47, 48, 104
Cystitis, bacterial, 85
Cytoplasmic membrane, 259

Dairy aspects, 31
Daunomycin, 19
Dehydroalanine, 103
Delvotest, 223
Demethylchlortetracycline, 19, 38, 39
Depsipeptides, 59
Destomycin, 19
Deuterofluoroalanine, 22, 38
Diamond back disease, 29
Diaveridine, 43
Diarrhoea, 200
Dicloxacillin, 4, 16
Diethylpyrocarbonate, 46
Diffusion, 104, 122
Dihydropteroic acid, 67
Diluent, 31, 182
Dimedone, 177
Diphenylioclonium Cl, 43
Disc assay, 223
DNA, 247
Dogs, 201
    (Beagle), 310
Double-blockade, 46, 67
Doxycycline, 16
Dry cow, 218, 219, 235, 251
Dyes, 32

Ear infections, 201
EDTA, 38
EDTA Fe, 42
Egg(s), 31
    sterile, 330
    yolk, 32
Eijkman reaction, 297, 327
Elastase, 109
Emtryl, 204
Enduracidin, 19
Enteric
    bacteria, 264
    fevers, 58
    infections, 323
Enteritis, 207
Enterococci, 58, 59
Eosin, 33, 297
Epicillin, 16
Erepsin, 109
Erysipelas, 201
Erysipeloid, 29
Erythromycin, 19, 21, 34, 38–40, 43, 46, 109, 179, 203, 295, 298
Erythritol, 35, 42
Ethambutol, 38
Ethanol, 37, 38
Ethidium bromide, 109
Ethionamide, 44
Ethyl violet, 34
Ethylene oxide, 36

Farm animal disease, 210
Farmer's lung organisms, 268
Fatty acids, 42, 245
Feed, 103
    antibiotic, 259
    growth promotion, 60
Ferric citrate, 33, 45
Ferrous sulphate, 45
Film
    impermeable, 153, 155
    permeable, 153, 155
Fish, 113, 116
Flavomycin, 204, 354
Floxapen, 4
Flucloxacillin, 4, 16
Fluoroadenosine, 36
Fluorouracil, 44
Folic acid, 64, 66
Folinic acid, 66, 74
Food, dried, 31
Formaldehyde, 177
Formamide, 37
Formic acid, 36, 37, 266, 267
Framycetin, 203
Fractional inhibitory concentration, 71
Freeze-drying, 132
Freezing injury, 35, 132
Fructose, 41
Fruit, 113, 275
    strawberries, 275
Fucidic acid, 19, 40
Fucidin, 38, 40
Fumagillin, 17, 19
Furazolidone, 203
    resistance, 328, 345
Furfural, 275, 282
Fusidic acid, 33, 44, 61, 298

Garlic, 41
Gas chromatography, 223
Gentamicin, 15, 19, 38, 39, 59, 89, 92, 338
Glucose, 36, 38
Glutamate decarboxylase, 136
Glutaraldehyde, 36, 44, 177
Glutathione, 104
Glycine, 32, 69
Gnotobiotic animals, 347
Grain, 265
Gramicidin, 19, 109, 179
Griseofulvin, 19
Groat, 115

Growth promoters, 124, 199, 204, 259, 315, 344
Guanine, 134
Gut distribution, 308

Hadacidin, 37
Ham, 115
Hamburgers, 116
Hamycin, 19
Hay, 267, 268
Heart, 242
Heat, 32, 35–7, 41, 42, 45, 275
  shock, 152
Heparin, 247
Hetacillin, 7, 16
Horses, 201
Humidity, 37
Hydrogen peroxide, 31, 36, 46, 251
Hygromycin B, 19

Ice-cream, 31
Immunoglobulins, 252
Indanyl sodium, 7
India, 338
Indole, 297, 327
Inosine, 69, 73
Intertest, 223
Intramammaries, evaluation, 204, 217
Iodide, potassium, 38
Iodoacetamide, 36
Irradiation, 35, 36, 41, 45, 52
Isobolograms, 71
Isoniazid, 38, 40, 44, 292

Josamycin, 19
Jouin photometer, 296

Kanamycin, 15, 19, 32, 34, 38, 39, 46, 89, 179, 298, 338
Kasugamycin, 19, 21
Keratin, 245
Kidney
  residue, 241
  test, 242

β-Lactam antibiotics, 3, 232
β-Lactamase, 12, 96, 177
  inhibitors, 61, 96
Lactation therapy, 219
Lactenins, 251
Lactic
  acid production, 148, 251
  D- and L- isomers, 148, 150
Lactoferrin(s), 251
Lactoperoxidase, 46, 251
Lanette wax, 183
Lanthionine, 103, 104
  β-methyl-, 103
Lasalocid, 19
Lecithin, 176, 177
Leprosy, 12
Leptospirosis, 201
Leucomycin, 19
Lincomycin, 15, 16, 19, 40, 203
Lipopolysaccharide, 251, 260
Lipoprotein, 260
Lithium chloride, 32
Liver, 243
Lividomycin, 19
Lubrol-W, 176
Lucensomycin, 19
Lymecycline, 16
Lysozyme, 136

Macarbomycin, 19
Macaroni, 115
MacConkey's agar, 297
Macrolide, 3, 124
Magnamycin, 29, 30
Maize, 267
Malachite green, 160
Mannitol Salt Agar, 32, 152
Mapharsen, 38
Maredamomycin, 19
Mastitis, 200, 206, 212, 232, 245
  acute clinical, 212
Meat, 113
  cooked, 323
  raw, 323
  soups, 113
Mecillinam, 9, 94
Media, microbiological, 32
Melting salts, 114
Membrane damage, 178, 262
Meningitis, 338
Mercaptopurine, 41, 64
Mercury
  compound, 37, 177
  succinimide, 38
Metabisulphite, 32
  potassium, 158
Methacycline, 16
Methicillin, 4, 16, 38–40, 298
Methionine, 45, 69
Methotrexate, 44
Methyl red reaction, 297
Methylene blue, 33, 34, 297
Metritis, 201
Mice, 29, 316
Microtitre technique, 325
Middlesborough, 338
Mikamycin(s), 19, 40
Miles–Misra count, 142
Milk, 31, 312, 330
  chocolate, 113
  evaporated, 31, 112, 113
  fermented, 31
  long life, 31

Milk (*cont.*)
    pasteurized, 31
    raw, 31
    roller dried, 31
    skim, 105
    spray dried, 31
    sterilized, 31
    sweet condensed, 31
Minimal effective concentration (MEC), 72, 284
Minimum bactericidal concentration, 90
Minimum inhibitory concentration, 70, 71, 93
Minimum salts–maximum growth, 296
Minocycline, 16
Mithramycin, 19
Mitomycin, 19
MK641/642, 22
Mocimycin, 19
Moenomycin, 19
Moisture meter, 269
Monensin, 19
Morpholine, 177
Most probable effective destruction dose, (MPED), 175
Most probable number technique, 136
Mucin, 29
Multiple resistance, 345
Murein layer, 259
Muscle residue, 124, 241
Mushrooms, 105, 113, 116
Mustard oil soap, 43
Mycoplasmas, 215
Mycotoxin(s), 41, 267

Naficillin, 4, 16, 97, 236
Naladixic acid, 33, 34, 38, 43
    resistance, 345
Neomycin, 19, 32–5, 38–40, 43, 44, 46, 109, 179, 203, 214, 239, 298, 318
    resistance, 345
Neonatal scours, 206, 207
Neutral red, 136
Neutralizers, 176
Nipagin-M, 183, 185, 186
Nisaplin, 110
Nisin(s), 19, 41, 42, 45, 103
    amino-acids, 118
    and pH, 121
    and spores, 125
    blood, 124
    inhibition, 119
    intestinal flora, 124
    muscles, 124
    resistance, 111, 117, 118
    urine, 124
    with heat treatment, 125
Nisinase, 108, 117

Nitrate, 38, 42
    potassium, 122
Nitrite, 42, 45, 46
Nitrofuran(s), 41
Nitrofurantoin, 43, 285, 291, 295, 298
Nitrovin, 204, 319, 354
Nocardiasis, 58
Nocardicin A, 13
Nosocominal infections, 338
Novobiocin, 18, 19, 32–4, 38, 46, 57, 179, 235, 298
Nystatin, 19, 183, 190

Oats, 267
Oleandomycin, 19, 32, 34, 38
Omadine Na, 37
Omadine Zn, 37
Opsonins, 252
Optimum ratio, 71
Orbenin, 4
Ormetoprim, 71
Osteogrycin(s), 40
Oxacillin, 4, 16, 18
Oxidation–reduction potential, 36
Oxygen, 42, 46
Oxytetracycline, 19, 21, 41, 183, 186, 239

Pancreatin, 109
Papaverine, 45
Paromomycin, 19, 32
Pasteurellosis, 200
Pasteurization, 42
Peaches, 115
Pears, 115
Peas, 105, 126
    green, 115
Penbritin, 4
Penicillin, 3, 9, 19, 34, 35, 37–40, 43, 44, 46, 89, 109, 203, 214, 220, 235, 236, 239, 286, 293, 298, 307
Penicillin V, 3, 19
Penicillinase, 9, 308
Penspek, 5
Pentachlorobenzene, 34
Pentamycin, 19
Pentanedione, 22
Peppers, 114
Pepsin, 109
Peptidoglycan, 259
Permeability, 58, 59, 108, 178
Persistance (resistance), 318, 321, 335, 349, 353
pH, 31, 35, 36, 41, 42, 45, 104, 141, 142, 282
Phage(s), 140, 346
    nisin, 110
Phanamycin, 33
Pharmacokinetic(s), 61, 70, 221, 229, 308
Phenacetin, 43

Phenbenicillin, 5
Phenethicillin, 5, 16, 18, 298
Phenols, 177, 179
Phenolics, 36
Phenoxyethanol, 38
Phenylalanine, 107
Phenylethanol, 37, 183
Phosphoromycin, 179
Phthalyl sulphathiazole, 43
Pigs, 201, 259, 270, 318, 323, 344
Pimaricin, 19
Pineapples, 115
Pinene, 42
Pivampicillin, 7, 16
Pivmecillinam, 9
Plasma, 78
  profile, 58
Plasmids, 322
Platinum, 44
Pneumonia, 200, 208
Polymyxin B, 19, 32–5, 37–40, 43, 44, 46, 57, 109, 179, 183, 203, 303, 304
  resistance, 345
Polyoxin(s), 19–21
Polypeptide, antibiotic, 261
Polyphosphates, 107
Polysorbate, 37
Pork
  raw, 330
  sausage, 157
Potatoes, 115
Potency, 284
Poultry, 259, 323, 344
  pastes, 116
Preincubation, 135
Preservatives, 51, 265
Pressure, 36
Pristinamycin, 19, 60
Procaine, penicillin, 236
Pro-drugs, 5
Proflavine, 109
Proguanil, 38, 65
Promin, 40
Propcorn *see* propionic acid
Propicillin, 5, 16
Propionic acid, 265
Propylene oxide, 36
Protease, 109
Protozoa, 18
Psittacosis, 200
Pterins, 66
Pteroylglutamic acid, 65
Ptyalin, 109
Pudding
  macaroni, 115
  rice, 115
  sago, 115
  semolina, 115
  tapioca, 115
Purines, 64
Puromycin, 109
Pyelonephritis, 201
Pyopen, 6
Pyrazinamide, 44
Pyrimethamine, 38, 43, 65
Pyrimidines, 64
Pyrrolnitrin, 19
Pyruvate, 32, 107

Quantities, addition of, 289
Quaternary ammonium compounds, 37
Quindoxin, 319

R-factors, 75, 315, 321
Radiation, 35, 36, 41, 44
  gamma, 44, 46, 110, 174, 180
Radio frequency, 37
Recovery, *see* resuscitation
Redox, 36
Residues
  antibiotic, 223, 239
  inhibitory, 223
Resistance, 49, 50, 76, 315
  multiple, 48, 76
  non-specific, 245
  reservoir, 322–30
Respiratory infections, 58, 201
Resuscitation, 31, 46, 47, 131, 132, 135, 174, 178, 181
Ribosome, streptococcal, 58
Ribostamycin, 19
Rice, 113, 269
Rifamide, 16
Rifampicin, 16, 17, 44, 179
Rifamycin, 15, 16, 19, 40
Rifamycin SV, 16
Rifazin, 16
Ristocetin, 17, 19
Rixapen, 5
Rollicycline, 16
Rose bengal, 34, 35, 282
Rotlauf, 29

Salicylanilides, 179
Salinomycin, 19
Salsify, 115
Salts, melting, 107
Sarkomycin, 19
Sauces, 115
Sauerkraut, 115
Sausages, 115, 157
  meat, 116
Selenite enrichment, 33, 35, 42
Senescence, 180
Sensitivity
  discs, 236
  testing, 212
Sequential drugs, 48
  blockade, 67

Serine, 104
Serotypes, 297, 320, 327–37
Serum, 34, 242
Sheep, 323
Shigellosis, 29
Siccanin, 19
Silage fodder, 116
Siomycin, 19, 92
Sisomicin, 19
Sodium chloride, 36, 41, 42, 45, 46, 150
  sulphite, 33
Sorbate K, 41, 46
Sorbic acid, 41, 42, 44, 114, 268
Sorbitol, 33
Sorghum, 267
Soups, 115
  fish, 115
  meat, 115
  mushroom, 115
Spaghetti, 113
Spectinomycin, 19, 40, 349
Spinach, 115
Spiramycin, 19
Spore, 105
Staphylomycin, 19, 40
Stendomycin, 18, 19
Stomacher, 239
Stop(s), 291
Strangles, 201
Streptomycin, 16, 19, 21, 29, 34, 35, 39, 40, 43, 44, 46, 89, 109, 179, 203, 214, 235, 236, 282, 293, 297, 298
  dihydro, 44
  resistant, 345
Stress, 46, 131, 132, 175
  heat, 133
Sub-lethal
  chemicals, 133
  heat, 131, 132, 174
  starvation, 134
  stress, 131
Subtilin, 37, 42, 124
Sulbenicillin, 16, 92
Sulfisoxale, 44
Sulphadiazine, 29, 32, 44, 65
Sulphadimethoxine, 71
Sulphadoxine, 71, 214
Sulphaguanidine, 43
Sulphamerazine, 44
Sulphamethoxazole, 40, 41, 44, 57, 62, 64, 82, 177
Sulphamezathine, 33
Sulphanilamide, 65
Sulphaquinoxaline, 65
Sulphathiazole, 34, 44, 66
  phthalyl, 43
Sulphetrone, 40
Sulphite, 32, 33
  sulphiting, 157
Sulphonamide, 29, 40, 43, 44, 46, 177, 203
  resistance, 345
Sulphones, 29, 177
Sulphur dioxide, 37, 42, 157
Survival days, 29
Swann committee report, 20, 199, 212, 323, 344
Swine dysentery, 200, 206
Synergism, 27, 28, 286
Synergistic, 28
  combinations, 9, 12, 229
Synergy, 57, 229

Talampicillin, 7
Teat canal, 245–51
Teichoic acid(s), 260
Tellurite, 32, 34
Temperature, 31, 35, 41, 42
Ternary acids mixture, 267
Terpineol, 43
Terramycin, 37, 38, 42
Tetracycline, 15, 16, 19, 21, 29, 34, 37–40, 46, 57, 177, 203, 297, 298, 319
  resistant, 345
Tetraethylthiuram, 37
Tetrapak, 31
Tetrathionate, 33
Tetrazolium, 33, 297
Thailand, 338
Thallous acetate, 33, 34
Thawing, 35
Thiocyanate, 33, 46, 251
Thioglycollate, 177, 178
Thionin(e), 34
Thiopeptin, 19, 21
Thiostrepton, 19
Thiosulphate sodium, 33
Thiry-Vella loops, 308
Threonine, 104
Thymidine
  phosphorylase, 69
  trifluoro, 73, 74
Thymidylate synthetase, 75
Thymine, 64, 69, 73, 177
Thymineless death, 73
Ticarcillin, 6, 8, 92
Tissue distribution, 308
Tobacco, 38
Tobramycin, 19, 92, 177
Tomato juice, 114
Tomatoes, 105, 113
Tongue, 115
Toxicity, nisin, 110, 111
Toxoplasmosis, 65
Transferable drug resistance, 316, 344
Tricarcillin, 16
Trichomycin, 19
Trifluorothymidine, 45
Trimethoprim, 12, 29, 41, 44, 57, 62, 64, 82, 177, 203, 214, 229
  resistance, 76
Triple combination, 297

Trypaflavine, 33, 43
Trypsin, 109
Trypticase soy broth, 135, 158
Tryptone, 32
  soy peptone, 183
Tryptophan, 37
Tryptose, 32
Tubercle bacilli, 292
Tuberculosis, 12, 57, 59
Tweens, 20, 42, 80, 176, 183
Tylosin, 19, 21, 42, 109, 124, 203, 354
  lactate, 41, 45
Tyrocidin, 179
Tyrothricin, 19, 35, 42

Ultrasonics, 36, 44, 116
Ultra violet, 36, 41, 42, 110
Undecylenic acid, 37
Urinary bladder, 16, 82
Urinary tract infection, 58, 59, 78
Urine, 74, 78, 241, 311

Vagina, 78
Validamycin, 19, 21
Vancomycin, 17, 19, 33, 34, 179
Variotin, 19
Veal
  calves, 331
Vegetables
  peas, 113
  soups, 113
Vietnam, 338
Vinblastine, 45
Vincristine, 45
Violet red, 136, 182
Viomycin, 19
Virginiamycin, 60, 204, 354
Viruses, 210, 215
Voges-Proskauer reaction, 297
Volatile fatty acids (VFA), 265

Water activity, 41, 42, 45, 132
Wheat, 267

Yeast(s), 268

Zinc bacitracin, *see* Bacitracin